Re-imagining Educational Futures in Developing Countries

Emmanuel Mogaji • Varsha Jain
Felix Maringe • Robert Ebo Hinson
Editors

Re-imagining Educational Futures in Developing Countries

Lessons from Global Health Crises

palgrave
macmillan

Editors
Emmanuel Mogaji
Department of Marketing, Events and Tourism
University of Greenwich
London, UK

Varsha Jain
Marketing
MICA
Ahmedabad, India

Felix Maringe
Wits School of Education
University of the Witwatersrand
Parktown, South Africa

Robert Ebo Hinson
Department of Marketing and Entrepreneurship
University of Ghana Business School
Accra, Ghana

Faculty of Management Science
Durban University of Technology
KwaZulu-Natal, South Africa

ISBN 978-3-030-88233-4 ISBN 978-3-030-88234-1 (eBook)
https://doi.org/10.1007/978-3-030-88234-1

This Palgrave Macmillan imprint is published by the registered company Springer Nature Switzerland AG.
The registered company address is: Gewerbestrasse 11, 6330 Cham, Switzerland

Contents

Notes on Contributors

Sylvia Arredondo is the general coordinator of Ideario Costa Rica Bicentennial National Dialogue, and coordinator and author of the UNA campaign at the service of Costa Rica and Communication Commission Vice-rectory for Research.

Nestor Asiamah is an international public health researcher whose research network extends to Africa, Europe, North America, and Oceania. His research interest focuses on physical activity, health research methodology, healthy ageing (social gerontology), and health management. He leads an international research team and serves as the executive director at the Africa Centre for Epidemiology (ACE). Asiamah is a PhD researcher with the University of Portsmouth, United Kingdom, and expects to graduate by September 2021.

Samia Chasi is a practitioner-scholar in higher education internationalisation with more than 20 years of experience in this field. She currently serves as strategic advisor to the International Education Association of South Africa (IEASA) and is a research fellow at the University of the Free State, South Africa. She is passionate about facilitating deeper understanding and connections between diverse people and institutions by creating spaces for critical engagement and constructive dialogue. Her research interests lie in Global South perspectives on higher education internationalisation, with a particular focus on South-North collaboration and partnerships.

Atish Chattopadhyay is an entrepreneur and an educator. Chattopadhyay is a keen proponent of globalisation of Indian business schools. He has previously held leadership positions at top institutions—SPJIMR Mumbai, MICA

Ahmedabad, and IMT Ghaziabad. Under his leadership, schools have initiated pioneering pedagogical innovations which won accolades globally, including AACSB's "Innovations that Inspire" award. As professor of Marketing, Chattopadhyay has published in top journals and consulted with top MNCs covering the Asia Pacific and Latin America. At Jagdish Sheth School of Management (JAGSOM), formerly IFIM Business School, he pioneered a study in association with industry to curate a graduate management curriculum that caters to the needs of Industry 4.0—which has won international accolades.

Otilia Chiramba holds a PhD in educational leadership, management and policy studies. At present, she is a post-doctoral research fellow at the University of Johannesburg in the Faculty of Education and an editorial board member for the *Journal of Education Studies*. Her research interest is in higher education specifically focusing on underprivileged groups of students like refugees, international students, and students from marginalised communities in South Africa and beyond. Her research work is informed by theories of resilience and social justice. She also teaches and supervises research up to PhD level. Chiramba has published two articles and eight book chapters in higher education and basic education in South Africa. Currently she is working towards publishing two co-edited books. She has been involved in grant-funded projects and has also been presenting her work at local and international conferences.

Freddy Veloz de la Torre is a professor at the Escuela Superior Politécnica del Litoral. He is currently director of the Technical Academic Secretary of ESPOL. He has a master's degree in management information systems. He was deputy director of the School of Design and Visual Communication (Edcom)—Escuela Superior Politécnica del Litoral. He was academic coordinator of the undergrade programmes in web design and information systems.

Ariana Daniela Del Pino Espinoza holds a Doctor of Art, Production and Research degree from the Polytechnic University of Valencia in Spain with a "cum laude" mention. Professor for more than nine years, she currently teaches at Escuela Superior Politécnica del Litoral (ESPOL) in Ecuador, the best public university in Ecuador. She has directed several projects for linkage for vulnerable groups and the popular and solidarity economy. She is currently developing a research project in digital branding and was advisor in the management of social communication and management of public affairs at

ESPOL. She has written several indexed articles and books and recently edited the book *Improving University Reputation Through Academic Digital Branding*.

Temitope Farinloye has a first degree from the University of Bedfordshire, Luton, and is presently working towards her master's degree at Kings College, London. She presently works at Questbury Research Services as a research associate. Her research interests are in the marketing of higher education, social media, and qualitative analyses of user-generated contents. She has published her works in reputable journal articles and as book chapters, and presented her work at conferences.

Damini Goyal Gupta holds a postgraduate diploma with specialisation in marketing (PGDM) from IMT Nagpur. She is a first-year, Fellow Program in Management research scholar at MICA, Ahmedabad, India. Her research interests are at the intersection of digital marketing, consumer behaviour, and luxury branding. She has over three years of industrial experience as a digital marketer working with Tata Motors, Bajaj Electricals, Dulux Paints, and many more. She has worked extensively in social media and digital innovation (AR, VR, experiential marketing). Gupta is a recipient of several awards for her campaigns and activations, including "Best Digital Innovation of the Year 2018" by Drivers of Digital Awards 2018.

Narce Dalia Ruiz Guzmán is a media and digital culture professor at Tecnologico de Monterrey. She has received a PhD in cultural industries by the Polytechnic University of Valencia and a master's degree in visual arts at Universidad Autonoma de Nuevo Leon. Producer and film festival programmer, she carried out research on the exhibition of Mexican films, gender studies, and digital platforms oriented towards the audiovisual ecosystem.

Robert Ebo Hinson is a professor, a marketing communications practitioner, turned scholar. He holds a DPhil in marketing from the University of Ghana and a PhD in international business from the Aalborg University Business School. Since turning scholar in 2003, Hinson has served as rector of the Perez University College, acting director of Institutional Advancement at the University of Ghana, and twice as head of the Department of Marketing and Entrepreneurship at the University of Ghana Business School. In 2019, Hinson was listed as one of the top 100 speakers in Ghana by the Speakers Bureau Africa.

Varsha Jain is a professor in integrated marketing communications and the doctoral programme and research co-chairperson at the MICA, India. She has authored over 100+ publications, including in the *European Journal of Marketing*, *International Journal of Information Management*, and many more. Jain is the recipient of more than 21 national and international awards and gold medals in scholarship. The recent award includes "JCB Reviewer of the Year Award 2020", *Journal of Consumer Behavior*, USA. In her research career, she is visiting guest at Emory Business School, Atlanta, USA, and visiting scholar and guest at The Medill School, North-western University, USA. Her research specialties lie in advertising, branding, digital marketing, luxury branding, and digital natives. Jain has recently co-authored the book *Consumer Behavior – A Digital Native* with Sheth and Schultz (Indian edition). Her forthcoming books include *Consumer Behavior: A Digital Native (African and Global edition)*, *Customer Relationship Management in the Digital Age*, *Higher Education in Emerging Countries in the Post Pandemic*, and *Qualitative Marketing Research in the Digital Age.*

Tawana Kupe is the vice-chancellor and principal of the University of Pretoria. Prior to his current position, he held various positions including being a head of department, head of school, executive dean, deputy vice-chancellor, and vice-principal. He holds a BA honours and master's degree in English from the University of Zimbabwe and a DPhil in media studies from the University of Oslo. In 2019 the Michigan State University bestowed upon him an honorary doctorate in humanities. Kupe is the Africa Co-Chair of the Australia-Africa Universities Network (AAUN) since 2019.

Ariana Andrea García León holds a master's degree in artistic production with specialisation in art and technology at the Polytechnic University of Valencia and a Bachelor of Arts in Graphic Design degree at ESPOL. She is professor and coordinator of the Degree in Graphic Design at the School of Art, Design, and Audiovisual Communication (FADCOM-ESPOL). Her area of expertise is in the research and evaluation of results in users on the influence of graphic design and the user experience in mobile applications on a specific product.

Mavis Thokozile Macheka is a lecturer for development studies in the Department of History, Archaeology and Development Studies at Great Zimbabwe University. She earned a DPhil in development studies from the University of KwaZulu Natal South Africa. She also obtained an MA and a Post-Graduate Diploma in Development Studies from Midlands State

University, Zimbabwe, and a BA from Masvingo State University (now known as Great Zimbabwe University), Zimbabwe. She is a political ecologist, research co-consultancy and a development practitioner. Her teaching and research straddle the fields of the rights of vulnerable groups of the society including women, differently abled persons, young people, and children. She also lectures modules in community development, livelihoods and sustainability, human rights, and development. With regard to vulnerable groups of the society, Macheka's research interests are on their inclusion and greater participation in project formulation, implementation, and evaluation of community development projects.

Felix Maringe is a full professor of higher education, former head of the school at the Wits School of Education, and assistant dean for internationalisation and partnerships at the Faculty of Humanities at Wits. He researches and publishes in the areas of globalisation, internationalisation, and the decolonisation of higher education.

Emmanuel Mogaji is a senior lecturer in advertising and marketing communications at the University of Greenwich, UK. His research interests are in higher education management. Mogaji has previously worked as a marketing communication executive, responsible for creative designs and managing marketing campaigns, liaising and building relationships with a range of stakeholders. He has previously edited three books on higher education published by Palgrave and Routledge. His publications have appeared in *International Journal of Information Management*, *Journal of Product and Brand Management*, *Australasian Marketing Journal*, and *International Journal of Bank Marketing*.

Sooraj Namboodiri is on the Fellow Program in Management (FPM), a doctoral-level program at MICA, Ahmedabad, India. He holds a Bachelor of Arts degree in psychology and a postgraduate diploma in marketing. His areas of interest include consumer behaviour, marketing theory, and history of marketing thought. Presently, his research broadly lies at the intersection of technology and consumer behaviour.

Nguyen Phong Nguyen is a lecturer in the School of Accounting at the University of Economics Ho Chi Minh City, Ho Chi Minh City, Vietnam. Nguyen is also a member of Certified Practising Accountants, Australia. His publications have appeared in the *Journal of Accounting and Public Policy*, *Industrial Marketing Management*, *European Journal of Marketing*, *Public*

Management Review, *Journal of Product and Brand Management*, *Asia Pacific Business Review*, and *Australasian Marketing Journal*.

Miguel De Freitas Noite is an experienced marketing manager with over ten years' experience in e-commerce and marketing. He seeks the growth of companies through creative and innovative marketing strategies. Noite is a keen researcher in the marketing, branding, and higher education areas, participating in industry conferences as a speaker. He holds an MA in marketing management and is presently a PhD student at the University of Greenwich, UK.

Adeyemi Oginni is an architect and research specialist with focus on thermal comfort and building performance, with budding interests in the urban planning issues in African cities. She obtained an undergraduate degree in architecture, graduating from the University of Lagos in 2004; a master's degree in environmental design in 2009; and a PhD from the Department of Architecture, University of Lagos, in 2018. Over these years she has worked with students on Urban Revitalization projects in Lagos, Architectural Design Studio projects, and Climatology Field Surveys for undergraduate and postgraduate students, as well as conducted research on thermal comfort and alternative building materials.

Antonio Pérez is the director of the Communication Area at the Polytechnic University of Valencia. He holds a Bachelor of Labour Sciences degree and a Master in Communication Management degree from the University of Barcelona. Since September 2010 he has been the head of the Communication Area of the Polytechnic University of Valencia, in charge of relations with the media, the web, social networks, and corporate image. He has given training courses in communication, reputation, social networks, and user service through digital media. Advisor on policies and institutional communication strategy of the National University of Costa Rica since April 2017, representing the Polytechnic University of Valencia in different entities of the television and communication field.

Maria Nuria Lloret Romero is the director of the CALSI international congress for 11 years. She is currently the director of the research project "Atenea: Women in Art and STEM" carried out by the Atenea International Congress. She is a member of the Gender Studies platform of the Spanish Universities, and director of the International Congress of Emerging Technologies since 2016. She is also co-director of the "Soundcool System for Collaborative Creation of Music Sound and Audiovisual". She has directed more of 50 research projects at national and European Union level and is an expert evaluator for the European Union since 1998 in the various Marcos programmes to the present. She has edited many books including *Systems Science and Collaborative Information Systems: Theories, Practices and New Research*, *Digital Tools for Academic Branding and Self-Promotion*, and *Improving University Reputation Through Academic Digital Branding*.

Nicolás Fernández Schatzer is the vice-chancellor of Universidad Internacional del Ecuador (UIDE), a private not-for-profit university with 7000 students across three campuses in Ecuador. At UIDE he leads the instiution's 400+% growth of international students and the transition to a new budgeting and financial KPI system. He holds a master's degree from the London Business School and a bachelor's degree from Webster University Vienna. He is presently studying on the Global Executive EdD programme at the University of South California, United States.

Himani Sharma is a third-year doctoral scholar in the Department of Media and Communication at MICA, India. She is a visiting scholar in the Department of Media, Society and Communication at the University of Innsbruck, Austria. Her current research is concerned with educational technology (EdTech) and its adoption in higher education. With a postgraduation in business administration (MBA) and mass communication (MJMC), she has previously worked as an assistant professor at a management school in Bengaluru, India. Her area of interest for research also includes educational leadership, digitisation in higher education, educational change and future of work (FoW), and issues of equity and inclusivity in higher education.

Pooja Sharma is a first-year Fellow Program in Management research scholar at MICA, Ahmedabad, India. She has completed a postgraduation in political science from Jawaharlal Nehru University, New Delhi. Her research interests broadly include political communication and marketing, gender and development, higher education, consumer behaviour, and behaviour change management. She has more than two years of experience in academic research.

Fortune Sibanda is a professor of religious studies in the Department of Philosophy and Religious Studies, Great Zimbabwe University, Masvingo, Zimbabwe. Sibanda has published book chapters and articles in referred journals. His research interests include new religious movements, religion and health, human rights issues, religion and the environment, law and religion. Sibanda is a member of a number of academic associations including the

American Academy of Religion (AAR), African Consortium for Law and Religion Studies (ACLARS), International Consortium for Law and Religion Studies (ICLARS), African Theological Institutions in Southern and Central Africa (ATISCA), Association for the Study of Religion in Southern Africa (ASRSA), and African Association for the Study of Religion (AASR).

Taiwo Soetan obtained his PhD from the University of North Dakota, Grand Forks, US; two master's degrees from the University of Manitoba, Winnipeg, Canada, and Strathclyde Business School, University of Strathclyde, Glasgow, UK; and his first degree from the University of Ibadan, Nigeria. He was a past vice chairman of the Canadian Institute of Marketing and he presently lectures in the Business Administration programme at the School of Business & Applied Arts, Red River College, Winnipeg, Canada.

Josiah Taru holds a Bachelor Science in Sociology degree and a Master of Science in Sociology degree from the University of Zimbabwe and a Social Anthropology and Doctoral degree in humanities from the University of Pretoria. Currently, Taru is based at Great Zimbabwe University. Taru is a member of the Human Economy Programme at University of Pretoria, South Africa. His research work focuses on Pentecostalism and state relations; Pentecostal consumption patterns; and precarity and subalternity studies. For the Zukonnect fellowship, Taru explores how a religious movement shapes and is shaped by urbanisation processes in Zimbabwe.

Gerald Wangenge-Ouma is a professor and the senior director of institutional planning, monitoring, and evaluation at the University of Pretoria. He has researched and published extensively in the area of higher education policy and funding. He has served on many ministerial task teams on various aspects of post-school education in South Africa, and currently serves on the board of the Partnership for African Social and Governance Research (PASGR).

List of Figures

List of Tables

Introduction

1

Reimagining Educational Futures in Developing Countries: An Introduction

Emmanuel Mogaji, Varsha Jain, Felix Maringe, and Robert Ebo Hinson

Introduction

Although all universities across the world are facing similar challenges due to the global pandemic, universities from emerging countries have inherent challenges that present an additional complexity to the way they can manage the impact of COVID-19 (Marinoni et al., 2020; Mogaji & Jain, 2020). There are challenges around the existing infrastructure; for instance, universities are underfunded by the government and have limited teaching resources. Admissions at public

E. Mogaji (✉)
Department of Marketing, Events and Tourism,
University of Greenwich, London, UK
e-mail: e.o.mogaji@greenwich.ac.uk

V. Jain
Marketing, MICA, Ahmedabad, India
e-mail: varsha.jain@micamail.in

F. Maringe
Wits School of Education, University of the Witwatersrand, Parktown, South Africa
e-mail: Felix.Maringe@wits.ac.za

R. E. Hinson
Department of Marketing and Entrepreneurship, University of Ghana Business School, Accra, Ghana
e-mail: rhinson@ug.edu.gh

E. Mogaji et al. (eds.), *Re-imagining Educational Futures in Developing Countries*,
https://doi.org/10.1007/978-3-030-88234-1_1

universities are growing more quickly than the government's capacity to finance these institutions (Iruonagbe et al., 2015; Olaleye et al., 2020).

Beyond the university itself, there are challenges with internet penetration and power supply. As many people must use the internet for online teaching and learning, poor internet connections pose a problem. Internet penetration in Nigeria stood at 42% in January 2020, and the average speed of mobile internet connections was 15.32 Mbps compared to the United Kingdom with 35.57 Mbps and Australia with 67.66 Mbps; in addition, 96% of mobile connections in Nigeria are prepaid (DataReportal, 2021). Countries in emerging economies also have an average speed of 10 Mbps (Hannata, 2019). The financial implications of using the internet are also an issue, as many people may have to buy more data to engage with teaching and learning.

The power supply in these countries poses a challenge that may affect the teaching and delivery of lectures. The World Energy Outlook special report recognises the persistent lack of access to electricity, and the unreliability of electricity supplies in emerging countries, including in the continent of Africa. This lack of access is a factor that is inhibiting the progress and development of the continent, as there are over 600 million people in Africa who do not have access to electricity (IEA, 2019) and 350 million people in developing Asia (Cozzi et al., 2018). While Africa has 20% of the world's population, it accounts for less than 4% of global electricity use (The Economist, 2019). This lack of access to electricity also provides challenges for universities, staff and students who may want to adopt online teaching. This is a peculiar challenge for emerging countries that may not apply in more developed locations.

Urbanisation, growing populations and economic conditions pose other challenges that are peculiar to emerging countries (Alhumaid et al., 2020). Even in many developed countries, there are still disadvantaged students from various backgrounds, including minority ethnic groups, and low-income, migrant and indigenous families, who have not benefitted from the internet and new technologies (Ng & Graham, 2018). If some individuals are still disadvantaged in developed countries, there are many more deprived students in emerging ones. Ho and Lau (2018) recognised the impact of the home literacy environment on student engagement including the educational levels of parents; the sociocultural and economic conditions of these countries also pose additional challenges. There are concerns around parents' abilities to support their children, and the availability of a conducive studying environment at home, especially when people live in high-density areas (Ijadunola et al., 2019; Rotas & Cahapay, 2020). Importantly, in emerging countries, parents also have lower literacy levels.

What We Set Out to Do: Aims and Objectives

Undoubtedly, HE, like any other sector, has been affected by the pandemic, but it is important we move beyond that and prepare for the 'new normal' (Lee et al., 2021). This book sets out to explore the impact of COVID-19 on HE in developing countries. We recognise that previous studies, like Crawford et al. (2020), have provided a timely map of the intra-period HE responses to COVID-19 across 20 countries; this was done through a desktop analysis of university and government data. Marinoni et al. (2020) also surveyed universities to understand the impact of COVID-19 on HE around the world, and Chan et al. (2021) edited a book on online teaching and learning in HE during COVID-19. However, none of these studies or projects explicitly explored COVID-19 in the context of the inherent challenges faced by HE in developing countries.

This edited book recognises this knowledge gap and looks beyond the present pandemic and gives a holistic view of the residual legacy of COVID-19 and how it has triggered the need to reimagine, re-evaluate and reposition the HE system, especially for students, the workforce and other stakeholders. We wanted to explore the struggles of universities, theoretically examine them and then provide relevant practical solutions to addressing their needs, adopting a custom-made approach and co-creating knowledge with stakeholders.

Specifically, the aim of this book was: first, to focus on the impact of the pandemic on HE; second, to explore the challenges faced by education providers, highlighting any relevant opportunities; and third, to present the openings that this pandemic brings and importantly address the call for research to understand and provide an insight into how to deal with the pandemic.

We wanted to bring an insight from different emerging economies and countries across different continents, sharing theoretical and practical insights into dealing with the aftermath of the pandemic (Vasudeva and Mogaji 2020). Furthermore, we made considerable efforts to achieve these objectives even though there were time constraints and issues around the quality of the research. We anticipate many HE practitioners and managers will find this relevant, as it is more likely to meet their needs, and it addresses their challenges unlike a generic book that just offers an insight into HE post the pandemic.

What We Did: Coverage and Content of the Book

Following a process of double-blind refereeing, 14 articles were selected that reflected some of the key challenges and themes of reimagining educational futures in developing countries; these represented a relevant area of research for scholars and practitioners. There are 30 contributing authors from different countries, ranging from Ecuador, India and Zimbabwe. The first chapter provides a background to the study and introduces the coverage and contents of the book, highlighting the different themes and chapters. The other chapters are grouped into four different themes. Theme I has four chapters with a focus on organisational resilience. There are four chapters in Theme II that explore the adoption of technology in universities. The third theme is about staff wellbeing explored over three chapters. The last theme in the third chapter is about reimagining the future.

In Chapter 2, Wangenge-Ouma and Kupe (2021) argue that while the exact parameters of COVID-19-inspired futures remain unknown, the pandemic has accelerated various incipient trends that have heightened disruption and complexity, meaning that many aspects of the status quo ante will change. Their chapter contends that for universities, the ultimate priority is not to cope with the short-term effects of the pandemic but to think carefully about how to reposition for long-term resilience and to ensure readiness to meet the challenges of the twenty-first century. They mapped out possible key pathways for rethinking or adapting HE strategies for a post-COVID-19 world.

The organisational resilience themes continue in Chap. 3, with Chiramba and Maringe (2021) calling for urgent strategic goals to be set in post-COVID-19 HE in South Africa. They acknowledged that the pandemic has exacerbated inequalities. They utilised the theory of organisational resilience based on the four elements of adaptive, adoptive, anticipative and transformative capacities to assess the extent to which universities have been grappling with abrupt closures and the prospect of reopening in the future. Furthermore, they specifically recommended strengthening the curricula, research, pedagogical and innovative interventions.

Chapter 4 from Chasi (2021) presented another perspective from South Africa on organisational resilience. The author explores how international HE partnerships can be reimagined in the aftermath of COVID-19 in South Africa. Chasi acknowledged that COVID-19 has affected the country's education system, and it was important to explore how lessons learnt from the pandemic can inform the reimagining of HE internationalisation. The author concluded that focusing on both people and technology, partnerships can be powerful tools in the process of reimagining internationalisation.

Chapter 5 presents a synthesised conversation with vice chancellors from three different universities across three different countries. In a global fireside chat, they reimagined HE in emerging economies in the wake of the global pandemic. The VCs' thoughts during the chat can be synthesised into seven key points—where we are, who we are, finances, challenges, opportunities, disruptions and future plans. Chattopadhyay et al. (2021) highlighted the need for universities in emerging economies to recognise their inherent challenges and explore opportunities for development, global partnerships, alternative sources of income and the digitalisation of teaching and learning.

The second theme of the book focuses on the influence of technology in redefining HE post the COVID-19 era. Chapter 6 focuses on the influence of technology on students' integrated learning for effective wellbeing in developing countries. Gupta and Jain (2021) attempted to understand and create a framework that integrates technological adaption into students' overall wellbeing in an inclusive and integrated learning environment. Their chapter looks at the implications of using the framework and how stakeholders and policymakers need to change their processes and approaches for future research on HE.

Chapter 7 maps out the global educational technology (EdTech) revolution during the pandemic from 'determinism' to 'solutionism'. Sharma (2021) recognised that EdTech came of age during the current global health crisis. This chapter reviews the success, growth, and challenges of the EdTech ecosystem uniquely endorsed by digitisation in HE. It builds upon the current discourse around the EdTech intervention in HE and suggests the dimensions critical for growth in the post-pandemic era.

When discussing teaching technology in this COVID-19 era, Zoom must be mentioned. Namboodiri (2021) in Chap. 8 explored students' engagement with online learning in HE and asked if we are 'Zoom-ing past "the new normal"'. Amidst a variety of distractions at home, achieving positive learning outcomes and student engagement during the class is imperative for a quality learning experience. The chapter provides a holistic view of student engagement from a stakeholder's perspective. It offers practical actionable insights into the key stakeholders enhancing students' engagement and offering quality online education.

Sharma et al. (2021) in Chap. 9 present prospects, challenges and recommendations for adopting artificial intelligence (AI) in universities in emerging economies. They recognised that AI in education (AIED) as one of the most prominent developments in the field of HE but questioned how universities in developing countries were positioned to adopt and benefit from it. Drawing upon the urgent discussions about the adoption of AIED in emerging economies, they identified the educational implications of AI by examining the challenges therewith and provided recommendations for adopting it.

Staff wellbeing was the third theme covered in the book. Three chapters focus on the preparedness of teachers in coping with the pandemic and action plan. The section starts with Chap. 10 exploring physical activity among African academics in a post-COVID-19 era. Asiamah (2021) noted that the new work patterns, necessitated by the outbreak of the pandemic and its social distancing measures, meant that interventions aimed at maintaining lecturers' physical health were necessary. This chapter showed the need for stakeholders to take specific actions to improve neighbourhood walkability and its utilisation for physical activities.

Espinoza et al. (2021) in Chap. 11 present a multinational survey of how university lecturers are coping with the switch to online teaching as an aftermath of the pandemic. Valid responses were collected from university lecturers at several universities in Costa Rica, Ecuador, Mexico and Spain. They concluded that understanding teaching staff's experiences would allow the creation of beneficial tools, the implementation of more strategic training plans and an improved understanding of the infrastructure needed to maintain and elevate current education levels in this new virtual paradigm.

Moving on from lecturers' experiences in South America and Europe, Macheka et al. (2021) in Chap. 12 presented the experiences of educators at Zimbabwean HE institutions. The chapter examines the experiences and preparedness of educators in adopting and adapting to emergency remote instruction (ERI) on the one hand and the availability of infrastructure that facilitates ERI on the other. Their findings revealed that most educators were not ready to adopt ERI in performing their duties and called for more support for lecturers.

The last section of the book, containing three chapters, focuses on reimagining the future for HE, exploring what universities must do moving forward to remain viable post the COVID-19 era. Leadership, financial empowerment and investment are considered in this section. Sharma and Jain (2021) in Chap. 13 present the role of culture in developing transformative leadership for HE. They acknowledge that the cultural fabric of institutions plays a significant role in interweaving fresh ideas and breakthroughs. They posited that transformational leadership could assist HE institutions to attain their purpose, focusing on integrated learning, collective goals, community-oriented objectives and collective wellbeing.

Nguyen and Mogaji (2021) explored universities' endowments in developing countries, highlighting perspectives, stakeholders and providing practical solutions. They recognised that the pandemic has exposed the need for new sources of funding in HE. Chapter 14 contextualises endowments in developing countries in the time of COVID-19 and provides practical recommendations for key stakeholders. They identified four stakeholders: the endowment provider, the endowed university, the endowment team and the endowment enablers and presented managerial implications for university managers who are exploring endowments as an additional source of income.

The last chapter focuses on reimagining the place of physical buildings in HE in a post-COVID-19 era. In Chap. 15, Oginni et al. (2021) question if universities should invest in physical teaching spaces considering more students and lectures are enjoying the prospects of online and hybrid teaching. They concluded that, ultimately, there is the need for physical teaching spaces, but this should be complemented with teaching technology. Universities, however, will have to explore their resources, student bodies and their pedagogical approaches to hybrid learning and strike the right balance between investing in the physical estate or the digital one.

What Is Outstanding? The Research Agenda for Reimagining Educational Futures in Developing Countries

Although we have attempted to provide a holistic view of reimagining educational futures in developing countries, we had challenges with the time constraints and the quality of chapter contributions that we received, and unfortunately, some of the key areas that we wanted to cover were not explored. While this may be considered a limitation, it opens an opportunity for future research, and we are using this section to highlight outstanding thoughts and research agendas.

These are unprecedented times that universities have not experienced before, and this calls for innovative solutions to meet these challenges. Although many universities in the developed world may be better equipped to face these challenges, there are inherent difficulties that universities in emerging countries will face; this raises the need for research around practice and policy—theoretically exploring these issues in the context of the challenges of these countries and providing contributions relevant for researchers, teachers and lecturers, university managers, policymakers, parents and other stakeholders (Kiraka et al. 2020; Pokhrel & Chhetri, 2021). Figure 1.1 below presents a conceptualised idea of reimagined educational futures in developing countries. While this is an inexhaustible area to explore, there are some

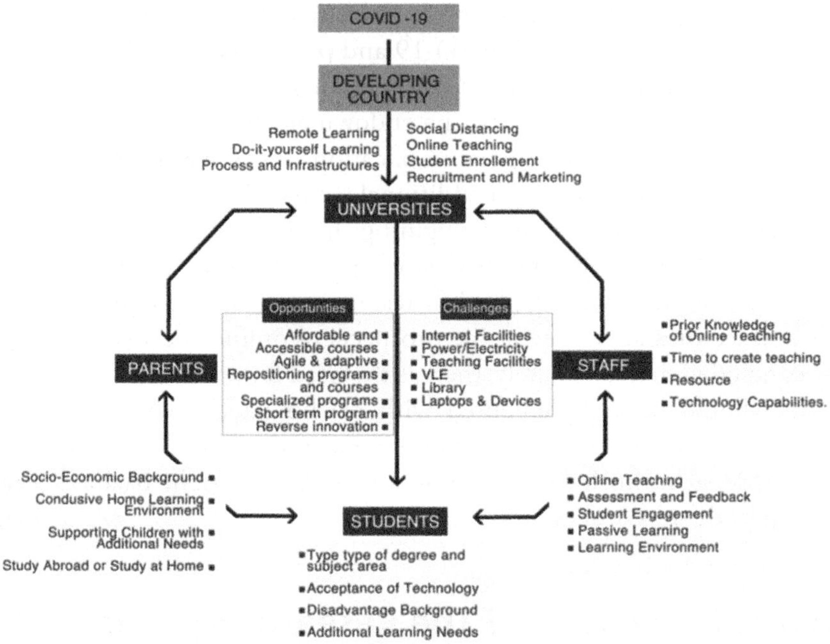

Fig. 1.1 Conceptualising the impact of the pandemic on higher education in developing countries. Adapted from Mogaji and Jain (2020)

research agendas that are worth exploring that will provide insights and perspectives to improve HE policy and practice at this time.

Future research can focus on four different strands: (1) universities—to understand how the pandemic is affecting them, the impact on their marketing strategies and the prospect of specialised and short-term programmes, MOOCs and vocational courses; (2) the staff—to better understand their prior knowledge and resources to deliver online lectures and their ability to support students in inclusive teaching and learning; (3) the students—they are the key stakeholders, and it is important to understand their willingness to acquire a university degree now or to defer to another academic year when universities may be better prepared; other factors affecting students' engagement with online teaching need to be considered too including their physical and mental wellbeing (Nurunnabi et al., 2020); (4) the parents—their roles as stakeholders cannot be ignored in redefining HE, (Ndofirepi et al. 2020) and future research should endeavour to examine the effects of socio-economic backgrounds on engagement and the impact of the home literacy environment on student engagement (Garbe et al., 2020).

Conclusion

Higher education in developing countries has to be reimagined as we plan for the post-COVID-19 era (Oloyede et al., 2021). There are no more excuses, and universities must take responsibility and work with their resources to improve the learning experience for their students (Nguyen & Mogaji, 2021). This introductory chapter presents an overview of the edited collection that explores the efforts and initiatives towards reimagining HE. We conclude that there are opportunities for universities in developing countries to improve the quality of education and collaborate and build partnerships, albeit virtually, with different universities around the world. Institutions must be agile and innovative and be able to reposition their programmes and courses.

References

Alhumaid, K., Ali, S., Waheed, A., Zahid, E., & Habes, M. (2020). COVID-19 & Elearning: Perceptions & attitudes of teachers towards e-learning acceptance in the developing countries. *Multicultural Education, 6*(2), 1–18.

Asiamah, N. (2021). Physical activity among African academics in a post-COVID-19 era: The terrain for action. In E. Mogaji, J. Varsha, F. Maringe, & E. Hinson (Eds.), *Re-imagining educational futures in developing countries: Lessons from global health crises*. Palgrave.

Chan, R. Y., Bista, K., & Allen, R. M. (Eds.). (2021). *Online teaching and learning in higher education during COVID-19: International perspectives and experiences*. Routledge: Oxon.

Chasi, S. (2021). Re-imagining international higher education partnerships in the aftermath of COVID-19. In E. Mogaji, J. Varsha, F. Maringe, & E. Hinson (Eds.), *Re-imagining educational futures in developing countries: Lessons from global health crises*. Palgrave.

Chattopadhyay, A., Kupe, T., Schatzer, N., & Mogaji, E. (2021). Fireside chat with three vice chancellors from three continents: Re-imagining higher education in emerging economies. In E. Mogaji, J. Varsha, F. Maringe, & E. Hinson (Eds.), *Re-imagining educational futures in developing countries: Lessons from global health crises*. Palgrave.

Chiramba, O., & Maringe, F. (2021). Organisational resilience as an urgent strategic goal in post-COVID-19 higher education in South Africa. In E. Mogaji, J. Varsha, F. Maringe, & E. Hinson (Eds.), *Re-imagining educational futures in developing countries: Lessons from global health crises*. Palgrave.

Cozzi et al., (2018). https://www.iea.org/commentaries/population-without-access-toelectricity-falls-below-1-billion. [Accessed 5 5 2020].

Crawford, J., Butler-Henderson, K., Rudolph, J., Malkawi, B., Glowatz, M., Burton, R., … Lam, S. (2020). COVID-19: 20 countries' higher education intra-period digital pedagogy responses. *Journal of Applied Learning & Teaching, 3*(1), 1–20.

DataReportal. (2021). Digital in Nigeria: All the Statistics You Need in 2021. Available at https://datareportal.com/reports/digital-2021-nigeria?rq=

Economist, (2019). More than half of sub-Saharan Africans lack access to electricity. [Online] Available at: https://www.economist.com/graphic-detail/2019/11/13/more-than-halfof-sub-saharan-africans-lackaccess-to-electricity. [Accessed 5 5 2020].

Espinoza, A., Guzmán, N., Torre, F., Romero, N., León, A., Pérez, A., & Arredond, S. (2021). Covid-19: Study of online teaching, availability and use of technological resources. In E. Mogaji, J. Varsha, F. Maringe, & E. Hinson (Eds.), *Re-imagining educational futures in developing countries: Lessons from global health crises*. Palgrave.

Garbe, A., Ogurlu, U., Logan, N., & Cook, P. (2020). Parents' experiences with remote education during COVID-19 school closures. *American Journal of Qualitative Research, 4*(3), 45–65.

Gupta, D., & Jain, V. (2021). Influence of technology on student's integrated learning for effective well-being in developing countries. In E. Mogaji, J. Varsha, F. Maringe, & E. Hinson (Eds.), *Re-imagining educational futures in developing countries: Lessons from global health crises*. Palgrave.

Hannata, (2019). https://seasia.co/2019/07/12/rank-of-countries-with-fastestandslowest-internet-in-the-world-2019 [Accessed 5 5 2020].

Ho, E. S. C., & Lau, K. L. (2018). Reading engagement and reading literacy performance: Effective policy and practices at home and in school. *Journal of Research in Reading, 41*(4), 657–679.

IEA. (2019). Africa energy outlook 2019. [Online]. Retrieved May 5, 2020, from https://www.iea.org/reports/africa-energy-outlook-2019

Ijadunola, M. Y., Ojo, T. O., Akintan, F. O., Adeyemo, A. O., Afolayan, A. S., & Akanji, O. G. (2019). Engendering a conducive environment for university students with physical disabilities: Assessing availability of assistive facilities in Nigeria. *Disability and Rehabilitation: Assistive Technology, 14*(4), 354–360.

Iruonagbe, C. T., Imhonopi, D., & Egharevba, M. E. (2015). Higher education in Nigeria and the emergence of private universities. *International Journal of Education and Research, 3*(2), 49–64.

Kiraka, R., Maringe, F., Kanyutu, W., & Mogaji, E. (2020). University league tables and ranking systems in Africa: Emerging prospects, challenges and opportunities. In E. Mogaji, F. Maringe, & R. E. Hinson (Eds.), *Understanding the higher education market in Africa*. Routledge.

Lee, K., Fanguy, M., Lu, X. S., & Bligh, B. (2021). Student learning during COVID-19: It was not as bad as we feared. *Distance Education, 42*(1), 164–172.

Macheka, M., Taru, J., & Sibanda, F. (2021). Emergency Remote Instruction (ERI) in times of Covid-19 pandemic: Experiences of educators at Zimbabwean higher education institutions. In E. Mogaji, J. Varsha, F. Maringe, & E. Hinson (Eds.),

Re-imagining educational futures in developing countries: Lessons from global health crises. Palgrave.

Marinoni, G., Land, H., & Jensen, T. (2020). *The impact of Covid-19 on higher education around the world*. IAU Global Survey Report. IAU.

Mogaji, Emmanuel., & Jain, Varsha. (2020). Impact of the Pandemic on Higher Education in Emerging Countries: Emerging Opportunities, Challenges and Research Agenda (June 8, 2020). Available at SSRN: https://ssrn.com/abstract=3622592 or http://dx.doi.org/10.2139/ssrn.3622592

Namboodiri, S. (2021). Zoom-ing past "the new normal"? Understanding students' engagement with online learning in higher education during the covid-19 pandemic. In E. Mogaji, J. Varsha, F. Maringe, & E. Hinson (Eds.), *Re-imagining educational futures in developing countries: Lessons from global health crises*. Palgrave.

Ndofirepi, E., Farinloye, T., & Mogaji, E. (2020). Marketing mix in a heterogenous higher education market: A case of Africa. In E. Mogaji, F. Maringe, & R. E. Hinson (Eds.), *Understanding the higher education market in Africa*. Routledge.

Ng, C., & Graham, S. (2018). Improving literacy engagement: Enablers, challenges and catering for students from disadvantaged backgrounds. *Journal of Research in Reading, 41*(4), 615–624.

Nguyen, P., & Mogaji, E. (2021). Universities' endowments in developing countries: The perspectives, stakeholders and practical implications. In E. Mogaji, J. Varsha, F. Maringe, & E. Hinson (Eds.), *Re-imagining educational futures in developing countries: Lessons from global health crises*. Palgrave.

Nurunnabi, M., Almusharraf, N., & Aldeghaither, D. (2020). Mental health and well-being during the COVID-19 pandemic in higher education: Evidence from G20 countries. *Journal of Public Health Research, 9*(Suppl 1).

Oginni, A., Mogaji, E., & Nguyen, P. (2021). Reimagining the place of physical buildings in higher education in developing countries in a post-COVID-19 era. In E. Mogaji, J. Varsha, F. Maringe, & E. Hinson (Eds.), *Re-imagining educational futures in developing countries: Lessons from global health crises*. Palgrave.

Olaleye, S., Ukpabi, D., & Mogaji, E. (2020). Public vs private universities in Nigeria: Market dynamics perspective. In E. Mogaji, F. Maringe, & R. E. Hinson (Eds.), *Understanding the higher education market in Africa*. Routledge.

Oloyede, A. A., Faruk, N., & Raji, W. O. (2021). COVID-19 lockdown and remote attendance teaching in developing countries: A review of some online pedagogical resources. *African Journal of Science, Technology, Innovation and Development*, 1–19.

Pokhrel, S., & Chhetri, R. (2021). A literature review on impact of COVID-19 pandemic on teaching and learning. *Higher Education for the Future, 8*(1), 133–141.

Rotas, E. E., & Cahapay, M. B. (2020). Difficulties in remote learning: Voices of Philippine University students in the wake of COVID-19 crisis. *Asian Journal of Distance Education, 15*(2), 147–158.

Sharma, H. (2021). Mapping the Global EdTech Revolution during the pandemic: From 'determinism' to 'solutionism'. In E. Mogaji, J. Varsha, F. Maringe, & E. Hinson (Eds.), *Re-imagining educational futures in developing countries: Lessons from global health crises*. Palgrave.

Sharma, P., & Jain, V. (2021). Role of culture in developing transformative leadership for higher education in emerging economies. In E. Mogaji, J. Varsha, F. Maringe, & E. Hinson (Eds.), *Re-imagining educational futures in developing countries: Lessons from global health crises*. Palgrave.

Sharma, H., Soetan, T., Farinloye, T., Mogaji, E., & Noite, M. (2021). AI adoption in universities in emerging economies: Prospects, challenges and recommendations. In E. Mogaji, J. Varsha, F. Maringe, & E. Hinson (Eds.), *Re-imagining educational futures in developing countries: Lessons from global health crises*. Palgrave.

Vasudeva, S., & Mogaji, E. (2020). Paving the way for world domination: Analysis of African Universities' mission statement. In E. Mogaji, F. Maringe, & R. Hidson (Eds.), *Understanding the higher education market*. Routledge.

Wangenge-Ouma, G., & Kupe, T. (2021). Seizing the COVID-19 conjuncture: Re-positioning higher education beyond the pandemic. In E. Mogaji, J. Varsha, F. Maringe, & E. Hinson (Eds.), *Re-imagining educational futures in developing countries: Lessons from global health crises*. Palgrave.

Wayne, T., Farinloye, F., & Mogaji, E. (2020). Analysis of African universities' corporate visual identities. In E. Mogaji, F. Maringe, & R. E. Hinson (Eds.), *Strategic marketing of higher education in Africa*. Routledge.

Theme I

Organisational Resilience

2

Seizing the COVID-19 Conjuncture: Re-positioning Higher Education Beyond the Pandemic

Gerald Wangenge-Ouma and Tawana Kupe

Introduction

COVID-19, which was declared a global pandemic in March 2020 by the World Health Organization (WHO), has disrupted society. It has claimed many lives (more than 4.6 million deaths by the end of September 2021), upended economies, and fuelled geopolitical tensions. It has heightened job losses, inequalities, and social deprivation. Universities had to close for some period, disrupting teaching, learning, and research, and many subsequently transitioned to online teaching and learning. The contagion has also accelerated key technology trends such as remote working, remote learning, 3D printing, and automation of jobs, while slowing down the momentum of trends such as globalisation and internationalisation mainly due to the closure of national borders and imposition of exacting travel requirements. It has exposed the limitations and, in some cases, lack of viability of existing ways of working and business models, as well as teaching and research, while simultaneously opening up new possibilities, for example the accelerated uptake of online education. Simply, COVID-19 has produced a new world whose contours we still do not comprehend fully, but to which universities and society at large have to adapt. Against this context, we argue that the COVID-19 pandemic has re-emphasised the role of universities as actors for the public

G. Wangenge-Ouma (✉) • T. Kupe
University of Pretoria, Pretoria, South Africa
e-mail: gerald.ouma@up.ac.za; tawana.kupe@up.ac.za

E. Mogaji et al. (eds.), *Re-imagining Educational Futures in Developing Countries*,
https://doi.org/10.1007/978-3-030-88234-1_2

good and can serve as a springboard for innovative possibilities aimed at re-positioning higher education.

This chapter examines the disruption and complexity caused by COVID-19 for higher education institutions (HEIs), the nexus between the challenges inspired or aggravated by the pandemic, and existing disruptive trends and crises, for example, digital transformation, economic crisis, demands for broadened access and participation by marginalised groups, and the pursuit of research that matters in transforming lives and communities. After unpacking the various COVID-19-related challenges which, in the context of many developing economies, are interwoven into existing socio-economic conditions ridden with poverty and deep, unsustainable inequalities, the chapter provides an overview of policy responses, specifically in relation to higher education in the South African context, followed by a mapping of key pathways for re-thinking or adapting higher education strategy for a post-COVID-19 world. The latter focuses on innovative possibilities with regard to teaching and learning, research, sustainability, and societal impact. Overall, the chapter argues that, whilst the exact parameters of COVID-19-inspired futures remain unknown, many aspects of the status quo ante will change. Thus, surviving and thriving in the post-pandemic environment calls for re-assessment, re-thinking, and adapting strategies by universities.

Theoretical Context

Universities, Complexity, and Uncertainty

Whilst the COVID-19 pandemic started as a public health challenge, it morphed into a multifaceted challenge that has caused and exacerbated significant social, economic, political, and technological disruptions, both at national and global levels. The pandemic can be described as a "wicked" problem that has caused turbulence, uncertainty, and complexity. For universities, which have a history of operating in environments that are unstable, unpredictable, and competitive, COVID-19 is the latest in a series of disruptive forces that universities have experienced in the past several decades. Globalisation, internationalisation, digital transformation, financial crises, demands for life-long learning, and new forms of knowledge, skills, and competences, are some of the major challenges that universities have had to respond to in order to remain relevant, competitive, and sustainable. These challenges have been exacerbated by COVID-19.

As Metcalfe (2020, p. 6) suggests, "attempting to make sense of the [COVID-19] pandemic can be understood … as academia's quintessential response to the unknown, coupled with a sector-wide existential crisis." Whilst, as argued in the preceding section, we still do not comprehend fully the implications of the pandemic for society, institutions, and public policy, we are beginning to comprehend its multi-layered implications for higher education.

Unlike the many challenges inherent in the university landscape, COVID-19 is unprecedented and a more formidable challenge. Even though there have been warnings of coronavirus outbreaks (Cheng et al., 2007; Hu et al., 2017), the outbreak of COVID-19 appears to have caught the world unprepared and has become a major public health crisis with multiple complex causalities. The scope and scale of COVID-19-related challenges are daunting. The challenges—health, economic, and social challenges—have multiple dimensions which are intertwined; and have a significant impact on existing challenges that universities have been dealing with. The uncertainty and turbulence created by these challenges make the COVID-19 emergency even more confounding: HEIs do not know how long the pandemic will last, the pace at which economies will grow, how this will affect public funding and public policy, if they will be able to meet enrolment targets, how the post-pandemic era will look like, and many other unknown unknowns.

Cohen (1999) and Grobman (2005), amongst others, postulate that the dramatic changes occurring in the structure and scope of organisations has put a premium on responsiveness to change. As open systems, organisations are affected by contingencies in their environment, which they have to respond to so as to enhance their adaptability. New demands, especially complex demands, require some form of reconfiguration in order to be more responsive and adaptable (Cohen, 1999). Ansell et al. (2020) posit that responsiveness to turbulent challenges such as COVID-19 call for cross-boundary collaboration, innovation, and robust governance strategies. These cannot be addressed fully by pre-defined plans or standardised, ready-made solutions, a point that is reiterated by Wangenge-Ouma and Kupe (2020, p. 2) in the context of universities as follows:

> the management of uncertainty … cannot be reduced to risk management procedures and protocols. Universities have to be innovative and proactive, they have to strengthen their capacity for sensing emerging developments and dealing with unknowns and, ultimately, orchestrating new directions and pathways towards the emerging futures.

The COVID-19 crisis, coupled with its complex causalities, can be described as a game changer for university responsiveness given the need for robust strategies to deal with the turbulence, uncertainty, and complexity (Ansell et al., 2020) and re-position for the yet unknown post-pandemic era. The pandemic has been characterised by abrupt changes that require HEIs to develop strategies to maintain their competitiveness and relevance, ensure their survival, and strengthen their impact on society.

COVID-19 caused a myriad of interconnected challenges for universities. Estimates by UNESCO (2020) indicate that, globally, more than 1.5 billion learners, across all levels of learning, were affected by the closure of educational institutions. The closure of universities, and the consequent inability to continue with face-to-face teaching and learning, led to the adoption of large-scale online teaching and learning, which often required the expansion of existing infrastructure and new infrastructure as well. As McCormack et al. (2021) point out, the abruptness of the shift meant that most institutions, students, and lecturers, were either unprepared or underprepared for the transition. In South Africa, given that the majority of the country's public universities are contact institutions, many of them did not have established capabilities for online education. However, some universities have been developing or experimenting with hybrid or blended learning models whereby contact sessions in traditional lectures, seminars, laboratories, and practicals are supplemented with online learning platforms, in which additional activities, notes, and other learning resources are provided online. This model has served these institutions well with the transition to emergency remote learning (Wangenge-Ouma & Kupe, 2020).

Globally, the migration to emergency online learning has sharpened existing socio-economic fault lines in higher education systems and society at large, mainly due to existing differential institutional resources and students' socio-economic circumstances that hamper their experience of the benefits of online education. A number of universities struggled with this transition mainly due to lack of the requisite information technology infrastructure, inadequate expertise for online pedagogies, and inability to provide computers and Internet bundles to their students. In higher education systems such as South Africa's, the historical resource differentials in the sector had significant implications: they accentuated existing equity challenges, impaired the ability of under-resourced universities to provide excellent education, and undermined their public good role (Wangenge-Ouma & Kupe, 2020). In addition to the broader economic impact of COVID-19, the pandemic is also having an impact on many elements of the finances of universities, amongst them:

1. Costs related to online teaching (learning management systems, purchases of computers/devices for students and staff, data, etc.);
2. Loss in revenue due to the cancellation of on-campus revenue-generating courses and programmes;
3. Ongoing financial hardship for families and loss of income as a result of retrenchments resulting in higher student debt levels—this is real in the context of stretched public finances and a battered economy. Financial hardship will require increased financial support;
4. Decline in third-stream income due to, amongst others, dramatic declines in financial markets and plummeting economies. These will affect returns on investments and will impact on donors, including alumni, who will face financial challenges of their own;
5. Research funding from private or government sources may decline;
6. Enrolments, especially for international postgraduate students, may decline;
7. Costs related to screening and testing of students and staff; and
8. Costs related to the purchase of personal protective equipment (PPEs) such as masks and gloves.

Universities are susceptible to larger economic and societal trends; large shifts in public funding levels and other government funding targeted at higher education institutions, increasing vulnerability of poor and working-class families, and the challenges in raising third-stream income. Universities must navigate fragmented funding streams, weather economic fluctuations, and contend with a variety of changes to traditional revenue sources. When resources are in a state of major flux, financial sustainability is compromised and organisational stability is threatened. Already, a number of colleges in the United States of America (USA) have closed permanently as a result of COVID-19-aggravated economic challenges.

The many negative effects of COVID-19 have put the spotlight on universities as actors for the public good. As of September 2021, more than 228 million people had been infected by COVID-19 and over 4.6 million lives had been lost. The economic impact of the pandemic, inter alia, accelerated job losses, low economic activity, and the collapse of many companies and businesses, and has had a negative impact on people's lives, leaving many households in a precarious position. Jayaram et al. (2020) predict that between 9 and 18 million jobs in Africa could be lost or made redundant due to COVID-19 and that 30 to 35 million jobs on the continent are at risk of reduction in salaries. Job losses, reduction in salaries, and the many other effects of the pandemic will exacerbate the already unacceptably high levels of poverty and inequality. It is estimated that the pandemic will push an additional 28–49 million people into extreme poverty (Namatovu & Larsen, 2021). The exacerbated inequalities and poverty levels are expected to linger long after the pandemic is over.

The foregoing is the milieu—an epidemic, loss of lives and livelihoods, increasing inequalities and economic disaster, turbulence and uncertainty—within which universities find themselves. It is a milieu that poses enormous challenges to the sustainability of universities and, simultaneously, requires universities to demonstrate their societal relevance. Inequalities in access, retention and student success are likely to increase, mostly affecting students from marginalised communities. Similarly, the health crisis has put pressure on universities to demonstrate that they are responsive to the contexts in which they are embedded by pursuing research that makes a positive impact on areas of great societal need.

Overall, organisations, including universities, are complex adaptive systems; "they gather information about their surroundings, themselves and their own behaviour and then use this information for adapting to and co-evolving with their environments" (Ashmos et al., 2000, p. 578). In other words, organisations continuously self-organise and co-evolve; they are "locked into perpetual co-evolutionary cycles of change in which the ever increasing turbulence of the environment leads to more flexible, innovation-driven organisational structures and processes" (Stead & Stead, 2013, p. 163). The COVID-19 emergency is cause to pause; universities have to make sense of its impact both in the short term and long term, and respond accordingly. The complex challenges caused and aggravated by the health crisis and the resultant uncertainty and turbulence call for innovative responses and proactive alignment with evolving societal realities. The scale and scope of the challenges demand a re-imagination of the university system, and the pursuit of bold responses to enhance the vitality, sustainability, and relevance of universities, and their contribution to societal advancement. The pandemic is a unique moment that behoves universities to think about the kinds of institutions that they want to be after the pandemic and their relationship with the state, society, industry and communities; re-think new pedagogical possibilities; and re-imagine a new future that addresses inequity and inequality.

National Policy Responses

This section provides an overview of national policy responses to the COVID-19 pandemic and how these responses affected universities. The focus is mainly on policy responses that are relevant to higher education. The analysis of national policy responses serves as a lead-in to the subsequent discussion on re-positioning HEIs. This is underpinned by the understanding that universities are embedded globally, nationally, and locally (Marginson & Rhoades, 2002), and this embeddedness influences the ways in which they mobilise their agency in response to complexity. Thus, whilst the preceding section foregrounds the analysis at the global level, this section highlights the importance of national and local dimensions. We also seek to contrast the short-term nature of most policy interventions to the pandemic, which are aligned with the trajectory of the pandemic and the various emergency response phases identified by Mann (2007), namely, preparedness, response, mitigation and recovery, with the need for re-imagining and re-positioning universities, discussed in the next section, which have a long-term horizon. Whilst there are similarities in the policy responses by countries across the world, the responses are mainly contextual. In this regard, we discuss South Africa's policy responses for illustrative purposes.

The South African government, like other governments, has been making decisions to manage COVID-19 and its consequences since WHO declared it a global pandemic in March 2020. Decisions on how to handle the crisis have followed the trajectory of the pandemic. The data used for this section were collected from government gazettes, budget statements, official reports, and public announcements made by national government leaders, mainly the president and cabinet ministers.

Declaration of a National State of Disaster

The first major policy intervention by South Africa was the declaration of a national state of disaster on 15 March 2020, by which time the country had 61 confirmed cases. The following are some of the key measures that were taken following the declaration of a national state of disaster (Ramaphosa, 2020):

1. Imposition of a travel ban on nationals from identified high risk countries such as the USA, Italy, Spain, South Korea, Iran, Germany, the United Kingdom, and China.
2. Discouragement of South African citizens from travel to or through high-risk countries.
3. Shutdown of land ports and sea ports.
4. Prohibition of gatherings of more than 100 people.

The measures above had a number of implications for universities, inter alia, cancellation of international travel and academic events such as conferences and workshops, and the suspension of academic programmes and graduation ceremonies. The latter decision was informed by the prohibition of gatherings of more than 100 people, which would prohibit the holding of lectures which often surpass 100 students. Because of the increasing number of infections, South African universities closed for early recess.

Lockdown

With the number of confirmed infections having increased six-fold since 15 March 2020, the South African government announced a nationwide lockdown on 23 March 2020 to contain the spread of the virus. The lockdown took effect on 26 March 2020. It imposed restrictions on the movement of people and goods, gatherings were prohibited, all businesses and other entities had to cease operations save for businesses involved in the manufacturing, supply or provision of an essential service, and all of the country's borders were closed (Minister of Cooperative Governance and Traditional Affairs, 2020). In light of the lockdown, universities, which had closed for early recess, extended their closure.

On 23 April 2020, the government introduced a graded alert level system, with full lockdown, as had been applicable from 26 March to 30 April 2020, representing Level 5. Subsequently, the president announced a move to Lockdown Level 4 from 1 May 2020. The various lockdown levels were determined mainly by the spread of the virus (number of infections) and the readiness of the country's health system as follows (Minister of Health, 2020, p. 4):

1. Alert Level 1: a low COVID-19 spread with a high health system readiness;
2. Alert Level 2: a moderate COVID-19 spread with a high health system readiness;
3. Alert Level 3: a moderate COVID-19 spread with a moderate health system readiness;
4. Alert Level 4: a moderate to a high COVID-19 spread with a low-to-moderate health system readiness; and
5. Alert Level 5: a high COVID-19 spread with a low health system readiness.

General regulations for each level of lockdown were published, with sector-specific regulations published by the respective ministers. For universities, the regulations included the percentage of students that they could accommodate across the various lockdown levels. For instance, for Lockdown Level 3, universities were permitted a maximum of 33% of the student population and 66% for Level 2. Universities were required to develop phased-in plans for each lockdown level, which had to be approved by the Department of Higher Education and Training (DHET). Universities were required to implement a screening and testing programme as employees and students returned to the campuses and also provide quarantine facilities for employees and students who tested positive. The 2020 academic year was also re-organised to enable its completion, which extended into early 2021 for some institutions (Minister of Higher Education, Science and Innovation, 2020a). The return of students to campuses did not mean the resumption of face-to-face teaching; it was to permit students to stay in the university residences, access Wi-Fi, and use laboratories and other university facilities.

Remote Multi-Modal Teaching and Learning

The declaration of a national state of disaster and the lockdown regime that followed meant that face-to-face teaching and learning could not take place. To ensure the continuity of teaching and learning under the lockdown conditions, all public universities were required to develop strategies for remote multi-modal teaching and learning in March 2020, for implementation from June 2020 until the return of full-contact teaching and learning. The main strategies for remote multi-modal teaching and learning were emergency online education and the physical delivery of learning materials (Minister of Higher Education, Science and Innovation, 2020a).

Mobile network operators zero-rated educational content sites of public universities and other public tertiary institutions. This meant that access to institutional websites was free. The DHET also negotiated with mobile network operators for discounted rates for students receiving funding support from the National Student Financial Aid Scheme (NSFAS). The students further received 10GB daytime and 20GB night-time data (Minister of Higher Education, Science and Innovation, 2020b).

Fees and Reprioritisation of Budgetary Allocations

The uncertainty over when the 2020 academic year would be completed raised concerns regarding tuition and accommodation fees. The concern was, if the 2020 academic year took longer than initially planned, would students be required to pay additional tuition and accommodation fees to cover the extended period? To address these concerns, the Minister of Higher Education, Science and Innovation (2020c, p. 6) directed that:

(a) In terms of tuition fees, the 2020 academic year was conceptualised as a "package" regardless of its length. Meaning that the cost of tuition would remain at the same level for the 2020 academic year regardless of the time frame for a student to complete and the mode of delivery for completion.
(b) The cost for university-owned accommodation would remain the same for the academic year, regardless of its length, capped to the end of March 2021.
(c) Where there were periods of non-occupation of accommodation, monthly payments could be reduced, based on a payment regime that spreads out the agreed costs over the 2020 academic year.

In response to the devastation caused by COVID-19, the South African government unveiled in April 2020 a R500 billion relief package which was to be funded partly by reprioritising R130 billion of expenditure from existing budgets, and borrowing from domestic and international lenders. The supplementary budget tabled on 24 June 2020, however, provided for a budget of R145 billion for COVID-19-related expenditure, of which R109 billion would be funded through the suspension of baseline allocations and reprioritisations. The budget reduced planned expenditure by R230 billion over the next two years (2021/22 and 2022/23) (National Treasury, 2020). Budget allocations for universities for 2020/21 were cut: infrastructure allocation for universities was reduced by R500 million while the block grant was reduced by R382.59 million (1.07%) (National Treasury, 2020). Similarly, the budget for the Department of Science and Innovation (DSI) was decreased by 16%. This cut will affect universities directly, inter alia, by reducing the number of postgraduate bursaries and PhD grants. The reduced funding also affected allocations to research chairs and centres of excellence. However, to assist universities to cover unplanned COVID-19 related expenses, the DHET asked universities to prepare campus readiness plans which were funded by reprioritising existing earmarked allocations such as Infrastructure and Efficiency Grant and University Capacity Development Grant. The total cost of the submitted plans was R1.85 billion. As would be expected, institutional requests varied considerably, ranging from R2.1 million to R402.8 million. According to the Minister of Higher Education, Science and Innovation, many of the items indicated in the readiness plans were unnecessary. The reprioritisation of funds into a COVID-19 Responsiveness Grant (CRG) supported universities to implement multi-modal teaching and learning through, for example, the provision of Internet bundles and laptops to students; and implementation of campus safety plans, which include screening, and purchase of PPEs and hand sanitisers (Minister of Higher Education, Science and Innovation, 2021).

COVID-19 Research and Development Activities

The Department of Science and Innovation (DSI) had by January 2021 invested over R68 million in COVID-19 research and development activities in the areas of diagnostics, therapeutics, vaccines, surveillance, and epidemiology (Minister of Higher Education, Science and Innovation, 2021). Some of the studies being supported include a study on plant-based manufacturing of antibodies for COVID-19, which aims to facilitate the rapid development of COVID-19 vaccines, therapeutic antibodies, and diagnostic reagents. There is also support for a study aimed at assessing the safety, immunogenicity, and efficacy of a COVID-19 vaccine candidate in South African adults living with HIV (Minister of Higher Education, Science and Innovation, 2021, p. 5).

The policy responses presented above represent immediate measures that were implemented by the South African government to manage the pandemic, ensure the health and wellbeing of staff and students, and ensure the continuity of teaching and learning. Measures were also implemented to address hardships experienced by students from disadvantaged socio-economic backgrounds by providing support with access to online education through the provision of devices and Internet bundles. The responses ranged from the imposition of strict measures, such as travel bans or restrictions, closure of HEIs, cancellation of face-to-face teaching and learning to the transition to emergency multi-modal, mainly online, teaching and learning, reprioritisation of budgets, and funding support for COVID-19-related research and development.

Catalyst for Re-imagining Higher Education

This section goes beyond the short-term measures discussed above and assumes a futuristic stance, underpinned by the idea of re-thinking and re-positioning higher education. Understandably, most efforts, such as the policy interventions discussed in the preceding section, are directed at containing the pandemic and dealing with its immediate effects. These include reducing the spread of the virus, treating the affected, vaccine development, managing the economic crisis that it has caused or aggravated, and ensuring continuity of learning at educational institutions. However, responses to the pandemic cannot be limited to its short-term effects and impacts only. As already mentioned, the health crisis is a unique moment that behoves universities to make sense of its impact both in the short term and long term, but, more importantly, seize the moment to learn, leverage it to be innovative and proactive, and adapt strategies for a post-COVID-19 world (Wangenge-Ouma & Kupe, 2020; Salmi, 2020). We argue that the uncertainty and complexity occasioned by COVID-19 are also catalysts for new ideas and innovative possibilities for HEIs; they are opportunities for recognition and exploitation that can support long-term success (Namatovu & Larsen, 2021) and enhancement of institutional vitality.

Before the pandemic, universities across the world were already grappling with challenges such as funding and institutional sustainability; widening participation for students from disadvantaged socio-economic backgrounds; providing innovative and flexible learning experiences; producing future-proof graduates; advancing the public good; deepening connections with communities, industry, and civil society; producing research that addresses the world's pressing problems; and embracing rapid technological change. COVID-19 has heightened some of these challenges, exposed the lack of viability of some institutional systems and processes, and accelerated various incipient trends which were heretofore regarded as future challenges. There are many elements underpinning a post-COVID-19 future-focused higher education. In this section we discuss innovations linked to the following elements: teaching and learning, research, sustainability, and societal impact. These four elements are derived from lessons learned from the responses (for example migration to online education and related innovations such as online assessments, provision of digital devices and data to students, telephone tutoring, and various COVID-19-related projects, including research my multidisciplinary teams, fundraising to support indigent students and collaborations with diverse actors, including industry, government departments, and communities) by universities to the pandemic, discussions in various forums on the implications of the pandemic for higher education, and the emerging literature on the subject.

Teaching and Learning

Throughout the world, the migration to emergency remote learning following the disruption of face-to-face teaching has been uneven. In unequal countries like South Africa, the transition has sharpened existing socio-economic fault lines, both in higher education and society at large, mainly due to existing differential institutional resources and students' socio-economic circumstances which hamper their experience of the benefits of online education. Notwithstanding the challenges with the migration to emergency remote teaching and learning, as noted by Salmi (2020, p. 9), "the pandemic has presented a great opportunity to scale-up innovations that enable many active, interactive, and experiential modes of education delivery". A good example of such innovations is hybrid or blended education. The various blended learning models—rotation, flipped classroom, and flex—provide multiple possibilities for innovation. For example, the rotation model where students alternate between contact classes and online learning could lead to cost reduction, especially for commuter students and also reduce demand for university accommodation. The flex model, where the majority of instruction takes place online with contact sessions as needed, is ideal for working students who can only study on a part-time basis with contact sessions being organised in block sessions (Wangenge-Ouma & Kupe, 2020). In addition, the hybrid or blended model, with a well-developed online dimension, provides opportunities for universities to tap into the burgeoning re-skilling and life-long learning markets.

The COVID-19 experience has arguably established online education as core to the strategies of universities for institutional resilience and academic continuity. More importantly, it presents opportunities for universities to rethink new digital, online, and pedagogical possibilities aimed at transforming the learning experience, and enact strategies for the development of the new generation of digital technologies such as cloud computing, machine learning, virtual reality, and augmented reality. Through these technologies, immersive and personalised education can be provided online at scale. Related is the use of virtual reality technologies to develop virtual laboratories, which can be shared amongst universities. Virtual laboratories are important not only in online contexts, but also as a response to the challenges related to traditional laboratories. Because of financial constraints, many universities cannot afford all the required laboratory equipment. The increasing number of students has also constrained the capacity of traditional laboratories with possible implications for the quality of learning. Virtual laboratories should not be viewed as a replacement for traditional laboratories. The utility of virtual laboratories varies depending on the subject and the intended teaching outcomes. In a blended learning context, virtual laboratories can be utilised as supporting material for lectures or for homework and also for pre-laboratory preparation. Through collaboration, universities can share virtual laboratories with a network of users, address some of the cost challenges, share content, and contribute to enhancing quality by including institutions that do not have the capacity to develop their own virtual laboratories in such networks.

Overall, the post-COVID-19 teaching and learning model should be able to respond more nimbly, flexibly, and successfully to crises and to evolving student and societal needs. This will require, inter alia, continuous strengthening of instructional design capabilities, pedagogical practices that promote active and interactive learning, innovations in assessments, investment in technology, continuous improvement of quality, and collaboration with other universities, locally and internationally, to design courses or share course content and offer joint programmes.

Research

The COVID-19 crisis has several implications for the future of research. One of them is the pursuit of research that matters in transforming lives and communities and addresses complex societal challenges. Such challenges include health, the environment, climate change, food security, poverty alleviation, and all the challenges related to the United Nation's Sustainable Development Goals. The need to combat the contagion, the treatment of patients, and the need to find a cure and a vaccine, have not only reified the importance of pursuing research that matters, but also the need to build transdisciplinary research capacity. The pandemic has shown how connected many issues are and the limitations of singular disciplinary approaches in addressing complex issues.

Whilst knowledge has over the years been fragmented into disciplines and sub-disciplines, societal challenges such as COVID-19 are inherently complex and require transdisciplinary responses. The call for transdisciplinary research is not new. It has, however, been heightened by pressure to solve complex societal challenges as well as the participation of multiple stakeholder collaboration in research (including social actors) and team science (Klein, 2015; OECD, 2020). As O'Rourke et al. (2016, p. 62) proclaim, "meeting grand challenges requires responses that constructively combine multiple forms of expertise… it requires cross-disciplinary expertise". The narrow scope of disciplines is simply inadequate to address complex societal challenges, especially those such as COVID-19 that are characterised by uncertainty and unpredictability. These challenges encompass multiple dimensions that disciplines handle separately (Klein, 2015; OECD, 2020). In other words, complex challenges have to be met with complexity in response (O'Rourke et al., 2016).

Linked to transdisciplinary research is the importance of collaboration across academic departments and faculties. This will require universities to re-think their academic structures and curricula to allow for more flexibility for departments and faculties to collaborate across disciplines. In other words, structures that inhibit transdisciplinarity have to be reformed. The pursuit of transdisciplinarity also requires that universities to re-think academic offerings, especially at the postgraduate level, towards more cross-disciplinary postgraduate programmes. Existing university structures are not the only impediments to the advancement of transdisciplinarity.

The pandemic has underscored the crucial need for multi-stakeholder scientific collaboration and partnerships, locally and internationally: international collaboration, transdisciplinary collaboration, inter-university collaboration, and collaboration between universities, government, industry, business, and communities. Collaboration is not antithetical to competitiveness, institutional autonomy, or differentiation. It is essential for post-pandemic reconstruction, research excellence, and effective responsiveness to the various disruptive trends impacting higher education and communities and navigating the complex, ever-evolving and, at times, contradictory relationship between higher education and its key publics. One of the silver linings of COVID-19 is the collaboration between scientists, governments, and other stakeholders that has resulted in policies and interventions that governments across the world have adopted to tackle the pandemic. As highlighted by Provenzi and Barello (2020), the pandemic is requiring that science and society work together to share needs, resources, actions, and solutions. This collaboration should be nurtured, strengthened, and sustained.

Sustainability

As already mentioned, the financial sustainability of universities is compromised when resources are in a state of major flux. Many universities have suffered significant financial losses due to the economic challenges wrought by COVID-19. The financial losses have resulted from the decline in tuition-fee revenue and government funding, loss of third-stream income, and the unexpected COVID-19-related expenses. Some countries such as Denmark, France, the United Kingdom, the USA, Finland, and Singapore approved economic rescue packages that included funds to help HEIs (Salmi, 2020). This intervention will go some way in cushioning HEIs from the economic hard knocks triggered by the pandemic. The financial challenge facing universities is mainly one of resource dependency. This is seen in the overreliance on a single source of income, mainly tuition fees or government funding; lack of financial diversification; and lack of endowment or reserves that could be used for unexpected expenses or to mitigate the decline in the main sources of income (Wangenge-Ouma, 2011; Wangenge-Ouma & Nafukho, 2011; Salmi, 2020).

Other than affecting HEIs, some of which have closed down as a result, the financial challenges are also expected to heighten affordability challenges for students which might result in lower enrolments. This is expected to affect mostly students from disadvantaged socio-economic backgrounds and those whose parents have lost their jobs. The enrolment of international students is also likely to be disrupted. Lower enrolments will result in lower tuition-fee income. Student debt is also expected to increase given the difficult financial circumstances.

The challenging context requires greater innovation going forward. The following questions are important in re-imagining resilient and sustainable universities: Are the business and funding models sufficiently flexible to evolve as circumstances change? What competitive and collaborative strategies should universities pursue in a post-COVID-19 world? What adaptive capacities should universities create to make them more resilient and prepared for a complex post-COVID-19 future? Universities have to maximise operational efficiencies, contain costs, and optimise multiple income streams. Collaborative alliances are an important sustainability strategy and have several advantages, including gaining access to new markets, sharing of research and development, learning new skills, and bolstering capacity and long-term sustainability (Wangenge-Ouma & Kupe, 2020). Such alliances include collaborative degree programmes, research partnerships involving multiple institutions such as the Gauteng Research Triangle (GRT) in South Africa, and shared services. The GRT is a research collaboration of the Universities of Pretoria, Johannesburg, and the Witwatersrand. It is intended to leverage the synergies of collaboration and transdisciplinary research to deliver mutually beneficial outcomes that none of the universities would be able to accomplish alone. Universities run a number of business functions such as information technology services, which are generally identical across the institutions. Many of the business services do not accrue any distinctiveness or special advantage to individual universities and are expensive. The costs of such activities, which draw resources away from the core academic focus of universities, can be managed through shared services arrangements.

Sustainability is not limited to financial dimensions; it also has important environmental and social dimensions. One of the silver linings of the COVID-19 pandemic is the reduction of carbon emissions, electricity, and water due to the closure of university campuses and suspension of travel. Globally, many universities have embraced environmental sustainability as an institutional imperative and have implemented various strategies related to carbon management; energy, water, and waste management; and recycling. The pandemic has placed sustainability at the intersection of the economy, environment, society, and human health. It is arguably a driver for re-inventing universities rooted in sustainability. This would include, amongst others, the development of ecologically sustainable infrastructure, integrating sustainability and smart campus principles in university operations, and embracing digital technologies for conferences and other academic engagements.

Societal Impact

The COVID-19 emergency has re-emphasised the role of universities as actors for the public good. Universities across the world continue to play a vanguard role in responding to the health crisis through research, public awareness campaigns, clinical trials and testing, and community outreach initiatives, amongst other efforts. These initiatives present an opportunity for universities to restore and strengthen trust in research and expertise and mobilise funding support, which has been declining. It is also an opportunity for universities to demonstrate that they are responsive to the contexts in which they are embedded. Higher education institutions remain, and had been even before COVID-19 emergency, under increasing pressure to demonstrate societal relevance. This is driven by factors such as the rise of the knowledge-based economy, the need for skills to drive economic growth and social development, shifts in the economy and the nature of the labour market, demographic trends, and the demands and expectations of interest groups (Pinheiro et al., 2015). Higher education, in this context, is regarded as a producer of relevant skilled professionals, knowledge, community service, and as a strategic resource for national competitiveness and development.

The concept of the "public good" has become a key lexicon in contemporary higher education debates. Arguments about higher education for the, and as a, public good make reference to the role of higher education in enabling lives of dignity and purpose, achieving dimensions that are central to creating a just and humane society, and the fulfilment of human beings and their communities (Leibowitz, 2012; Mtawa & Wangenge-Ouma, 2021). The loss of jobs and general workplace insecurity and closure of universities, amongst other COVID-19-related developments, are a strong reminder of the crucial role of higher education to society, communities, and individual lives. Universities are thus called upon to strengthen their commitment to serve the public good; act as a bulwark against inequality by expanding access and eliminating differential success and graduation rates based on race, gender, and class; and support post-COVID reconstruction by, amongst others, expanding opportunities for skills development and life-long learning.

In the South African context, universities since the collapse of apartheid have been called upon to play a lead role in advancing the transformation and development imperatives of the post-apartheid dispensation; that is, to reflect and serve their new milieu. It is in this context that the White Paper for Post-School Education and Training (DHET, 2013), for example, sets an enrolment target of 1.6 million for South African universities by 2030 and, in accord with the National Development Plan (NDP) (National Planning Commission (NPC), 2011), identifies the scarce and critical skills needs for South Africa's economic development as an important priority. Further, the two policy documents call for an increase in research and innovation for effective participation in a global knowledge economy. The country's high levels of inequality are a challenge with which South African HEIs must contend. The unacceptably high levels of inequality in the country are linked to factors such as the lower skill levels among marginalised communities. In this regard, an integral part of the public mission of South African universities has to be enhancing access, equity, and social justice. Providing educational opportunities to students from diverse communities and undoing the regressive effects of socio-economic background on educational achievement are important imperatives which universities must continue to address.

Conclusion

The COVID-19 outbreak has highlighted the underlying weaknesses in HEIs and higher education systems globally, and opportunities for higher education to re-invent itself. The systemic flaws are neither new nor previously unknown. Given the uncertainty caused by the COVID-19 pandemic and its exposure of the underlying weaknesses of HEIs, it is natural to seek to understand possible response trajectories to the dramatic shifts that the pandemic has either caused or accelerated. The pandemic has galvanised HEIs to embrace new possibilities, speed up change, and re-think and re-position themselves to strengthen their relevance, vitality, and transformation of society. The ultimate priority, therefore, is not to cope with the short-term effects of the pandemic, but to think carefully of how to reshape higher education for long-term resilience and to ensure HEIs' readiness to meet the challenges of the twenty-first century. It is about maximising higher education's value proposition by being innovative, flexible and adaptive to respond to societal needs, and advance equity and inclusivity, while guaranteeing sustainability. The post-pandemic university has to strengthen its engagement with and impact on society, optimise innovative pedagogical possibilities, embrace blended learning, support excellence in transdisciplinary research, utilise digital technologies and platforms, produce outstanding graduates who make a difference in society, and strengthen partnerships, collaborations, and global engagement.

References

Ansell, C., Sørensen, E., & Torfing, J. (2020). The COVID-19 pandemic as a game changer for public administration and leadership? The need for robust governance responses to turbulent problems. *Public Management Review*. https://doi.org/10.1080/14719037.2020.1820272

Ashmos, D. P., Duchon, D., & McDaniel, R. R. (2000). Organisational response to complexity: The effect on organisational performance. *Journal of Organisational Change Management, 13*(6), 577–594.

Cheng, V. C., Lau, S. K., Woo, P. C., & Yuen, K. Y. (2007). Severe acute respiratory syndrome coronavirus as an agent of emerging and reemerging infection. *Clinical Microbiology Reviews, 20*(4), 660–694.

Cohen, M. (1999). Commentary on the organisation science special issue on complexity. *Organisation Science, 10*(3), 373–376.

Department of Higher Education and Training (DHET). (2013). *White paper for post-school education and training. Building an expanded, effective and integrated post-school system*. DHET.

Grobman, G. M. (2005). Complexity theory: A new way to look at organisational change. *Public Administration Quarterly, 29*(3/4), 350–382.

Hu, B., Zeng, L.-P., Yang, X.-L., Ge, X.-Y., Zhang, W., Li, B., Xie, J. Z., Shen, X. R., Zhang, Y. Z., Wang, N., Luo, D. S., Zheng, X. S., Wang, M. N., Daszak, P., Wang, L. F., Cui, J., & Shi, Z. L. (2017). Discovery of a rich gene pool of bat SARS-related coronaviruses provides new insights into the origin of SARS coronavirus. *PLOS Pathogens, 13*(11). https://doi.org/10.1371/journal.ppat.1006698

Jayaram, K., Leke, A., Ooko-Ombaka, A., & Sun, Y. S. (2020). *Tackling COVID-19 in Africa-An unfolding health and economic crisis that demands bold action*. McKinsey Analysis. https://www.mckinsey.com/featured-insights/middle-east-and-africa/tackling-covid-19-in-africa

Klein, J. T. (2015). Reprint of "discourses of transdisciplinarity: Looking back to the future". *Futures, 65*, 10–16.

Leibowitz, B. (2012). Introduction: Reflections on higher education and the public good. In B. Leibowitz (Ed.), *Higher Education for the public good: View from the South*. SUN Press.

Mann, T. (2007). Strategic and collaborative crisis management: A partnership approach to large-scale crisis. *Planning for Higher Education, 36*(1), 54–64.

Marginson, S., & Rhoades, G. (2002). Beyond national states, markets, and systems of higher education: A glonacal agency heuristic. *Higher Education, 43*, 281–309.

McCormack, T. J., Lemoine, P. A., Waller, R. E., & Richardson, M. D. (2021). Global higher education: Examining response to COVID-19 pandemic using agility and adaptability. *Journal of Education and Development, 5*(1). https://doi.org/10.20849/jed.v5i1.848

Metcalfe, A. S. (2020). Visualising the COVID-19 pandemic response in Canadian higher education: An extended photo essay. *Studies in Higher Education, 46*(1), 5–18.

Minister of Cooperative Governance and Traditional Affairs. (2020). *Disaster Management Act, 2002: Amendment of regulations issued in terms of Section 27 (2)*. Published in Government Gazette, No. 43148.

Minister of Health. (2020). *Directions issued in terms of regulation 3(3) of the regulations made under section 27(2) of the Disaster Management Act, 2002 (act no. 57 of 2002): Criteria to guide the determination of alert levels*. Published in Government Gazette, No. 43599.

Minister of Higher Education, Science and Innovation. (2020a, May 23). *Statement on the implementation of measures by the post school education sector in response to COVID-19*.

Minister of Higher Education, Science and Innovation. (2020b, July 8). *Joint statement on measures implemented by the National System of Innovation and higher education in response to the covid-19 epidemic*.

Minister of Higher Education, Science and Innovation. (2020c, October 5). *Directions for national framework for tuition and accommodation fees for academic year 2020 in the public higher education institutions*.

Minister of Higher Education, Science and Innovation. (2021, January 18). *Statement on plans for the reopening of post school education and training institutions and the contribution of science and innovation in the fight against COVID-19*.

Mtawa, N. N., & Wangenge-Ouma, G. (2021). Questioning private good driven university-community engagement: A Tanzanian case study. *Higher Education*. https://doi.org/10.1007/s10734-021-00685-9

Namatovu, R., & Larsen, M. M. (2021). Responding to COVID-19: Insights from African firms. *African Journal of Management*. https://doi.org/10.1080/23322373.2021.1878809

National Planning Commission (NPC). (2011). *National development plan. Vision 2030*. NPC.

National Treasury. (2020). *Budget review 2020*. National Treasury.

O'Rourke, M., Crowley, S., & Gonnerman, C. (2016). On the nature of cross-disciplinary integration: A philosophical framework. *Studies in History and Philosophy of Biological and Biomedical Science, 56*, 62–70.

OECD. (2020). *Addressing societal challenges using transdisciplinary research*. OECD Science, Technology and Industry Policy Papers, No. 88. OECD.

Pinheiro, R., Wangenge-Ouma, G., Balbachevsky, E., & Cai, Y. (2015). The role of higher education in society and the changing institutionalized features in higher education. In J. Huisman et al. (Eds.), *The Palgrave international handbook of higher education policy and governance*. Palgrave Macmillan.

Provenzi, L., & Barello, S. (2020, June 5). The science of the future: Establishing a citizen-scientist collaborative agenda after Covid-19. *Public Health*. https://doi.org/10.3389/fpubh.2020.00282

Ramaphosa, C. (2020). *Measures to combat Coronavirus COVID-19 epidemic*. The Presidency.

Salmi, J. (2020). *COVID's lessons for global higher education. Coping with the present while building a more equitable future*. Lumina Foundation.

Stead, G.S., & Stead, W.E. (2013). The coevolution of strategic management in the global marketplace. *Organisation and environment, 26*(2), 162–183.

UNESCO. (2020). *Global Monitoring of School Closures caused by COVID-19*. https://en.unesco.org/covid19/educationresponse

Wangenge-Ouma, G. (2011). Managing resource dependence difficulties in African higher education: The case of multiple exchange relationships. *Higher Education Policy, 24*, 167–184.

Wangenge-Ouma, G., & Kupe, T. (2020). *Uncertain times: Reimagining universities for new, sustainable futures*. Universities South Africa Working Paper. Universities South Africa. https://www.usaf.ac.za/wp-content/uploads/2020/09/Uncertain-Times-Paper.pdf

Wangenge-Ouma, G., & Nafukho, M. F. (2011). Responses to conditions of decline: The case of Kenya's public universities. *Africa Education Review, 8*(1), 169–188.

3

Organisational Resilience as an Urgent Strategic Goal in Post-COVID-19 Higher Education in South Africa

Otilia Chiramba and Felix Maringe

Introduction and Background

This chapter provides a largely theoretical contribution towards understanding the efficacy of responses by universities in South Africa to the ongoing COVID-19 pandemic and assessing what needs to be done to build them into resilient organisations. To this end, the chapter uses an organisational resilience framework to explore the strengths and weaknesses of the universities in relation to their key responsibilities at the curriculum, pedagogy, research, and innovation and societal engagement levels. By so doing the framework promotes proactive organisational decision making. The chapter specifically has two aims:

1. To explore using the adoptive, adaptive, anticipative, and transformative framework of organisational resilience in relation to the nature and efficacy of South African universities' responses to the COVID-19 pandemic.
2. To examine ways in which universities could build resilient frameworks for strengthening their role around four core responsibilities of the curriculum, pedagogy, research, and innovation and societal impact.

O. Chiramba (✉)
University of Johannesburg, Johannesburg, South Africa

F. Maringe
Wits School of Education, University of the Witwatersrand, Parktown, South Africa
e-mail: Felix.Maringe@wits.ac.za

E. Mogaji et al. (eds.), *Re-imagining Educational Futures in Developing Countries*,
https://doi.org/10.1007/978-3-030-88234-1_3

Methodologically, the chapter utilises a theoretical approach that benefits from empirical evidence of research by others and our own research at the University of the Witwatersrand (Maringe et al., 2020). We came to this problem as engaged researchers and practitioners in a university which is part of the HE sector in South Africa and which provides leadership across many dimensions in the sector. This was achieved, in part, through the findings from a ZENEX-commissioned research (Maringe et al., 2020) which explored the quality of home learning in low-income family households during the COVID-19 pandemic.

The COVID-19 pandemic has uncovered hidden weaknesses in our higher education (HE) institutions. It has laid bare the real extent of the inequalities that universities do not always feel comfortable to admit still exist 25 years after the attainment of democracy in 1994 in South Africa. These inequalities have their roots in the colonial and apartheid system. Over the years, despite the legal, constitutional, and strategic intentions to dismantle them, the inequalities have persisted. The COVID-19 pandemic has, in many ways, exposed the real extent of these inequalities.

As universities turned to online teaching and learning, the foundations for delivering equality of epistemological access, especially to students in low-income families, revealed serious structural, pedagogical, technological, and ethical defects previously taken for granted in the more sanguine and traditional face-to-face modalities that universities generally operate under. The transition to online teaching and learning is a multifaceted concept whose impact has not received enough attention in South Africa and more so in the context of the COVID-19 pandemic.

We discuss how South Africa, despite the attainment of democracy, is still trapped in the colonial and apartheid past. We further argue that the COVID-19 pandemic helps to exacerbate the challenges already in existence. Such challenges include the social, political, and economic discrimination, and inequalities of class, gender, and race (Maringe et al., 2020).

We also highlight efforts made to transform HE sectors in South Africa. We argue that there has been extensive use of transformational language in the post-apartheid policies, but up to now, we have only succeeded in attaining a few physical changes like the establishment of a single HE system, increasing access for previously disadvantaged students from poor communities into HE institutions, and other changes such as the renaming of buildings, university roads, laboratories, and other physical facilities (Maringe, 2017). Beyond this, universities still pose inequalities in epistemological access to students from diverse backgrounds in HE.

We trace back the notion of inequality to colonialism and coloniality. We argue that there is a deeply embedded culture of inequality in Africa, through sets of repressive laws based on racial and class superiority where Africans were marginalised, oppressed, and victimised as second-class citizens in their countries of birth. We discuss how the notion of decolonisation is hamstrung by coloniality, and we explore the concept in its three forms: the coloniality of knowledge, the coloniality of being, and the coloniality of power (Quijano, 2000; Mignolo, 2011).

We also explore how COVID-19 has exacerbated the already existing problems. We argue that the abrupt turn to online teaching and learning was the only noble idea to ensure continuity of learning, however, it has resulted in the further widening and deepening of inequalities of epistemological access amongst students in HE.

We then propose a four-framework theory of organisational resilience in building resilient universities for the post-COVID-19 era in South Africa. We use the theory to understand how much improvement has been made and how much further the universities can improve in their critical elements of curriculum, pedagogy, research, and innovation and community engagement through the four capacities of adoptive, adaptive, anticipative, and transformational resilience.

Colonial and Apartheid Antecedents of HE in South Africa

Higher education is a key sector in the developmental matrices of countries the world over. Through HE, nations build human capacities for effective participation in key sectors of the economy, labour, and employment markets. HE sectors are also central to the development of new knowledge through post-graduate research, training, and innovation, including through research conducted by staff. In South Africa, however, HE is in a state of crisis, largely due to its colonial and apartheid legacy, diminished funding, and what we could call transformation inertia, despite pronouncements to the contrary (Maringe, 2017). We argue in this chapter, along with other scholars (see for example Heleta, 2016; Mamdani, 1998; Ndlovu-Gatsheni, 2015), that HE in South Africa remains locked in the colonial and apartheid past and, as such, is not fit for the purposes of the new democratic dispensation.

Following the above argument, Heleta (2016) noted that these universities (formerly White-only universities) were basically allowed to continue with business as usual when it came to the maintenance of whiteness, hegemonic institutional cultures, and degradation and dehumanisation of Black South Africans through the Eurocentric curriculum.

This view had earlier been expressed by Mamdani (1998) when he observed that students in South Africa are being taught a curriculum which presumes that Africa has no intelligentsia worth reading and that the only worthwhile knowledge is that which stems from the Western canon.

The current COVID-19 pandemic has cruelly exposed the highly sedimented inequalities that were deliberately created in and through the agency of HE in South Africa. The poorly resourced homes for the students who have been previously disadvantaged could not provide adequate access to learning. As all post-colonies around the world demonstrate, there exists a pervasive coloniality of knowledge in South African HE through which the sector has virtually remained untransformed despite intentions to do so. As the pandemic hit the shores of the country in early 2020, South Africa closed its HE institutions in line with the global prescriptions built around the need for social distancing to reduce cross infections. Students were thus sent home, and universities adopted a new technology-driven remote teaching and learning strategy to replace the traditional face-to-face teaching and learning, a strategy largely beneficial to middle- and upper-middle-class students who have access to social, financial, and technological resources and capital. However, students from low-income households who tend to reside in economically, socially, and technologically deprived communities tend to experience a sense of inadequacy and incapacity in a technology-driven teaching-learning environment, which also takes away the power of social engagement through isolation (Maringe et al., 2020).

Colonialism and apartheid established an unequal, segregated, and racially differentiated system of HE (Heleta, 2016) where the Black majority had severely limited access to universities, where they were taught inferior forms of curricula designed to make them unquestioning labourers in the lower rungs of the economy, and where the resources available to them were substantially inferior compared to those available to White students. Today, despite the gallant efforts to democratise HE in South Africa, especially in terms of increasing access to formerly disadvantaged groups, the university curricula and the pedagogies have not transformed to reflect the demographic shifts that have happened in HE since 1994 (Fataar, 2018). Due to this, poor students from low socioeconomic backgrounds and low-income households continue to experience the lowest learning outcomes, tend to drop out before completion of studies in higher numbers, are inclined to find it most difficult to transition into the employment markets, and also tend to study degrees with relatively low-status subjects (Heleta, 2016).

Post-1994 Transformation of HE in South Africa

There has not been a shortage of ambition and desire to transform HE in South Africa since the attainment of democratic rule in 1994. To dismantle the social, political, and economic discrimination and inequalities of class, gender, and race that remained pervasive in South Africa and in HE especially, the South African Constitution of 1996 (Constitutional Court of South Africa, 1996) and the Education White Paper of 1997 directed the state to lead change in HE. This was to be facilitated through principles and values of human dignity, the achievement of equality, and the advancement of non-sexism and non-racialism through the creation of a single coordinated HE system for all, the restructuring of programmes and institutions, and the advancement of all forms of knowledge in keeping with international best practices in the global sectors of HE (Department of Education (DOE), 1997). Since 1994, much transformation has happened in the HE sectors, including the establishment of a single system, increased access for previously disadvantaged students from poor communities into HE, and pro-poor funding mechanisms, amongst others. It can be argued that the HE system has been highly successful in promoting and achieving physical access and in tinkering with the more cosmetic, though necessary changes such as the renaming of buildings, university roads, laboratories, and other physical facilities.

In the global context, and on the African continent more specifically, South Africa's HE system is ranked very highly, if not the highest (Maddock & Maroun, 2018). Its global status and visibility are largely maintained by five formerly all-White universities: University of Cape Town (UCT), University of the Witwatersrand (WITS), University of Pretoria (UP), University of Stellenbosch (SU), and University of Johannesburg (UJ), many of which appear consistently in the top echelons of the world's best universities. Both in terms of curricula traditions and the pursuit of knowledge, these universities have maintained White privilege in ways that make it hard to differentiate them from some of the top Western universities. In the same universities, despite the policies designed to attract more Black participation, which have resulted in substantially increased Black student participation, the statistics of performance, degree quality outcomes, wastage and dropout, progression and transition to higher levels of learning and employment, continue to trace the contours of race, privilege, and class in South Africa (Badat, 2010). If anything has changed in terms of the indices of inequalities in HE in South Africa since 2010, it has been in the widening, rather than the narrowing, of inequalities in the system which has been laid bare by the onslaught of the COVID-19 pandemic.

The Nature and Persistence of Inequalities in HE in South Africa

To understand the nature and persistence of inequalities in HE in South Africa and indeed in other post-colonial countries, we turn to the concept of coloniality. Following hundreds of years of colonial rule by Western imperialist nations of Europe, African nations embarked on the decolonisation project resulting in gradual political independence starting with Kwame Nkrumah's Ghana in 1957 (Wilburn, 2012) and ending with democratic attainment in Nelson Mandela's South Africa in 1994 (Beck, 2000). Colonialism had established an entrenched system of inequality in Africa, through sets of repressive laws based on racial and class superiority where Africans were marginalised, oppressed, and victimised as second-class citizens in their countries of birth. This allowed colonising countries to loot resources, minerals, and raw materials at will in service of their European empires. Three different forms of violence were unleashed on the African natives.

The first was violence on African knowledge systems. Systematically, African knowledge systems were decimated and replaced by watered-down versions of the Western canon, through which the world was to be understood, interpreted, valued, and operationalised. Students who succeeded through the colonial education systems, albeit always maintained in small numbers, were generously rewarded with opportunities to good jobs which were well paid. This created an insatiable affinity to Western knowledge as the only way out of the drudgery of poverty and deprivation. To date, the desire for Western knowledge and the affinity and its promotion in HE institutions, including its preference by the labour markets, has maintained its dominance over anything that comes in the name of indigenous local knowledge in many parts of the continent's school and HE systems.

The second form of violence unleashed on local African populations was cultural violence, which defines the state of being in the world of any group of people. The whole spectrum of the cultural identity of Africans was systematically violated starting with the marginalisation of African languages in school and university curricula, the denigration of African traditional practices and beliefs, and even the hatred of the colour of the African skin. In Zimbabwe, Ambi, a skin lightening cream was heavily promoted with the promise that Africans 'May Be Improved' (Davids et al., 2016). To be Black was seen as a curse, and the more the Africans embraced whiteness, the better servants they would become in different layers of settler economies. It is not unusual to hear the average African celebrating when their children are able to speak in English and to express pride at the fact that their child can barely speak in the indigenous language but can speak in English. In high school, boys who had strong rural backgrounds (SRBs) were derided by girls as SRBs and often did not find favour with the females.

The third form of violence Africans endured is the general sense of being made to feel powerless and hopeless if one did not embrace the Western values, thought, and behaviours. Settler power was exerted on the local population through economic, military, legal, social, psychological, recreational, and a host of other processes. In Zimbabwe, as indeed in South Africa, many places were reserved for Whites only. Blacks and dogs were often signalled for no entry to some shops and places of entertainment. Africans who had achieved a minimum level of Western education were sometimes allowed in White-only spaces, reinforcing the impression that being White was to be privileged. These kinds of violence during colonialism bred long-standing patterns of power which manifest through coloniality.

Coloniality is a term that came into the lexicon through the works of Quijano (2000), Mignolo (2011), Maldonado-Torres (2012), Dussel (2008), and Ndlovu-Gatsheni (2013). Although these authors define it differently, the central meaning of coloniality is a tendency of previously colonised nations to retract back to the colonial condition despite the independent status of the nation. It speaks to the elevation of the Western canon as the blueprint for global development, to which everyone in the world must utilise and conform. It highlights the tendency to use Western values and standards as the authentic benchmarks for global progress and development as it represents a kind of reproduction of the economic, intellectual, cultural, administrative, and leadership formations which were intended as dominant prescriptions for the aspired modernity and liberal world order.

Understanding inequalities in HE in South Africa, thus, necessitates an appreciation of the three forms of coloniality: the coloniality of knowledge; the coloniality of being; and the coloniality of power. The COVID-19 pandemic brutally exposed the state of the coloniality of HE in South Africa.

COVID-19 and the Turn to Online Remote Teaching and Learning

As universities went under lockdown in March 2020 due to the COVID-19 pandemic, the idea of continuity of learning became a pervasive strategic priority across HE sectors in the world, including in South Africa. The transition from traditional face-to-face teaching has resulted in the further widening and deepening of inequalities of epistemological access amongst students in HE (Morrow, 2007).

The online teaching and learning modality was introduced abruptly in universities across the world, as a reaction to the national lockdowns caused by the COVID-19 pandemic. Online teaching and learning had previously been used in universities, to a lesser extent, to supplement traditional face-to-face teaching and learning. However, in the effort to curb the spread of the pandemic and in response to the national lockdown, universities have completely turned to online teaching and learning. Since its introduction in the last decades in some institutions, this modality proved to be a very significant new pedagogical mode, which enhanced effectiveness in teaching and learning (Beck, 2010; Stacey, 2007). It has been proven that students who use the online modality perform better than those who use the face-to-face modality (Johnson et al., 2000). This is so because online teaching and learning has significant spaces, for example, learning management systems, which allow several activities, such as the provision of lecture notes, resources, and self-assessment to happen anytime, anywhere (Stacey, 2007). It is also effective in facilitating collaborative learning through computer-mediated communication for peer interaction and group activities, where this was once only possible in face-to-face learning situations (Beck, 2010). One of its greatest advantages is that it allows flexibility (Johnson et al., 2000). Students may learn in the spaces in which they feel most comfortable. However, it becomes a huge barrier if one does not have such spaces at home. Although the online modality has several and significant advantages for teaching and learning, it might not give equal access to learners, especially in terms of hardware, software, and internet connectivity within their spaces and given the situation that advantaged students already possess better experience in using smartphones and laptops, than their colleagues from disadvantaged backgrounds. Therefore, online teaching and learning, unlike traditional on-campus learning, will likely widen the inequality gap between the rich and the poor, especially in developing countries like South Africa which only attained its democracy in 1994.

A synthesis of the key ideas emerging from all the challenges associated with transitioning from the face-to-face to online modalities may equip universities with an understanding of how they might build resilience around teaching and learning. We believe building resilience starts with understanding issues and challenges related to this transition.

Building Resilient Universities for the Post-COVID-19 Era in South Africa

We frame the chapter within the theory of organisational resilience with the hope that resilience theory will help us recognise how the reproduction and deepening of educational inequalities in the post-COVID-19 era might be disrupted. Kerr (2015 p. 3) argued that organisational resilience is the capacity of any organisation to 'anticipate, prepare for, respond and adapt to incremental change and sudden disruptions to survive and prosper.' He further argued that organisational resilience goes beyond risk management towards a more holistic view of health and success. Although Kerr's argument is focused on the business world, it may also be applicable and relevant to educational institutions in today's increasingly complex and ever-changing HE sectors. Just like organisations in the business world, a resilient HE system is the one that not 'merely survives over the long term, but also flourishes—passing the test of time' (Kerr, 2015 p. 4).

Before the COVID-19 pandemic, the education systems and specifically HE systems in Africa in general and South Africa in particular were already exposed to some other difficulties such as inequality. These emanate from colonial and apartheid antecedents, as discussed in the previous section. As previously argued, COVID-19, therefore, exacerbates the inequalities that already exist. Building resilient universities requires universities' leadership to be aware of today's complex, dynamic, and interconnected world and rethink a strategic imperative for HE sectors to prosper in such circumstances. Kerr (2015) argued that organisational resilience cannot be a one-off or short-term exercise, but it is most likely to be achieved over time and in the long term. Some of the strategies for mastering organisational resilience require the adoption of high-quality habits and best practice to ensure improvement in HE sectors by building competence and capability across the staff and all other aspects of an organisation (Kerr, 2015). Thus Kerr (2015) further argues that competence and capability allow leaders to take measured risks with confidence, making the most of opportunities that present themselves.

In tandem with scholars such as Bahadur et al. (2015) and Jeans et al. (2017), we, as authors, believe that resilience involves the ability to bounce back when faced with adversities. They provided a lens through the concepts of adoptive, adaptive, anticipative, and transformative capacity to examine and show how universities and students may thrive in challenging circumstances. This involves taking deliberate roles in adjusting to adverse circumstances (OECD, 2014). We have learned that resilience may be used significantly as great capital to build effective universities capable of offering worthwhile experiences to their students (Chiramba, 2020). As a result, utilising the four concepts as outlined by Bahadur et al. (2015) and Jeans et al. (2017), we explored how universities might achieve resilience through these concepts. Below is a brief description of what each capacity entails:

1. Adoptive capacity—a passive form of resilience which nevertheless ensures stability
2. Adaptive capacity—allows incremental change and involves university leaders making deliberate efforts to adjust, especially in adverse circumstances
3. Anticipative capacity—ability to stay prepared and plan for an unseen challenge
4. Transformative capacity—universities' leadership making deliberate efforts to perform systemic and structural changes

We hope that the theory in its four dimensions equips universities and individuals with means to disrupt the reproduction and deepening of educational inequality, caused by both the COVID-19 pandemic and the colonial and apartheid antecedents. In the following section, we discuss the role of the universities in building the four capacities.

The Role and Purpose of the University

The role and purpose of the university have evolved over time. According to Trow (1973), the elite university, designed to preserve leadership of societies in the hands of the privileged, has effectively been replaced by the mass university, in line with the social justice imperative for widening participation in many parts of the world. Essentially, universities have always been custodians of the knowledge and values of their societies and the engines for economic development through their knowledge and innovation responsibilities. With the rise of globalisation, universities have been adopting a more universal perspective, driven by a desire to strengthen their international capital and leading the knowledge and innovation needs of a rapidly globalising world. In all this, the most enduring role of the university is captured in the German Humboldtian model of the modern university (Qin, 2011), which places research as its most important function and on which the world's best universities, such as Yale, Harvard, Oxford, and Cambridge, amongst others, are modelled.

However, because of the persistent coloniality of knowledge, of being, and of power, universities in the developing world benchmark their progress and aspirations for excellence along the trajectories of these tried-and-tested models. We think that universities in the less developed world need to re-imagine new roles and purposes for themselves which not only reflect the developmental priorities of their nations and regions, but also champion the dismantling of coloniality to reflect greater relevance for their contexts.

As organisations, universities play these roles through four main organisational pillars: the curriculum, pedagogy, research, and innovation and societal engagement (van Wyk, 2009). By curriculum, we mean the designed, planned, and implemented course components by the universities (Richards, 2013). This includes teaching and learning which we further define as the totality of student's experiences viewed in terms of the educator's or school's instructional goals (Richards, 2013). The second organisational pillar involves the concept of pedagogy which refers not only to the methods that are used to transmit the curriculum but also to the theories that determine the decision for transmitting the curriculum (Young, 2013). The third pillar is about research and is the most significant purpose for which universities have been created. Research is delivered in two main ways: firstly through the work of the academics who are expected to publish to create innovations which stimulate growth and development and secondly through the production of doctoral graduates who become the new knowledge creators of the future (Young, 2013). The last pillar is innovation and societal engagement and it involves trying to find ways in which to engage the people in matters of development rather than only informing them about matters of development (Lee, 2020).

In the section that follows, we assess the extent to which universities in South Africa have been trying to build some resilience around the four dimensions and especially in the context of the COVID-19 pandemic (Table 3.1).

Discussion and Conclusions

Resilient universities are the ones able to cope with abrupt changes, such as those occasioned by the COVID-19 pandemic in 2020. However, this is not enough as the universities need to prepare themselves for often uncertain futures to maintain a sustainable role across their key responsibilities to societies. We deployed an organisational framework comprising of the need to build four capacities.

Table 3.1 A model of organisational resilience at curriculum, pedagogy, research, and innovation and societal engagement levels

Dimension of organisational resilience (Bahadur et al., 2015; Jeans et al., 2017)	Meanings	Evidence of development in institutions	Tendencies towards coloniality
Adoptive	A capacity around universities defined by efforts to stabilise	**Curriculum** Adopt the principle of continuity of learning (Gedifew & Muluneh, 2020) Highlight the need for not changing the curriculum (Bryson & Andres, 2020) **Pedagogy** Switch to remote teaching (Gewin, 2020) **Research** Emphasis placed on research methodology encouraging data collection through online means (Gewin, 2020) **Innovation and societal engagement** Innovation minimalist and societal engagement affected by COVID-19 protocol of social distancing (Bryson & Andres, 2020)	Little or no effort from the universities to accommodate all learners, including those from lower economic households (Bryson & Andres, 2020).

(*continued*)

Table 3.1 (continued)

Dimension of organisational resilience (Bahadur et al., 2015; Jeans et al., 2017)	Meanings	Evidence of development in institutions	Tendencies towards coloniality
Adaptive	A capacity defined by universities and students to allow flexibility in the effort to improve students' experiences	**Curriculum** Put all the curriculum requirements on universities' teaching management systems (Moorhouse, 2020) **Pedagogy** Poor students provided with laptops, smartphones, and negotiation with the service providers for zero-rated platforms (Moorhouse, 2020) **Research** Members of staff who did not have laptops were given these by universities Supervision of post-graduate students was done online, and they also submitted projects for final examination online Virtual graduations (Hill & Jochim, 2020) **Innovation and societal engagement** Paralysed because of social distancing and minimalist innovation (Mutero & Govender, 2020)	Universities remain rigid and still follow the Western way in the curriculum, research and pedagogy (Hill & Jochim, 2020).

(*continued*)

Table 3.1 (continued)

Dimension of organisational resilience (Bahadur et al., 2015; Jeans et al., 2017)	Meanings	Evidence of development in institutions	Tendencies towards coloniality
Anticipative	A capacity that allows one to be proactive and stay prepared for unseen challenges	**Curriculum** Nothing much happened to inform about what is anticipated (Camargo 2020) **Pedagogy** Centres of teaching and learning have taken a useful lead in offering support to staff through webinars (Hill & Jochim, 2020) Not much is done in thinking about various ways to deliver the curriculum in times of a pandemic (Maringe et al., 2020) **Research** Trying to go back to the old ways of doing things (Camargo Jr, 2020) **Innovation and societal engagement** Innovative, but not predictive, meant to solve existing problems. Societal engagement paralysed because of COVID-19 protocols of social distancing (Mutero & Govender, 2020)	Rather reactive and abrupt turn to Western ways of solving problems, in the process increasing the gap between the haves and have-nots (Maringe et al., 2020)

(*continued*)

Table 3.1 (continued)

Dimension of organisational resilience (Bahadur et al., 2015; Jeans et al., 2017)	Meanings	Evidence of development in institutions	Tendencies towards coloniality
Transformative	A capacity to engineer universities' efforts towards systemic and structural change	**Curriculum** Few attempts at systemic and structural change (Maringe et al., 2020) **Pedagogy** Fire-fighting techniques and strategies rather than being proactive (Camargo Jr, 2020) **Research** Little or no evidence of transformation (Camargo Jr, 2020) **Innovation and societal engagement** Universities continue to be hamstrung by Western ideas as well as COVID-19 protocols for social distancing (Mutero & Govender, 2020)	Change is evident in policy, and not much is evident on the ground. Legacy of colonialism and apartheid still apparent (Mutero & Govender, 2020)

The Adoptive Capacity

As the pandemic spread around the world, the first capacity universities required was an adoptive capacity. This largely comprised organisational responsiveness to a crisis and an ability to act quickly to circumvent the spread and effects of the virus, while at the same time ensuring continuity of the core business of the organisation (Gedifew & Muluneh, 2020). Key decisions, made in line with government advice, were to immediately close all universities, but at the same time to ensure continuity of learning. Students from low-income households were faced with the immediate closure of the university and with no easy access to money for travel and some with no ready homes to go to, found themselves scrambling for money at short notice, which was highly problematic.

A lesson for universities is the need to have an emergency fund that can be accessed on a means-tested basis, so that poor students are not always left to their own devices in times of emergency and crisis. The decision to ensure teaching and learning continuity resulted in the abrupt transition from face-to-face to remote teaching and learning modalities. However, again students bore the brunt as they lost substantial learning time while universities were arranging for the purchase of teaching and learning technologies which would be loaned to students from low socioeconomic households. When these eventually arrived, the students from low socioeconomic households had to grapple with issues of poor internet access, load-shedding, and weak signals due to bandwidth problems in locations where many of them reside (Maringe et al., 2020).

While the adopted solution had resonance and agency for the wealthier middle-class students, it nevertheless posed substantial challenges for the poor students who are in the majority in most of the universities in the country. Perhaps solutions might have been considered, which would have included the use of the repackaging of curricula on traditional non-internet-based technologies, such as memory sticks, to remove the barriers imposed by internet-based learning (Devlin, 2020).

The Adaptive Capacity

The adaptive capacity of an organisation refers to its ability to provide flexibility in learning, in terms of time for attendance, the variety of learning materials, submission formats, assessment flexibility, and task completion times (Karlsen & Pritchard, 2013). To a large extent, such considerations were given little attention in the new online modalities, thus placing substantial strain on students, especially those from low-income households who faced electricity load-shedding at crucial learning times amongst other challenges. Overall, although universities embedded principles of leniency, this tended to be nowhere near enough to cover the extent of unanticipated challenges faced by students in the new remote teaching and learning modalities. Equally, although universities migrated courses onto institutional teaching and learning management systems, the courses were mostly copied and pasted without sufficient, if any, adjustment. There was an assumption of pedagogical and curricula transferability between face-to-face and remote modalities of teaching and learning (Mavhunga, 2016). Universities were thus only marginally able to embed an adaptive capacity in the transition to online teaching and learning. We think that a substantial amount of work needs to go into this aspect of building resilient universities and also prioritise lecturers' and students' readiness and competency in using online strategies in South Africa.

The Anticipative Capacity

Although discourses of blended and online teaching and learning have been gaining momentum in HE even before the onset of the pandemic, they remained largely at theoretical levels and tended to be applied in small isolated courses (Hill & Jochim, 2020). In addition, universities tend to work best in stable environments. Even though they are frequently touted as engines of change and innovation, there is a general apathy when it comes to changing things that seem to work well. The sector does not seem to have a strong tradition in anticipating futures and so tends to focus on the here and now, leaving questions of posterity largely unattended to (Hill & Jochim, 2020). The onset of the COVID-19 pandemic cruelly exposed this weakness.

As authors, we believe that any viable sector or organisation has to constantly interrogate three areas that define its existence. These are the past, the present, and the future. In South Africa, as in many other post-colonial spaces, the past is either not accessible in its pure form, or when it is available, the past is presented in bastardised and distorted forms based largely on only those things the colonisers want the rest of the world to know about the colonised. The present tends to be moulded around the values, knowledge systems, economic models, and lifestyles of the same Western colonisers as those of the indigenous people have been made invisible and are largely irretrievable. As indicated earlier, HE institutions generally do not have a strong tradition in imagining their own futures (Gidley, 2012). In the context of the current pandemic, there also appears to be an overwhelming sense of a desire to return to the old normal, which, as Devlin (2020) suggests, must be resisted. This is, however, peppered with a re-emergence of the discourse of blended teaching and learning. What we do not see in sufficient amounts are the strategic approaches and the new budgetary lines to operationalise this envisaged future. As always, an idea that is not put into practice remains but an idea.

The Transformative Capacity

Linked to the above, the transformative university is one with a capacity to work effectively under different circumstances, one with a deep sense of a shared identity towards which all strategies are directed and one which has a capacity to turn the lives of its citizens in equally beneficial ways (Devlin, 2020). Transformative universities are thus deeply democratic institutions with embedded principles of social justice, equality, and equity to the extent that they measure their success based on the progress and achievement of their most vulnerable students. They emphasise support more than performance. They recognise that physical access alone is not an end in and by itself. The focus needs to turn to cognitive access, which must be achieved equitably for all. Beyond cognitive access, transformative universities constantly ask questions about which knowledge is of the greatest worth for teaching, learning, and research endeavours within the sector. As indicated previously, the tendency to default to the Western canon is endemic in the university sectors, especially those in the post-colonial world. Transformation in universities is, therefore, hamstrung by several factors, including fear of becoming deskilled, apprehension about the need to reinvest in new learning, inadequate budgets to support change, weak infrastructures to support change, the romantic appeal of and attachment to the Western canon, persistent pressure by the West to exert its power and influence over local decisions, and the subtle use of force and economic power to maintain dominance and leadership in the academy (Maringe, 2017).

We turn now to a discussion of the extent to which the four core university responsibilities have been impacted by the ongoing pandemic.

Creating Resilient Organisations Around Four Core University Responsibilities

Given the four universal functions of the university and based on the observations we made about the state of the resilience of the institutions in the face of the pandemic, we end the chapter with some suggestions about how the four areas of curriculum, pedagogy, research, and innovation and societal engagement can be strengthened (Maringe, 2017). We see the pandemic both as having presented universities with sets of unique challenges, but also as having created a substantial opportunity for universities to re-imagine their future. Although the suggestions we make below relate specifically to South African universities, we are confident that the issues we raise will have sufficient resonance with the needs of other post-colonial institutions and more broadly with other universities on the global stage.

Curricula Resilience

The curriculum is the mainstay of any university as it provides a way to conceptualise everything that goes on in the university, including that which is meant to create value for students, staff, the organisation, and society. Looked at this way, and not from narrow perspectives where the curriculum is seen as syllabuses or course outlines, the term provides a broad focus on the purposes and goals of universities, the nature of the worthwhile knowledge that they should be producing and developing, the ways in which the university should go about its business, and the approaches the university uses to demonstrate the progress it is making towards the achievement of its goals. There are two fundamental problems with the curricula of universities in South Africa. Their purposes and goals have barely changed from those handed down by the colonial administrators of the past. The most successful universities in South Africa tend to closely reflect the templates of universities in the global north in terms of their developmental trajectories and ambition.

We think that universities in the developing world must look in three places to begin a process of transforming their purposes and goals. The past, present, and future framework we described earlier, for goal setting and purpose determination should be utilised as a basis for deciding which knowledge is most valuable for these institutions and as a basis for re-imagining new futures for themselves.

Pedagogical Resilience

We use the term pedagogy broadly in this chapter to refer to frameworks for delivering the curriculum. Of course, we note the fact that pedagogies are not simply technical and enabling tools in universities. They also have a knowledge and theoretical base of their own. Based on the principles of social justice, equality, equity, and non-discrimination, new pedagogical forms need to be developed in universities. If such had been in place, the abrupt turn to online teaching and learning adopted at the onset of the COVID-19 pandemic would have been brought under the microscope before implementation. The possibilities of enhancing inequalities and inequities in HE would have been debated before implementation, and this might have forced universities to rethink this strategy. As usual, our Africa has always been quick to adopt whatever works in universities in the global north. Possibilities of using television, radio, and Wi-Fi-less technologies as alternatives to online teaching and learning might have been given consideration to create the necessary equity and equality of access, especially by students from low-income households (Chiramba & Maringe, 2020). What our universities in South Africa tend to forget is that there is a new majority in our contemporary institutions, namely the working-class students. The universities are by far still pandering to middle-class values for which they were created and handed down to us by colonialism and more specifically by apartheid in South Africa. Ideas for developing pedagogies of the working class could be inspired by the Freirean notion of the pedagogy of the oppressed (Freire, 1971) and ideas of the pedagogies of the poor (Rehmann & Baptist, 2011).

Research Resilience

Research in universities in South Africa tends to trace the prescriptions of the Western canon, in nearly every respect including its theoretical basis, its methodological processes, and the ways it is subjected to scrutiny and valued. There is no strong indigenous theoretical tradition to help researchers reflect more relevantly, appropriately, and effectively on research issues. For example, to reflect on leadership issues in education and HE, we tend to use Western theories of leadership and often end up forcing data to behave according to these frameworks. In the same ways, despite traditional Africa's excellent record of living harmoniously with nature, conservation of natural resources, and the recycling of waste into usable forms, our contemporary understanding of and thinking around issues of climate change are driven largely by Western models of thought around these issues. In the context of the current pandemic, traditional African ways of dealing with disease outbreaks and mitigation are rarely given space, if at all, in the conceptualisation of national responses to pandemics. In the area of research ethics, we maintain strict adherence to principles of confidentiality and anonymity which have a place in protecting participants' rights and safety from harm, but which nevertheless entrench the marginalisation of the vulnerable and less powerful people, through whom we create knowledge. The entire model of creating perfect knowledge for others needs to be brought to scrutiny as it is largely responsible for entrenching power and privilege in the hands of the already more powerful in societies, while effectively further disempowering the vulnerable and less privileged. There is, therefore, a basis on which to build a case for the decolonisation of research in the African university and in others in the less developed world, including in post-colonial societies.

Innovation and Societal Impact Resilience

The credibility and efficacy of African solutions continue to be measured by the extent to which Western powers have been involved in their development. This, in part, has led to the increasing importance of partnerships, which, despite the potential they have to develop world-class knowledge and solutions, tend to be driven by interests and leadership of the northern partners. Needless to say, most north-south knowledge and innovation partnerships are funded by organisations which are deeply immersed in Western traditions. Without furthering the desires and interests of the funder, knowledge production can easily be curtailed. A case in point is how no COVID-19 vaccine has been developed on the African continent following the outbreak of the pandemic. If Africa has participated at all in the development of these vaccines, it has been through trials done on the continent in partnerships with institutions in the northern hemisphere. Consequently, Africa's solutions continue to be dictated by the rich countries of the north. New ways of conceptualising partnerships, their funding, and the location of the basic science processes should be imagined in ways that enhance the efficacy of solutions on the African continent.

Towards a Conclusion

Given the purposes of the chapter and the theoretical and empirical evidence we have drawn on, we offer the following tentative conclusions. We describe them as tentative because we think that they need to be subjected to further scrutiny, testing, and research. The proposals we make, however, call for bold responses to interrogate what we describe as persistent coloniality of the South African HE sector.

Universities in South Africa have shown substantial weaknesses as resilient organisations in the face of the ongoing pandemic. Although they demonstrated some resilience in both their adoptive and adaptive capacities, serious weaknesses were evident in regard to failures to assess the efficacy of strategies dictated to them by the responses of universities in wealthy countries. The adoption of online teaching and learning is a case in point, as the impact on poor students was only given attention after the fact.

Within the four-framework theory of organisational resilience utilised in this chapter, the universities showed the greatest weaknesses in the anticipative and transformational capacities. There does not seem to exist a strong tradition within the universities of anticipative research. The greatest preoccupation of the universities is on the here and now. Yet if universities cannot invest in futuristic research, the sector will always be caught unprepared in the face of new disasters and disease outbreaks. Their transformative capacity remains hamstrung in coloniality, and, as such, South African universities might be described as models for the continuance of the colonial ambitions of Western nations. The need for developing university goals and purposes deeply embedded in carefully selected knowledge in the spaces of the past, the present, and the future is both urgent and crucial in South Africa.

The influence of the Western canon across all the core responsibilities of our universities is very strong. As long as our universities do not assume leadership in the re-engagement of indigenous theories to underpin research endeavours, and as long as we default towards Western theorisation frameworks for the solution of Africa's problems, African universities will forever remain on the peripheries as second-class knowledge producers in the global academy.

We hope that this chapter has raised important issues. We consider it to be a small contribution towards a re-theorisation of organisational resilience which provides important insights into re-imagining the post-COVID-19 African university.

References

Badat, S. (2010). The challenges of transformation in higher education and training institutions in South Africa. *Development Bank of Southern Africa, 8*(1), 1–37.

Bahadur, A. V., Peters, K., Wilkinson, E., Pichon, F., Gray, K., & Tanner, T. (2015). *The 3As: Tracking resilience across BRACED* (BRACED Knowledge Manager working paper). London: Overseas Development Institute (ODI).

Beck, R. B. (2000). *The history of South Africa*. Greenwood Publishing Group.

Beck, V. S. (2010). Comparing online and face-to-face teaching and learning. *Journal on Excellence in College Teaching, 21*(3), 95–108. Retrieved May 14, 2020, from https://www.learntechlib.org/p/74546/

Bryson, J. R., & Andres, L. (2020). Covid-19 and rapid adoption and improvisation of online teaching: Curating resources for extensive versus intensive online learning experiences. *Journal of Geography in Higher Education, 44*(4), 608–623.

Camargo, K. R. D., Jr. (2020). Trying to make sense out of chaos: Science, politics and the COVID-19 pandemic. *Cadernos De Saude Publica, 36*, e00088120.

Chiramba, O., & Maringe, F. (2020). Social justice for refugee students in higher education in sub-Saharan Africa: Policy disjunctures. In A. P. Ndofirepi & M. Musengi (Eds.), *Inclusion as social justice* (pp. 57–70). Brill Sense.

Chiramba, O. F. (2020). *Biographical narrative study of refugee students' lived experiences at a selected South African university* (Unpublished Doctoral dissertation). University of the Witwatersrand.
Constitutional Court of South Africa. (1996). Bill of rights. Retrieved November 12, 2013, from https://www.google.com/search?q=Constitutional+Court+of+South+Africa+(1996).+Bill+of+rights.+Retrieved+November%2C+12%2C+2013+from+xxx+.&rlz=1C1SQJL_enZA924ZA925&oq=Constitutional+Court+of+South+Africa+(1996).+Bill+of+rights.+Retrieved+November%2C+12%2C+2013+from+xxx+.&aqs=chrome..69i57j69i60.2263j0j7&sourceid=chrome&ie=UTF-8
Davids, L. M., Van Wyk, J., Khumalo, N. P., & Jablonski, N. G. (2016). The phenomenon of skin lightening: Is it right to be light? *South African Journal of Science, 112*(11/12). Art. #2016-0056, 5 pages. https://doi.org/10.17159/sajs.2016/20160056; https://globalpressjournal.com/africa/zimbabwe/illegal-skin-bleaching-creams-flood-market-zimbabwe/
Department of Education. (1997). *Education White Paper 3: A programme for the transformation of higher education*. Government Gazette, No 18207 of 15 August 1997. Pretoria: Department of Education.
Devlin, S. (2020). What new agency comes from a complete global reset? Retrieved February 10, 2020, from http://www.diplomainprofessionalstudies.com/202021/the-new-normal
Dussel, E. (2008). *Twenty theses on politics*. Duke University Press.
Fataar, A. (2018). Decolonising education in South Africa: Perspectives and debates. *Educational Research for Social Change, 7*, vi–ix.
Freire, P. (1971). To the coordinator of a "cultural circle". *Convergence, 4*(1), 61.
Gedifew, M., & Muluneh, G. S. (2020). Building a change adaptive university: A system of composite indicators to measure and facilitate pervasive changes. *Higher Education Quarterly*. https://doi.org/10.1111/hequ.12279
Gewin, V. (2020). Five tips for moving teaching online as COVID-19 takes hold. *Nature, 580*(7802), 295–297.
Gidley, J. M. (2012). Re-imagining the role and function of higher education for alternative futures through embracing global knowledge futures. In A. Curaj, P. Scott, L. Vlasceanu, & L. Wilson (Eds.), *European higher education at the crossroads* (pp. 1019–1037). Springer.
Heleta, S. (2016). Decolonisation of higher education: Dismantling epistemic violence and Eurocentrism in South Africa. *Transformation in Higher Education, 1*(1), 1–8.
Hill, P. T., & Jochim, A. (2020, October 29). Can public education return to normal after the COVID-19 pandemic? *Brookings*. Retrieved May 14, 2020, from https://www.brookings.edu/blog/brown-center-chalkboard/2020/10/29/can-public-education-return-to-normal-after-the-covid-19-pandemic/
Jeans, H., Castillo, G. E., & Thomas, S. (2017). *Absorb, adapt, transform: Resilience capacities*. Oxfam International.

Johnson, S. D., Aragon, S. R., & Shaik, N. (2000). Comparative analysis of learner satisfaction and learning outcomes in online and face-to-face learning environments. *Journal of Interactive Learning Research, 11*(1), 29–49.

Karlsen, J. E., & Pritchard, R. M. (Eds.). (2013). *Resilient universities: Confronting changes in a challenging world.* Peter Lang.

Kerr, H. (2015). *Organizational resilience: Harnessing experience, embracing opportunity.* BSI Group.

Maddock, L., & Maroun, W. (2018). Exploring the present state of South African education: Challenges and recommendations. *South African Journal of Higher Education, 32*(2), 192–214.

Maldonado-Torres, N. (2012). Decoloniality at large: Towards a trans-Americas and global transmodern paradigm (Introduction to second special issue of "Thinking through the Decolonial turn"). *Trans Modernity: Journal of Peripheral Cultural Production of the Luso-Hispanic World, 1*(3).

Mamdani, M. (1998). Is African studies to be turned into a new home for Bantu education at UCT? *Social Dynamics, 24*(2), 63–75.

Maringe, F. (2017). Transforming knowledge production systems in the new African university. In *Knowledge and change in African universities* (pp. 1–18). Brill Sense.

Maringe, F., Chiramba, O., Pournara, C., Ndlovu, N., & Magabane, A. (2020). *The quality of home learning in low-income family households.* A Zenex Foundation Learning Brief.

Mavhunga, E. (2016). Transfer of the pedagogical transformation competence across chemistry topics. *Chemistry Education Research and Practice, 17*(4), 1081–1097.

Mignolo, W. (2011). *The darker side of western modernity: Global futures, Decolonial options.* Duke University Press.

Moorhouse, B. L. (2020). Adaptations to a face-to-face initial teacher education course 'forced' online due to the COVID-19 pandemic. *Journal of Education for Teaching, 46*(4), 609–611.

Morrow, W. (2007). *Bounds of democracy; Epistemological access in higher education.* HSRC Press.

Mutero, I. T., & Govender, I. G. (2020). Advancing the exploration of engaged creative-Placemaking amongst universities and communities for social cohesion in South Africa. *Journal of Asian and African Studies, 55*(3), 429–445.

Ndlovu-Gatsheni, S. J. (2013). *Coloniality of power in postcolonial Africa.* African Books Collective.

Ndlovu-Gatsheni, S. J. (2015). Decoloniality as the future of Africa. *History Compass, 13*(10), 485–496.

OECD. (2014). *Guidelines for resilience systems analysis: How to analyse risk and build roadmap for resilience.* OECD publishing.

Qin, Z. H. U. (2011). The Humboldtian model and the future of research universities. *Comparative Education Review, 9*(1).

Quijano, A. (2000). Coloniality of power and Eurocentrism in Latin America. *International Sociology, 15*(2), 215–232.

Rehmann, J., & Baptist, W. (2011). *Pedagogy of the poor: Building the movement to end poverty*. Teachers College Press.
Richards, J. C. (2013). Curriculum approaches in language teaching: Forward, central, and backward design. *RELC Journal, 44*(1), 5–33.
Stacey, E. (2007). A study of face-to-face and online teaching philosophies in Canada and Australia. *Journal of Distance Education, 22*(1), 19–40.
Trow, M. (1973). Problems in the transition from elite to mass higher education. Policies for higher education. In *The general report of the Conference on Future Structures of Postsecondary Education*. Paris: Organization for Economic Co-operation and Development.
Van Wyk, J. M. (2009). *The progress examination as an assessment tool in a problem-based learning curriculum: A case study of the Nelson R. Mandela School of Medicine* (Unpublished Doctoral dissertation). University of KwaZulu-Natal.
Wilburn, K. (2012). Africa to the world! Nkrumah-era philatelic images of emerging Ghana and Pan-Africanism 1957–1966. *African Studies Quarterly, 13*(1/2).
Young, M. (2013). Overcoming the crisis in curriculum theory: A knowledge-based approach. *Journal of Curriculum Studies, 45*(2), 101–118.

4

Re-imagining International Higher Education Partnerships in the Aftermath of COVID-19

Samia Chasi

'Every misfortune is a blessing.'
—African proverb

Introduction

In public discourse, the COVID-19 pandemic is generally referred to as a crisis. It is a health crisis, a socio-economic crisis, a humanitarian crisis. COVID-19 has, as one of the key characteristics of crises, clearly had 'a profound influence on people, organisations, or even countries' (Keown-McMullan, 1997, p. 9). Highlighting the magnitude of the ongoing pandemic, the United Nations Development Programme (UNDP) considers it 'the defining global health crisis of our time and the greatest challenge we have faced since World War Two' (UNDP, n.d.).

Having severely disrupted higher education institutions (HEIs) around the globe, COVID-19 is also an education crisis. It has significantly changed a wide variety of aspects of higher education (HE), including internationalisation. Border and campus closures have affected internationalisation activities of universities in unprecedented ways, bringing traditional mobility endeavours to a grinding halt. In causing such disruption, the pandemic threatens the financial sustainability of programmes and institutions. At the same time,

S. Chasi (✉)
Faculty of Education, University of the Free State, Bloemfontein, South Africa

E. Mogaji et al. (eds.), *Re-imagining Educational Futures in Developing Countries*,
https://doi.org/10.1007/978-3-030-88234-1_4

it provides us with an opportune moment to pause and critically reflect on internationalisation concepts, models, and practices.

This chapter understands crisis as 'an unstable or crucial time or state of affairs in which a decisive change is impending', as defined by the Merriam-Webster dictionary.[1] It is based on the assumption that 'a crisis is not always bad or negative' (Keown-McMullan, 1997, p. 4) and follows Roy (2020) in saying that 'The pandemic is a portal', an opportunity for people to 'break with the past and imagine their world anew' (Roy, 2020, para. 48). The author agrees with Neuwirth, Jović, and Mukherji (2020, p. 3), who, referring to the rapid transition from face-to-face instruction to virtual classrooms in response to COVID-19, highlight that life after the pandemic will not be 'a *return to normal*, but rather that it will be a *new normal* [emphasis in original]'. Furthermore, their proposition that the mode to be in regarding online learning 'is *not resumption*, but rather *re-envisioning* and *re-imagining* [emphasis in original]' is extended to the context of HE internationalisation and partnerships.

Re-imagining HE internationalisation, this chapter highlights the contribution international partnerships can make towards more equitable and inclusive HE environments. It does so from the perspective of South Africa, an emerging country reeling from the economic and social impact of COVID-19. It does so at a time when the pandemic is still a moving target, as South Africa is experiencing a heightened COVID-19 crisis at the beginning of 2021. The country, where the emergence of a mutated SARS-COV-2 lineage was reported in December 2020 (NICD, 2020), is in the grip of a second wave, which saw numbers of infections and deaths rise to levels higher than ever before. In this context, the chapter is an exercise in writing *from the pandemic*, rather than *about* it. Reflecting on experiences so far, it offers a cautious look into a future that seems increasingly difficult to predict.

Impact of COVID-19 on Higher Education in South Africa

The impact of the COVID-19 pandemic on the HE sector in South Africa has been profound. As noted by the Minister of Higher Education, Science and Innovation, it 'dominated our minds and hearts in the year 2020… and brought unprecedented challenges for the leadership and management of both our PSET [Post School Education and Training] sector and our national

[1] See: https://www.merriam-webster.com/dictionary/crisis.

system of innovation' (DHESI, 2021, p. 2). Before exploring this in more detail, it is useful to briefly outline how the South African government has responded to the global pandemic.

Overall, the national response to COVID-19 has been based on a risk-adjusted approach, taking into account several factors such as the level of infections, the rate of transmissions, the capacity of health facilities, as well as the economic and social impact of implemented measures and restrictions. This approach includes an alert system of five levels, determining the extent to which restrictions are to be applied during different phases of the national state of disaster. The system ranges from lockdown level 5, indicating the highest spread and lowest health system readiness, to lockdown level 1, with the lowest spread and highest health system readiness.[2]

The president of South Africa first declared a national state of disaster in March 2020, and the country has been in a continuous lockdown since then, with varying levels being implemented at different times. Towards the very end of 2020, the lockdown alert level was raised from level 1 to an adjusted level 3 in an attempt to curb the 'second wave' of the pandemic marked by alarmingly rising numbers of COVID-19-related infections and deaths.

For most of 2020, the activities of universities in South Africa were adversely affected by the nation-wide implementation of COVID-19-related measures, including campus closures and comprehensive travel restrictions under lockdown level 5. The phased return of students and staff to campuses under lockdown levels 4, 3, and 2, and the adherence to social distancing and health protocols under lockdown level 1 allowed for a continuation of activities, but was a far cry from normalcy. The following sections will briefly address the situation universities find themselves in as of early 2021, with specific consideration given to the implications of the pandemic on academic calendars as well as the human and financial resources of South African HEIs.

The 2020 academic year was marked by extraordinary challenges caused by severe disruptions to the teaching, learning, research, and service functions of universities in the wake of unprecedented, nation-wide university closures. This disruption was of such magnitude that its consequences continue to be felt in 2021. For example, while January generally marks the start of a new academic year in South Africa, the country's universities are facing a special challenge, which sees them having to deal with the demands of two academic years. The opening of the 2021 academic year has been delayed by several months to March or April, as universities are expected to first complete the

[2] More detailed information about the alert levels is published by the South African government and available at: https://www.gov.za/covid-19/about/about-alert-system

2020 academic year by February or March 2021 (DHESI, 2021). The 2020 academic year ran over, mostly due to COVID-19-related restrictions that brought teaching and learning activities to a grinding halt and necessitated universities to move their activities online. Implementing emergency remote learning measures took institutions, depending on available infrastructures and resources, from several weeks in the case of some research-intensive universities to several months in the case of disadvantaged institutions.

Until the end of February 2021, work on completing one academic year while preparing to open another was done under the conditions of an adjusted lockdown level 3, which stipulated, among others, strict requirements for hygiene and social distancing as well as restrictions regarding the movement and gatherings of people. Since March 2021, South Africa is on an adjusted alert level 1. Managing the demands of two academic years at the same time requires careful consideration for the time being. However, the COVID-19 pandemic is likely to have even more far-reaching consequences for the human and financial sustainability of the South African HE sector in the mid to long term.

As of mid-November 2020, South Africa's 26 public universities reported to have lost 58 people to the pandemic, a total made up of 48 staff members and 10 students (DHESI, 2021). While each of these deaths is a tragic loss to the families, friends, classmates, and colleagues of the individuals concerned, their collective loss robs South African HE of years and decades of knowledge, experience and expertise, which negatively affects the human resource capacity of the sector as a whole.

Provided that it can, as often assumed, take up to 20 years before someone becomes a full professor, replacing senior academics and researchers lost to the pandemic becomes a long-term endeavour. Losing such staff in considerable numbers poses a challenge not only to the institutions at which they were employed, but to South African HE in general. Loss of life, skills, and experience is particularly disconcerting in a sector that is struggling to achieve ambitious targets as outlined in the National Development Plan, including improving qualifications of academic staff and increasing the number of doctoral graduates and scientists by 2030 (National Planning Commission, 2012).

The economic impact of COVID-19 on the South African HE sector, which is already financially constrained, is also far-reaching. In 2020, the Department of Higher Education, Science and Innovation (DHESI) invested almost R69 million in activities regarding COVID-19-related research and development (DHESI, 2021). These funds did not constitute additional spending, but were reprioritised from the previous allocation (ibid.). The chief executive officer (CEO) of Universities South Africa (USAf), an organisation representing all public universities in the country, is reported to have serious concerns about the impact of COVID-19-related expenditure on the financial wellbeing of universities, as institutions incurred considerable expenses for preparing to switch to remote learning, keeping campuses safe, and dealing with defaults in the payment of tuition fees, upon which universities rely as a major income stream (Nordling, 2021). At the same time, the demand for funding support continues to rise. Applications for the 2021 academic year to the National Student Financial Aid Scheme (NSFAS), a scheme through which the South African government provides financial aid to poor undergraduate students, grew by 25%, as compared to the previous year (DHESI, 2021). Furthermore, there are concerns about the potential of an even bigger financial crisis looming in 2021, based on expected cuts to the national budget and subsidies for HE (Nordling, 2021).

Lessons for Internationalisation from the Ongoing COVID-19 Pandemic

Having briefly considered the general impact of COVID-19 on HE in South Africa, the following sections reflect on lessons that can be learnt from the pandemic with a particular focus on HE internationalisation. These reflections on lessons learnt are, as indicated earlier, not written from an 'after-the-fact' perspective. Rather, they draw on experiences so far and are based on the understanding that, with the pandemic in full force, our ground is still shifting.

It is important to note in this regard that HE landscapes are generally dynamic, and that universities are resilient institutions that have existed for centuries and have adapted to ever-changing environments. In the twenty-first century, as highlighted by Weber (2016), the survival of HEIs around the world depends on their capacity to respond to the challenges they face, including internationalisation, competition, the increased pace of scientific and technical progress, and the emergence of the knowledge economy. Related to this, Sledge and Fishman (2014) reflect on the fast-changing landscape in American HE, particularly regarding technological advances and new models of learning, and consider implications for how universities and other organisations can adapt to a new era of lifelong learning in the digital age. Apart from global trends and developments, universities are also affected by changes in their local environments. Chasi (2020c, p. 10) points out in that regard that the South African HE sector has, since the end of apartheid, 'faced several disruptive events including the university mergers of 2005 as well as the nation-wide student protests of 2015 and 2016.'

However, it goes without saying that the challenges COVID-19 poses to HE are unparalleled. In the wake of campus closures and other lockdown restrictions, universities around the globe were confronted with a 'tsunami of changes', including:

> ...an immediate pivot to online teaching and learning; rapid rethinking of pedagogy, assessment and curricula; emergency investment in digital infrastructure; re-evaluation of real estate; a blockage in the flow of international mobility; and behavioural changes among students and staff. (Brink, 2021, para. 4)

This 'tsunami' included changes concerning internationalisation activities of universities. Most notably, challenges in that regard were linked to the impact of the pandemic on student mobility flows, which, in turn, negatively affected mobility-based income streams of universities. In its modern understanding, internationalisation is a relatively recent phenomenon that has increasingly gained prominence since the 1980s. In these past 40 years, there has not been a pandemic that compares to COVID-19 in terms of its global reach and magnitude, leading to unprecedented closures of HEIs all around the world and bringing mobility to a halt at a global stage. However, this does not mean that there is nothing to be learnt from reflecting on the past.

As far as the relevance of past pandemics to the ongoing COVID-19 crisis is concerned, Kretchmer (2021) suggests taking the following key points into consideration: (1) an increase in global health cooperation, (2) an increase in unpredictability, (3) an expansion of the state, (4) an acceleration of technologies and economies, and (5) an increased burden on the poor. While all five of these points are relevant from a South African perspective, three of them seem particularly pertinent to a discussion on what can be learnt from COVID-19 in the context of HE internationalisation: global cooperation, acceleration of technology, and a burden on the poor. Taking these points into account, the sections that follow consider the pandemic a phenomenon that simultaneously reaffirms the importance of HE internationalisation, functions as an accelerator of innovation, and has the potential to deepen existing inequalities.

Reaffirming the Need for and Importance of Higher Education Internationalisation

As far as internationalisation is concerned, COVID-19 presents both a threat and an opportunity. Apart from threatening the financial wellbeing of HEIs, the pandemic gave rise to racist rhetoric and xenophobic sentiments, which, in turn, are reported to have incited discrimination and violence particularly against people of Asian descent in a number of countries around the world, including South Africa (HRW, 2020). In the wake of such incidents, the United Nations (UN) published a set of recommendations to address and counteract hate speech and discrimination and to promote inclusion, solidarity, and international human rights (UN, 2020).

International education can make a contribution towards countering intolerance and discrimination and fostering inclusion and social cohesion. It does so by highlighting the value of diversity of cultures, experiences, and viewpoints and by facilitating international and intercultural dialogue and cooperation. In light of COVID-19 as a global challenge, the Network of International Education Associations (NIEA) issued a statement reaffirming the 'importance of international higher education to our mutually beneficial and sustainable future, as international collaboration is essential to finding solutions to global problems, which manifest differently in our local contexts' (NIEA, 2020, p. 1). From a South African perspective, the pandemic:

> ...can be used as a powerful argument for the importance of internationalisation, as it illustrates that grand challenges such as a global pandemic cannot be solved by any one institution, nation or region alone but require collaboration that transcends borders and disciplines. (IEASA, 2020, p. 3)

South African 'scientists continue to work with their international counterparts to ensure that knowledge is pooled in order to bring COVID-19 under control' (DHESI, 2021, p. 7), thus making a clear case for the importance of international collaboration and partnerships, particularly in the areas of COVID-19-related research, vaccine development, and clinical trials. The role universities play in such endeavours cannot be underestimated as HEIs are important stakeholder in South Africa's national system of innovation.

Accelerating Innovation

In South Africa, COVID-19 has acted as an accelerator of innovation. From the start of the pandemic, many South African universities have confronted the various challenges arising in the wake of COVID-19 head-on:

> They are at the forefront of vaccine research and clinical trials. They are, to extents that are unparalleled in this context, delivering academic programmes online and conducting virtual graduation ceremonies. They are developing apps and innovative solutions to produce hand sanitisers, face shields, antimicrobial coatings and tracking devices. (Chasi, 2020a, para. 31)

Such contributions highlight the important role universities play in addressing societal and, indeed, global challenges. They give expression to a 'profound change [that] is taking place in our understanding of the mission of higher education' (Brink, 2021, para. 5), with a shift from curiosity-driven knowledge production and research to demand-led research (Brink, 2021).

Another deep realisation emerging from the experience of COVID-19 is that change is not only possible, but can, if necessity requires, be brought about quickly. The pandemic has led to profound changes in the way we interact, learn, and work. Universities were prompted to develop or increase their capacity to work online and remotely in the shortest possible time, and they did so in periods spanning from weeks to months. In an attempt to both 'save lives and at the same time save the academic year' (DHESI, 2021, p. 22), all South African universities 'had to adapt their systems and teaching methods to provide remote support' (ibid.). However, differences in the availability of institutional infrastructures and resources led to varying degrees of implementation readiness. In this regard, the pandemic holds another important lesson, putting a spotlight on inequality.

Entrenching Inequality

In a recent report published by Oxfam (2021), COVID-19 is referred to as the 'inequality virus', suggesting that the pandemic will be remembered 'as the first time since records began that inequality rose in virtually every country on earth at the same time' (Oxfam, 2021, p. 9). The report also acknowledges that the 'coronavirus crisis has swept across a world that was already extremely unequal' (Oxfam, 2021, p. 10). Global inequalities manifest, for example, in COVID-19-related vaccine development and roll-out, where poorer, emerging countries like South Africa are at risk of being left behind. At the same time, 'a small group of rich nations, representing just 14% of the world's population, has bought up more than half the supply of leading COVID-19 vaccine contenders' (Oxfam, 2021, p. 33).

In South Africa, COVID-19 has starkly highlighted the differentiated nature of the country's HE system, where, as a legacy of apartheid, historically advantaged institutions (HAIs), as distinguished from historically disadvantaged institutions (HDIs), are generally better equipped to deal with COVID-19-related challenges (IEASA, 2020). It has also illustrated that the burden of the pandemic is primarily placed on the poor. When institutions implemented remote teaching activities, students at the highest risk of being left behind were those who lived in poverty and in conditions not 'conducive to online learning, without access to computers and laptops, affordable data, reliable internet connectivity, electricity or a dedicated physical space in which to study' (IEASA, 2020, p. 2). In this sense, the pandemic feeds off and exacerbates inequality.

Inequality is not only a characteristics of HE, but also of HE internationalisation in South Africa, as it has not been advanced evenly across the country's universities (IEASA, 2020). The first national internationalisation policy framework, whose adoption was formally announced in November 2020, notes that internationalisation has not benefitted South African institutions equally, as HDIs 'still have very low levels of international relations and are not yet, therefore, benefitting from internationalisation to the degree that they could' (DHET, 2019, p. 21).

Apart from disparities within the South African HE sector, internationalisation is, in the global context, generally characterised by inequality in so far as it is 'dominated by Northern perspectives in terms of its definitions, concepts and practices' (Chasi, 2020b, para. 8). Student mobility and income flows tend to favour institutions in the North, and partnerships between HEIs in the Global North and the Global South are often considered challenging due to imbalances in power, resources, and knowledge (Chasi, 2019).

From the perspective of South Africa as a representative of the Global South, HE internationalisation is inherently problematic, as it does not benefit Southern institutions as much as their Northern counterparts. If applied uncritically, within dominant paradigms, internationalisation can therefore further entrench existing inequalities. To help mitigate this potential, internationalisation efforts of South African universities 'should be permeated by an agenda that focuses on inclusion and social justice' (IEASA, 2020, p. 4). This is particularly important in light of challenging times ahead, where internationalisation activities are at risk of being de-prioritised and de-funded when universities face cuts on budgets and resources. In this context, it is critical that internationalisation is not a goal in itself, but aligned to relevant institutional and national goals, contributing to HE transformation, nation building, and the public good (ibid.).

Following from the above, neither COVID-19 nor internationalisation are equalising forces for the South African HE sector. Both have been shown to not only bring existing inequalities to the fore, but to 'further deepen existing divides between those who have—for example, opportunities to benefit from online teaching or study abroad places—and those who do not' (IEASA, 2020, p. 3). With this in mind, it is worth exploring how lessons learnt from the pandemic can inform the re-imagining of internationalisation, particularly in the context of international HE partnerships.

International Higher Education Partnerships Re-Imagined

The COVID-19 crisis as experienced in the South African HE sector does not exist in a vacuum. More broadly, it is 'connected to a wider set of crises; of social inequality, of climate change, of technological disruption, and linked to all of the above: a crisis of the global capitalist system' (DHESI, 2021, p. 2). At the same time, it is a crisis that places us at a 'pivotal point in human history', urging us to act to bring about positive change:

> We cannot return to the brutal, unequal and unsustainable world that the coronavirus found us in. Humanity has incredible talent, huge wealth and infinite imagination. We must put these assets to work to create a more equal and sustainable economy that benefits all, not just the privileged few. (Oxfam, 2021, p. 54)

What does the above mean for HE internationalisation? How can we create more equal and sustainable international partnerships? Tackling such questions, it is worth drawing on debates and literature that have addressed challenges in international HE partnerships, highlighting in particular that these partnerships are often imbalanced and that the benefits of internationalisation are not evenly shared between institutions in emerging countries and their counterparts in the Global North (Chasi, 2019).

In the *Nelson Mandela Bay Global Dialogue Declaration* (IEASA, 2014), for example, representatives of a variety of national, regional, and other organisations working in international HE highlight the 'importance of decision-making and practices in the development of internationalisation activities that are imbued with ethical considerations and inclusivity' (IEASA, 2014, p. 2). Furthermore, they note that 'internationalisation must be based on mutual benefit and development for entities and individuals in the developed, emerging and developing countries' (ibid.). Regarding international HE partnerships, Jooste (2015) points out that they should play an equalising role and proposes that partners operate in alignment with the concept of a 'global commons'. Hagenmeier (2015) considers the lack of equality a key threat to partnerships and highlights the importance of substantive equality for mutually beneficial and reciprocal partnerships. Similarly, De Wit (2015) notes that partnerships have the capacity to entrench and perpetuate inequalities and asymmetries in HE and that it is important for the future of partnerships that they are transformational in character and operate on equal terms.

Sensibly predicting the future of HE and HE internationalisation is made difficult by the many uncertainties that exist at the start of 2021 (De Wit, 2021). In this context, it is 'more important than ever to follow the developments closely in the coming period, pay attention to critical concerns such as inequality, as well as to positive signs of innovation' (De Wit, 2021, para. 13). With this in mind, the following sections explore the role of internationalisation in promoting inclusion and social justice. More specifically, they focus on how international partnerships can be re-imagined to help mitigate inequalities in the South African HE sector. In doing so, consideration is given to two key elements: people and technology.

People

Partnerships depend on people. If partnerships are to be more equal and facilitate inclusion and social justice, the people who are engaged in these partnerships have to be committed to supporting such causes. While these causes are not new, what seems to have changed is that the awareness of inequality and injustice around the world is growing, accelerated by the collective experience of COVID-19. The pandemic has, although manifesting differently in local contexts, affected all universities around the globe in ways no other crisis seems to have done before. This realisation has provided a collective opportunity to pause and reflect, a process which has been aided by social movements fighting for liberation and justice by targeting discrimination, violence, white supremacy, and black pain, including #BlackLivesMatter and #RhodesMustFall.

Amongst HE internationalisation practitioners and scholars, particularly those based in the Global North, growing awareness can lead to growing willingness to engage and confront such issues, which are often difficult and sensitive. As an example of encouraging signs, a webinar entitled 'Decolonising international partnerships',[3] hosted by the Canadian Bureau for International Education (CBIE) in October 2020, provided participants, mostly international relations officers, with an opportunity to critically reflect on personal and institutional partnerships practices.

In the context of international HE partnerships, particularly those between institutions in the Global North and the Global South, inequalities can be addressed using a decolonial lens (Chasi, 2019). In this regard, decolonisation is understood as 'both an attitude and a practice aimed at rehumanising the world' (Chasi, 2020b, para. 5). It provides a tool for tackling unequal power dynamics and working towards greater balance, equality, and justice in partnerships (ibid.), thus working towards the possibility of a more socially just world.

As noted earlier, HE internationalisation has an important role to play in promoting inclusion, social cohesion, and justice by bringing diverse people, institutions, and cultures into conversation and providing them with opportunities to learn about and from each other. At a conference hosted jointly by the International Education Association of South Africa (IEASA) and the African Network for Internationalisation of Education (ANIE) in October 2020,[4] Professor Thuli Madonsela, South Africa's former public protector, emphasised this role in her keynote address and urged African universities to foster internationalisation driven by the African philosophy of *Ubuntu* and care for each other, which speaks to our interconnectedness and collective humanity. Professor Madonsela also called on African universities to use the opportunities presented by COVID-19 for positive transformation and enhancement of internationalisation. Many such opportunities are linked to the use of technology.

Technology

In the age of the Fourth Industrial Revolution, technological disruptions and advances are the proverbial order of the day. However, COVID-19 has accelerated change in that regard, making technology an even greater component of our everyday lives, especially regarding the way we interact. When campus

[3] The webinar recording is available at: https://cbie.ca/event/decolonizing-international-partnerships/

[4] The conference, entitled "Innovation and Resilience in Higher Education Internationalisation in an Era of COVID-19 & Beyond", was held virtually on 1 and 2 October 2020. More information is available at: https://ieasa.studysa.org/virtual-conference-2020/

closures and a national lockdown were announced with only a few days' notice in South Africa, universities had to move their activities online, literally overnight. As HE has become more virtual in the wake of the pandemic, it is now widely expected that the future provision of academic and administrative services alike will be based on blended approaches, combining both physical and virtual activities.

On the one hand, HEIs are waiting to return to 'normal' activities including travel and classroom teaching. On the other hand, 'online teaching and learning as well as online research collaboration and networking will definitely increase, and that is a positive development for the environment' (De Wit, 2021, para. 8). A reduction in physical mobility, especially air travel, will lessen internationalisation's carbon footprint and make a valuable contribution to combatting climate change. Furthermore, reducing physical mobility and replacing it with virtual mobility has the potential of addressing inequalities inherent in many traditional international partnerships, especially those focussing on the exchange of students and staff.

For example, traditional student exchanges, particularly those facilitated within North-South partnerships, tend to be imbalanced and benefit Northern universities more than their Southern counterparts. Funding constraints often make such arrangements elitist and exclusionary by benefitting only a select few (Chasi, 2019). To address this, the use of online technologies can inspire re-imagined partnerships efforts that allow for greater access and inclusion of previously disadvantaged individuals and institutions, who were unable to participate in traditional partnership opportunities for socio-economic reasons. Such can be achieved by placing greater emphasis on the exchange of knowledge than on the mobility of people, thus facilitating equality and mutual benefit in international partnerships (IEASA, 2020).

In re-imagining student exchange and collaboration, universities do not have to reinvent the wheel. For example, Collaborative Online International Learning (COIL) is a relatively new area of interest and focus in internationalisation that might gain considerable momentum through the COVID-19 pandemic. The *iKudu* project,[5] which is coordinated by a South African university and funded by the European Union (EU) in the framework of Erasmus+, is a university partnership that is already under way and can serve as an example in that regard. Recognising that South African students face severe socio-economic challenges preventing them from participating in physical mobility opportunities, the project partners aim to rethink internationalisation by developing a contextualised South African approach to

[5] More information about the project is available at: https://www.ufs.ac.za/ikudu

internationalisation of the curriculum (IoC) through COIL. Using technology, COIL is considered 'a fertile space in which to promote openness to knowledge pluralisation through diverse learners interacting and sharing knowledge perspectives' (Wimpenny et al., 2021, para. 10). The project aims to 'move beyond the rhetoric of openness, pluralism, tolerance, flexibility, and transparency towards ways in which decolonisation and internationalisation are reflected in educational practice' (Wimpenny et al., 2021, para. 16).

The use of online technologies and pedagogies can inspire re-imagined internationalisation efforts to counteract some of the challenges of traditional internationalisation models that negatively impact the environment and bring about unequal benefits for universities. A series of challenging conversations titled 'Unleashing the new global university',[6] hosted by the University of Cape Town (UCT) between June and September 2020, provided a platform for the exchange of experiences and generation of ideas in that regard (UCT, n.d.). The aim of the series was to rethink HE internationalisation and reflect on the role of technology in re-imagining ways in which universities engage in teaching, learning, and research as well as networking and collaboration. Recognising that travel restrictions and lockdowns have opened up global connections by removing distance as a barrier, one of the core questions considered was if internationalisation experiences can be made more equitable by going virtual. Spanning a broad spectrum of university activities, speakers considered online meetings, workshops, conferences, as well as virtual alternatives to classroom teaching, supervision, mentoring, and peer support.

Regarding international student experiences, for example, there was general consensus that virtual mobility can never replace physical mobility in terms of providing a fully immersed, lived experience of another institution, country or culture. However, it was equally agreed that virtual mobility offers alternatives for more equitable and inclusive engagements by increasing affordability as well as access. Access refers both to the increased diversity of participants as well as to resources and expertise from elsewhere.

Technology-driven change, accelerated by COVID-19, comes at a time where South Africa has, for the first time, adopted a national *Policy Framework for Internationalisation of Higher Education in South Africa* (DHET, 2019). Going forward, South African universities should consider how what they have learnt from their responses to COVID-19 can inform the implementation of this policy and contribute to the re-imagining of HE

[6] More information about the webinar series is available at: https://www.news.uct.ac.za/features/the-new-global-university/

internationalisation more broadly. This applies particularly to investments made in online technologies and lessons learnt regarding the mitigation of inequalities in the digital economy. It also relates to the adaptability and resilience South African universities have shown in working in less resourced and constrained environments. Such resilience relates to challenges in responding to COVID-19 as much as those linked to advancing internationalisation in South Africa for over two decades.

Re-imagining the future of HE and HE internationalisation requires boldness and courage. As Brink (2021, para. 41) notes, 'If we have the will and the energy, our response… could yet prove to be not only an example of academic responsibility, but an inflection point in the changing mission of higher education'. The same can be said regarding the changing nature of HE internationalisation.

Conclusions

This chapter has explored COVID-19 as both a threat and an opportunity in the context of HE in South Africa, where neither the pandemic nor internationalisation are equalising forces. While COVID-19 threatens HE internationalisation as we know it, this is not, in itself, a bad thing. With particular reference to traditional internationalisation activities focussing on physical mobility, it has been highlighted that HE internationalisation was already suffering a crisis of inequality before the arrival of COVID-19, especially from a Global South perspective.

Reflecting on how lessons learnt from the pandemic can help mitigate inequalities in HE and HE internationalisation, this chapter argues for COVID-19 to be taken as a turning point. Considering changes regarding both people and technology, international HE partnerships can be a powerful tool in re-imagining HE internationalisation in South Africa and elsewhere and in creating a global HE community that is more inclusive and socially just.

It is difficult to know what the future holds and what the residual legacy of COVID-19 will be. From the perspective of HE in an emerging country like South Africa, 'Nothing could be worse than a return to normality', as observed by Roy (2020, para. 47), if that implies a continued use of dominant HE internationalisation models and practices. Regarding mobility, for example, it is not desirable to fully return to activities and programmes that require physical travel. On the contrary, it is pertinent to change minds and to continue using blended approaches in the provision of academic and administrative services to increase access to internationalisation initiatives that have traditionally hindered participation of people from resource-constrained institutions, countries, and regions.

In light of universities having moved their activities swiftly online in the wake of COVID-19, geographical distance and lack of funding should no longer function as barriers to international engagement and exchange. What we have experienced so far in terms of online teaching, learning, collaboration, and networking should serve as a 'laboratory' for further exploration of alternative approaches to mobility and internationalisation more broadly. The use of existing and new technologies should continue to be at the forefront of re-imagining HE internationalisation. With this in mind, the pandemic becomes, in the words of Roy (2020), a 'portal', as it provides practitioners and scholars around the world with an opportunity to break with the past of imbalanced partnerships and imagine HE internationalisation anew.

References

Brink, C. (2021, January 21). Academic responsibility: The changing mission of HE. *University World News* (Africa ed.). Retrieved January 25, 2021, from https://www.universityworldnews.com/post.php?story=20210119052730285

Chasi, S. (2019). *North-South partnerships in public higher education: A selected South African case study*. PhD Thesis, University of the Witwatersrand, Johannesburg. Retrieved January 29, 2021, from http://wiredspace.wits.ac.za/handle/10539/28064

Chasi, S. (2020a, April 9). COVID-19 has put HE internationalisation under review. *University World News* (Africa ed.). Retrieved January 19, 2021, from https://www.universityworldnews.com/post.php?story=20200408093750683

Chasi, S. (2020b, August 27). Decolonisation—A chance to reimagine North-South partnerships. *University World News* (Africa ed.). Retrieved January 19, 2021, from https://www.universityworldnews.com/post.php?story=20200826111105105

Chasi, S. (2020c). Embracing resilience in internationalisation. In International Education Association of South Africa (Ed.), *Study South Africa—The guide to South African higher education* (19th ed., pp. 9–10). Pretoria: IEASA.

De Wit, H. (2015). Partnerships for the future: Trends, challenges and opportunities. In N. Jooste, H. De Wit, & S. Heleta (Eds.), *Higher education partnerships for the future* (pp. 95–101). Unit for Higher Education Internationalisation in the Developing World.

De Wit, H. (2021, January 16). It's getting harder to predict the future of HE. *University World News* (Global ed.). Retrieved January 21, 2021, from https://www.universityworldnews.com/post.php?story=20210115105133419

Department of Higher Education and Training [DHET]. (2019). *Policy framework for internationalisation of higher education in South Africa*. Retrieved January 29, 2021, from https://www.dhet.gov.za/Policy%20and%20Development%20Support/Policy%20Framework%20for%20Internationalisation%20of%20Higher%20Education%20in%20South%20Africa.pdf

Department of Higher Education, Science and Innovation [DHESI]. (2021). *Statement on plans for the reopening of post school education and training institutions and the contribution of science and innovation in the fight against COVID-19*. Retrieved January 20, 2021, from https://www.dhet.gov.za/SiteAssets/Media%20Advisory%20and%20Statements%202021/STATEMENT%20-%20PSET%20reopening%20and%20DSI%20COVID-19%20developments.pdf

Hagenmeier, C. (2015). Ensuring equality in higher education partnerships involving unequal universities in divergent contexts. In N. Jooste, H. De Wit, & S. Heleta (Eds.), *Higher education partnerships for the future* (pp. 41–46). Unit for Higher Education Internationalisation in the Developing World.

Human Rights Watch [HRW]. (2020, May 12). Covid-19 fueling anti-Asian racism and Xenophobia worldwide. National Action Plans Needed to Counter Intolerance. *HRW News*. Retrieved January 27, 2021, from https://www.hrw.org/news/2020/05/12/covid-19-fueling-anti-asian-racism-and-xenophobia-worldwide#

IEASA. (2020). *Higher education internationalisation in South Africa in the context of the COVID-19 pandemic—Impact on international students* (Position Paper). Retrieved January 27, 2021, from https://ieasa.studysa.org/wp-content/uploads/2020/05/IEASA-position-paper_COVID-19_May2020_Final.pdf

International Education Association of South Africa [IEASA]. (2014). *Nelson Mandela Bay declaration on the future of internationalisation of higher education*. IEASA. Retrieved April 15, 2021, from https://www.aieaworld.org/assets/docs/Press_Releases/nelson_declaration.pdf

Jooste, N. (2015). Higher education partnerships for the future: A view from the South. In N. Jooste, H. De Wit, & S. Heleta (Eds.), *Higher education partnerships for the future* (pp. 11–21). Unit for Higher Education Internationalisation in the Developing World.

Keown-McMullan, C. (1997). Crisis: When does a molehill become a mountain? *Disaster Prevention and Management: An International Journal, 6*(1), 4–10. https://doi.org/10.1108/09653569710162406

Kretchmer, H. (2021, January 11). COVID-19 and geopolitics—5 lessons from past pandemics. *World Economic Forum—The Davos Agenda 2021*. Retrieved January 18, 2021, from https://www.weforum.org/agenda/2021/01/covid-19-geopolitics-lessons-pandemics-history/

National Institute of Communicable Diseases [NICD]. (2020, December 18). The emergence of a mutated SARS-CoV-2 lineage in South Africa. Retrieved April 14, 2021, from https://www.nicd.ac.za/the-emergence-of-a-mutated-sars-cov-2-lineage-in-south-africa/

National Planning Commission. (2012). *National Development Plan 2030. Our future—Make it work*. Retrieved January 26, 2021, from https://www.gov.za/sites/default/files/gcis_document/201409/ndp-2030-our-future-make-it-workr.pdf

Network of International Education Associations [NIEA]. (2020). *Statement on the importance of international higher education and research*. Retrieved January 27, 2021, from https://ieasa.studysa.org/wp-content/uploads/2020/07/NIEA-Statement-on-the-importance-of-international-higher-education-and-research.24-July-2020.pdf

Neuwirth, L. S., Jović, S., & Mukherji, B. R. (2020). Reimagining higher education during and post-COVID-19: Challenges and opportunities. *Journal of Adult and Continuing Education*. https://doi.org/10.1177/08/09653569710162406

Nordling, L. (2021, January 21). "Deep concerns" over South African university funding. *Research Professional News*. Retrieved January 22, 2021, from https://www.researchprofessionalnews.com/rr-news-africa-south-2021-1-deep-concerns-over-south-african-university-funding/

Oxfam. (2021). *The inequality virus. Bringing together a world torn apart by coronavirus through a fair, just and sustainable economy*. Retrieved January 25, 2021, from https://oxfamilibrary.openrepository.com/bitstream/handle/10546/621149/bp-the-inequality-virus-250121-en.pdf

Roy, A. (2020, April 3) The pandemic is a portal. *Financial Times*. Retrieved January 29, 2021, from https://www.ft.com/content/10d8f5e8-74eb-11ea-95fe-fcd274e920ca

Sledge, L., & Fishman, T. D. (2014). *Reimagining higher education—How colleges, universities, businesses, and governments can prepare for a new age of lifelong learning* (A GovLab report). Deloitte University Press. Retrieved April 5, 2021, from https://www2.deloitte.com/content/dam/insights/us/articles/reimagining-higher-education/DUP_758_ReimaginingHigherEducation.pdf

United Nations [UN]. (2020). *United Nations guidance note on addressing and countering COVID-19 related hate speech*. Retrieved January 27, 2021, from https://www.un.org/en/genocideprevention/documents/Guidance%20on%20COVID-19%20related%20Hate%20Speech.pdf

United Nations Development Programme [UNDP]. (n.d.). *COVID-19 pandemic—Humanity needs leadership and solidarity to defeat the coronavirus* [online]. Retrieved January 29, 2021, from https://www.undp.org/content/undp/en/home/coronavirus.html

University of Cape Town [UCT]. (n.d.). *Unleashing the new global university. A series of challenging conversations* [online]. Retrieved January 22, 2021, from https://www.news.uct.ac.za/features/the-new-global-university/

Weber, L. E. (2016). The university in the 21st century. In L. E. Weber & J. J. Duderstadt (Eds.), *University priorities and constraints* (pp. 203–214). Economica.

Wimpenny, K., Hagenmeier, C., Jacobs, L., & Beelen, J. (2021, January 21). Decolonisation through inclusive virtual collaboration. *University World News* (Africa ed.). Retrieved January 25, 2021, from https://www.universityworldnews.com/post.php?story=20210121054345601

5

Fireside Chat with Three Vice Chancellors from Three Continents: Re-imagining Higher Education in Emerging Economies

Atish Chattopadhyay, Tawana Kupe, Nicolás Fernández Schatzer, and Emmanuel Mogaji

Introduction

It is no longer news that the COVID-19 pandemic has affected every facet of human lives. The global pandemic has forever changed how humans live and engage in activities (Mogaji, 2021). Things we thought were not possible are now being done with ease out of the necessity to reinvent and reposition our lives. From mobility restrictions, working patterns and the usual interactions, things have changed, and we need to accept this and start planning for what lies ahead.

Authors' names "Atish Chattopadhyay, Tawana Kupe, and Nicolás Fernández Schatzer" are arranged alphabetically.

A. Chattopadhyay
Vijaybhoomi University, Karjat, Maharashtra, India

T. Kupe
University of Pretoria, Pretoria, South Africa
e-mail: tawana.kupe@up.ac.za

N. F. Schatzer
International University of Ecuador, Loja, Ecuador
e-mail: marcelof@usc.edu

E. Mogaji (✉)
Department of Marketing, Events and Tourism, University of Greenwich, London, UK
e-mail: e.o.mogaji@greenwich.ac.uk

E. Mogaji et al. (eds.), *Re-imagining Educational Futures in Developing Countries*,
https://doi.org/10.1007/978-3-030-88234-1_5

Higher education has been impacted by this global pandemic (Crawford et al., 2020). Previously, higher education was delivered through interpersonal relationships and engagement between tutor and student, often in a face-to-face setting. However, with the emergence of this global pandemic there were disruptions, and many universities were thrown in at the deep end and had to survive, adjusting their teaching styles and student engagement (Ali, 2020). Online classes became the norm and students had to study at home, with faculties, likewise, teaching from home. While many of the developed countries may have had access to technology and other infrastructure to allow them to adjust, there were inherent challenges for many other universities around the world, who may not have much access (Mogaji & Varsha, 2020; Al-Ataby, 2020).

The global pandemic was no respecter of geography (Cheater, 2020). This was not a pandemic affecting the developed countries alone but also the emerging economies, who were still struggling with socio-economic development (Aristovnik et al., 2020; Agormedah et al., 2020). Many of their universities are not funded enough, they do not have access to technology, an internet connection is not often guaranteed, and homes may not even be conducive to learning (Olaleye et al., 2020; Ndofirepi et al., 2020). These are some of the challenges faced by many students in the emerging economies. The struggle is real, and yet their education is important (Mogaji & Varsha, 2020).

To further discuss the impact of the global pandemic, to look beyond the present situation and to re-imagine higher education in emerging economies, a global fireside chat was organised by Dr Emmanuel Mogaji of the University of Greenwich to bring together different vice chancellors (VC) from the emerging economies and have a conversation about where we are with higher education in emerging economies and where we plan to go. Three vice chancellors from three different continents were involved in this conversation. Representing Asia was Professor Atish Chattopadhyay from India, the vice chancellor of Vijaybhoomi University, Mumbai; representing the African continent was Professor Tawana Kupe, vice chancellor at the University of Pretoria, South Africa; while Mr Nicolás Fernández, vice chancellor at the International University of Ecuador, Ecuador, represented South America.

The chat aimed to explore impacts, preparedness, during-pandemic measures, recovery measures and long-term strategies (Zhang et al., 2021) for universities in emerging economies. Questions to these VCs were in three strands. First, higher education post-COVID (before March 2020), when we could consider things to be normal, and to understand the higher education system in their country and possibly their continent. Second, higher education during COVID (March 2020 to March 2021), asking questions about their experience during the pandemic, to understand how the pandemic has affected their students, teaching staff and other professional staff/ non-teaching staff and to explore how the pandemic has affected their relationship with other stakeholders, such as funders, regulatory bodies and other universities, in their country. Third, higher education post-COVID (April 2021 onwards). The VCs were asked about their projections for higher education post-COVID, to understand lessons that had been learnt from all these experiences, what they plan to do differently and how they see the future of higher education in their continent post-pandemic.

Considering limited knowledge is available regarding managing higher education in a pandemic, experts' and thought leaders' opinions presented in this chapter are relevant to understanding difficult issues in challenging times like this (Zhang et al., 2021). Having this global fireside chat with these VCs, as the leaders of their respective universities, allows us to have a holistic view of the challenges and direction in which things are going. The conversation with the VCs highlighted their initiatives to support student experiences, the challenges they face, especially leading a university in emerging economies, and the prospect of technology, bridging the gap between students and quality education.

This chapter presents an overview of the whole conversation. It is presented as a form of communique and intensified thought from all the speakers. The aim of the chapter is to present a different perspective to the ongoing discussion around the impact of the pandemic in higher education. Primarily, it presents experts' and thought leaders' opinion on the understanding of the impact of the global pandemic on higher education in emerging economies. These insights are from the leaders of universities in emerging countries: they are experiencing the challenges, have direct responsibilities for directing the affairs of the universities and can provide leadership and direction in the face of adversity.

The remainder of this chapter presents the seven key points of re-imagining higher education in emerging economies; they are presented in this chapter and, subsequently, by a concluding section. This study presents a theoretical contribution to the study of higher education management and leadership, especially in these challenging times and in emerging economies. In addition, it provides managerial implications relevant to university administrators around the world, recognising the impact of the pandemic and enhancing their existing measures to re-imagine the future of higher education in their universities and countries.

Re-imagining Higher Education in Emerging Economies

This section of the chapter presents the seven key points of re-imagining higher education in emerging economies. The fireside chat with the university leaders was intended to solicit views regarding the impact of COVID-19 on higher education, how their universities prepared for the pandemic, measures that were taken during the COVID-19 pandemic and projections for their universities and higher education post-pandemic. Their comments and conversation during the fireside chat was synthesised into these seven points by the moderator of the chat (fourth author), and quotes from the three VCs were integrated to support each point.

Where We Are

In redefining the future of higher education in emerging economies, it is important for university administrators to contextualise the country in which they operate and how to propose a country-centred approach towards education development. Importantly, the right definition of location and its inherent challenges needs to be recognised. There was the idea of how best to describe emerging economies, as some will consider them emerging economies, third world or the Global South (Sharma et al., 2021). These are just geographical inclinations, which may not necessarily provide a full context.

Therefore, irrespective of the geographical label, universities must recognise the need to meet the immediate educational needs of their countries, while still recognising their challenges (with students, funders and even global partners), reflecting on what makes universities in emerging economies different, and how these differences and challenges can be harnessed collectively to develop the sector. No doubt the role of the government and policy makers cannot be ignored, but universities will have to come together collectively and redefine higher education in their country.

Who We Are

Following on from the country context, this point recognises the unique features of a university and how it operates among other universities in the higher education sector in their country and on the global stage (Ndofirepi et al., 2020; Kieu et al., 2020). There are different types of universities around these emerging economies, each with its own unique features and responsibilities (Farinloye et al., 2020). There are small private universities, where it is easier to get to know the students on a personal level, where leaders get involved in teaching and engage with students' parents and, likewise, there are huge public universities with different funding structures, student bodies and courses being offered. University administrators are expected to reflect on the unique position of their universities, recognise their strengths and weaknesses and make the effort to refine their education offering with regard to their student bodies, the courses being offered and student engagement (Watermeyer et al., 2021).

Finances

This is one of the inherent challenges of higher education in many of the emerging economies, where the structure of the funding differs across countries and universities (Mogaji & Varsha, 2020, Oginni et al., 2021). No doubt we recognise the role of the government in funding higher education, but, in most cases, these are not always enough. Universities have lost revenue through non-payment of tuition fees, empty student accommodation, catering and conferencing, costs associated with COVID-19 testing and making the environment COVID compliant (Foley & Piper, 2021). Coupled with government challenges of dealing with COVID and money being diverted towards the health crisis, funding of higher education will be affected (Oleksiyenko et al., 2020). University leaders are going into the future with the financial burdens of COVID-19 unlikely to ease up, and this suggests the need to be more versatile, prudent and creative in raising and spending money. The financial management of higher education will become prominent in re-imagining higher education. There is contemplation around investment in technology or physical buildings, using artificial intelligence to replace some human tasks, cutting jobs and working with partners to reduce costs and share resources (Oginni et al., 2021; Sharma et al., 2021).

Challenges

With finance being the main challenge, there are other key challenges in higher education in emerging economies that are worth exploring in an attempt to re-imagine the sector (Wangenge-Ouma & Kupe, 2021). First is the limited number of universities and, therefore, the limited number of spaces for prospective students. There are many students who are willing to attend university but there are not enough university spaces for them; universities are not being funded enough to cater for this growing need (Adefulu et al., 2020; Farinloye et al., 2020). While private universities are filling the gap, it is not surprising to see many students exploring universities outside their home countries (Olaleye et al., 2020). Second, for those who are still studying in their country, there are challenges with infrastructure, especially in the wake of this pandemic. Many students struggled with having laptops and conducive learning environments, and it was not surprising to see universities providing laptops and internet access for their students in order to aid the digitised learning (Mogaji & Varsha, 2020). Third, there are challenges around the pedagogical developments of universities post-pandemic (Crawford et al., 2020): to develop a curriculum and modules that are relevant and can be taught post-pandemic and will enhance employment.

Opportunities

While challenges may abound in emerging economies, the opportunities are also enormous, especially when looking at the future (Mogaji & Varsha, 2020). It is therefore left to university administrators to recognise these opportunities and use it to their advantage. Technology has broken barriers and has given access to education around the world. There are opportunities for cross-collaboration between universities, and students learning from beyond their shores (García-Peñalvo et al., 2021; Bao, 2020). These are times motivating change and re-imagining how education is being delivered and consumed. Students can now learn at their own pace and engage with learning. Students' enrolments can also expand and meet that growing need for higher education, albeit not physically on campus but through virtual learning. There are opportunities for global partnerships, such as International Visiting Scholars allowing researchers and faculty staff in diaspora to contribute to universities in their home countries. Universities can create curriculums and teaching facilities to attract and offer a quality education to prospective students who may have otherwise travelled abroad. The need to decolonise the curriculum will also take more prominence moving into the future, as students recognise a diversified teaching team and teaching material is needed in a redefined higher education (Chiramba & Maringe, 2021; Chasi, 2021).

Disruptions

These opportunities are bound to bring disruption into the higher education provision. University managers need to be aware of these possible disruptions and be prepared to take advantage. They should not be caught unaware about what to do (Wangenge-Ouma & Kupe, 2021; Chasi, 2021). There are growing possibilities for students to pick and choose what they want to study. They can co-create their own learning and take more responsibility, as learning is now beyond the walls of the classroom (Chattopadhyay & Hommel, 2021). Importantly, this also challenges universities to step up their game, redefine their value proposition and position themselves as a redefined higher education (Hinson & Mogaji, 2020). Students will have options to choose where and what to study and, therefore, the well-positioned universities are more likely to have the chance to attract these students (Mogaji & Yoon, 2019). While ranking may remain important for understanding positioning of the universities, students will become more demanding as they make informed decisions about their university, based on employability, experience and engagement (Kiraka et al., 2020; Wangenge-Ouma & Kupe, 2021). Faculties may also be in more demand; students can choose to study a course or degree in any part of the world. Renowned lecturers can open their online classes for international enrolments; these lecturers become more in-demand, become their own brand outside their universities and can create a niche for themselves (Chattopadhyay & Hommel, 2021).

Future Plans

Universities must prepare for the future, which is now here. The negative impact of COVID on higher education has been well reported, and it is therefore important to build on the positive experiences and prepare for the future. Technology will play an important role and, consequently, investments in digital technologies to aid teaching and learning will be paramount. This is looking beyond Zoom and Microsoft Teams and adopting artificial intelligence to understand the students, and shape teaching and learning (Dwivedi et al., 2021; Sharma et al., 2021). Staff, including academic and professional services, will also need to deal with the integration of technology into their work (Chattopadhyay & Hommel, 2021). Faculties are becoming more like media producers and content creators, communicating with students on more interactive levels. Universities will plan for the digitalisation of teaching, learning and administrative tasks and will train staff to work with these technologies. Data and analytics will become more important to understand the student and ease the co-creation of knowledge (Dwivedi et al., 2021). Universities will have to start forming partnerships and alliances between themselves and other global bodies to enhance research and development (Wangenge-Ouma & Kupe, 2021; Chasi, 2021).

In all this, the finance needs to be improved. Universities need to start considering endowment and alternative sources of income to achieve their target (Nguyen & Mogaji, 2021). Importantly, empathy will become necessary. In the face of technology advancement and possible limited physical engagement, university administrators and staff need to show more empathy to the students and other stakeholders (Sharma et al., 2021). This is a trying time for everybody, and it is a learning process as we move into the future (Wangenge-Ouma & Kupe, 2021). Universities need to recognise this is an adaptation period and be more understanding. This could be in the form of submission deadlines, type of assessment or even tuition fees assistance. It is a new time for everyone.

Conclusion

This study reflects and synthesises a conversation with vice chancellors, from three different universities across three different countries, in a global fireside chat on re-imagining higher education in emerging economies, in the wake of the global pandemic. The VCs shared their experiences of the impact of the pandemic on their universities and what they think are important for present and future consideration in redefining higher education. This is an attempt to gain information in order to inform globally relevant research and policy-making agendas (Zhang et al., 2021). University leaders were asked to share their activities pre-pandemic, during the pandemic and post-pandemic within their own universities. Leaders' thoughts about the pandemic, future changes in higher education and possible action plans were captured during the chat and synthesised into seven key points, as discussed.

This study provides additional theoretical insight into higher education management (Ndofirepi et al., 2020; Mogaji & Varsha, 2020), especially post-pandemic, by providing insights from experts and thought leaders. In congruence with Crawford et al.'s (2020) analysis of university and government sources across 20 countries to map out higher education responses to COVID-19, we recognise that higher education providers and leaders have had diverse experiences and approaches in dealing with the impact of the pandemic. The study highlights the inherent challenges of higher education in the emerging economies and presents an additional theoretical understanding about the experiences of stakeholders in those countries. In addition, this study provides holistic top-to-bottom insights from the different countries in which these universities operate, the specific universities and the impact on staff, students and other stakeholders.

Managerial implications relevant to university administrators, managers and staff are also presented in this chapter. Firstly, the universities must recognise their inherent challenges and explore opportunities for development, global partnership, alternative sources of income and digitalisation of teaching and learning (Wangenge-Ouma & Kupe, 2021; Chasi, 2021). Secondly, university administrators need to put measures in place to harness the positive impact of COVID in redeveloping their curriculum, improving their teaching, training staff and supporting students (Chiramba & Maringe, 2021; Sharma et al., 2021). Thirdly, university faculties need to recognise that the tide is changing, and they should take responsibility for their training, personal development, research activities and their brand as academic staff. Higher education is being disrupted, and only the prepared will excel (Mogaji, 2021; Chattopadhyay & Hommel, 2021).

This study has several limitations, which suggest potential areas for further research. The synthesis was from an informal fireside chat and not from a research data-gathering perspective. As a result, the data collected may not fully represent the universities, countries or continents of the vice chancellors. We also acknowledge that the study concentrated on one university in one country, and therefore the findings may not be generalised, and also, therefore, findings should be interpreted in that context. Future research could empirically explore the role of university leaders in dealing with the impact of COVID in higher education. In addition, further research can explore the role of technology in shaping teaching and learning across emerging economies. This includes the use of artificial intelligence, machine learning and chatbots. The role of staff in engaging with these technologies and adapting to a redefined higher education can also be explored.

References

Adefulu, A., Farinloye, T., & Mogaji, E. (2020). Factors influencing post graduate students' university choice in Nigeria. In E. Mogaji, F. Maringe, & R. E. Hinson (Eds.), *Higher education marketing in Africa – Explorations on student choice*. Springer.

Al-Ataby, A. (2020). Technology-Enhanced Learning and Teaching in COVID-19 Era: Challenges and Recommendations. *International Journal for Innovation Education and Research, 8*(10), 317–331.

Agormedah, E. K., Henaku, E. A., Ayite, D. M. K., & Ansah, E. A. (2020). Online learning in higher education during COVID-19 pandemic: A case of Ghana. *Journal of Educational Technology and Online Learning, 3*(3), 183–210.

Ali, W. (2020). Online and remote learning in higher education institutes: A necessity in light of COVID-19 pandemic. *Higher Education Studies, 10*(3), 16–25.

Aristovnik, A., Keržič, D., Ravšelj, D., Tomaževič, N., & Umek, L. (2020). Impacts of the COVID-19 pandemic on life of higher education students: A global perspective. *Sustainability, 12*(20), 8438.

Bao, W. (2020). COVID-19 and online teaching in higher education: A case study of Peking University. *Human Behavior and Emerging Technologies, 2*(2), 113–115.

Chasi, S. (2021). Re-imagining International Higher Education Partnerships in the Aftermath of COVID-19. In E. Mogaji, V. Jain, F. Maringe & R. Hinson (Eds.), *Re-imagining Educational Futures in Developing Countries*. Cham: Palgrave.

Chattopadhyay, A., & Hommel, U. (2021). De-institutionalization of management education in the post-pandemic world: East-West perspectives. In H. Chaturvedi & A. Dey (Eds.), *The new normal: Challenges of managing business, social and ecological systems in the post COVID 19 era* (pp. 306–322). Bloomsbury.

Cheater, S. (2020). Health inequalities – Covid-19 will widen the gap. *International Journal of Health Promotion and Education, 58*(4), 223–225.

Chiramba, O., & Maringe, F. (2021). Organisational resilience as an urgent strategic goal in post-COVID-19 Higher Education in South Africa. In E. Mogaji, V. Jain, F. Maringe & R. Hinson (Eds.), *Re-imagining Educational Futures in Developing Countries*. Cham: Palgrave.

Crawford, J., et al. (2020). COVID-19: 20 countries' higher education intra-period digital pedagogy responses. *Journal of Applied Learning & Teaching, 3*(1), 1–20.

Dwivedi, Y. K., et al. (2021). Artificial Intelligence (AI): Multidisciplinary perspectives on emerging challenges, opportunities, and agenda for research, practice and policy. *International Journal of Information Management, 57*(4), 101994–101995.

Farinloye, T., Adeola, O., & Mogaji, E. (2020). Typology of Nigeria universities: A strategic marketing and branding implication. In E. Mogaji, F. Maringe, & R. E. Hinson (Eds.), *Understanding the higher education market in Africa*. Routledge.

Foley, L., & Piper, N. (2021). Returning home empty handed: Examining how COVID-19 exacerbates the non-payment of temporary migrant workers' wages. *Global Social Policy*. https://doi.org/10.1177/14680181211012958

García-Peñalvo, F. J., Corell, A., Abella-García, V., & Grande-de-Prado, M. (2021). Recommendations for mandatory online assessment in higher education during the COVID-19 pandemic. In *Radical solutions for education in a crisis context* (pp. 85–98). Springer.

Hinson, R., & Mogaji, E. (2020). Co-creation of value by universities and prospective students: Towards an informed decision-making process. In E. Mogaji, F. Maringe, & R. Hinson (Eds.), *Higher education marketing in Africa* (pp. 17–46). Palgrave Macmillan.

Kieu, T., Mwebesa, C., Sarofim, S., Soetan, T., & Vululleh, S. P. (2020). Marketing higher education in Africa: Moving from research to practice. In E. Mogaji, F. Maringe, & R. Hinson (Eds.), *Strategic marketing of higher education in Africa* (pp. 221–237). Routledge.

Kiraka, R., Maringe, F., & Kanyutu, W. (2020). University league tables and ranking systems in Africa: Emerging prospects, challenges and opportunities. In E. Mogaji, F. Maringe, & R. Hinson (Eds.), *Understanding the higher education market in Africa* (Routledge Studies in Marketing). Routledge. ISBN 978-0367344382.

Mogaji, E. (2021). Academic staff using university website profile page for academic digital branding. In *Improving university reputation through academic digital branding* (pp. 30–46). IGI Global.

Mogaji, E., & Yoon, H. (2019). Thematic analysis of marketing messages in UK universities' prospectuses. *International Journal of Educational Management, 33*(7), 1561–1581.

Mogaji, E., & Varsha, J. (2020). *Impact of the pandemic on higher education in emerging countries: Emerging opportunities, challenges and research agenda.*

Ndofirepi, E., Farinloye, T., & Mogaji, E. (2020). Marketing mix in a heterogenous higher education market: A case of Africa. In E. Mogaji, F. Maringe, & R. E. Hinson (Eds.), *Understanding the higher education market in Africa*. Routledge.

Nguyen, P., & Mogaji, E. (2021). Universities endowments in developing countries: Perspectives, stakeholders and practical implication. In E. Mogaji, J. Varsha, F. Maringe, & E. Hinson (Eds.), *Re-imagining educational futures in developing countries: Lessons from global health crises*. Palgrave.

Oginni, A., Mogaji, E., & Nguyen P. (2021). Reimagining the Place of Physical Buildings in Higher Education in Developing Countries in a Post-COVID-19 Era. In E. Mogaji, V. Jain, F. Maringe & R. Hinson (Eds.), *Re-imagining Educational Futures in Developing Countries*. Cham: Palgrave.

Olaleye, S., Ukpabi, D., & Mogaji, E. (2020). Public vs private universities in Nigeria: Market dynamics perspective. In E. Mogaji, F. Maringe, & R. E. Hinson (Eds.), *Understanding the higher education market in Africa*. Rotledge.

Oleksiyenko, A., Blanco, G., Hayhoe, R., Jackson, L., Lee, J., Metcalfe, A., … Zha, Q. (2020). Comparative and international higher education in a new key? Thoughts on the post-pandemic prospects of scholarship. *Compare: A Journal of Comparative and International Education*, 1–17.

Sharma, H., Jain, V., & Mogaji, E. (2021). Defining developing countries in higher education context. *Research Agenda Working Papers, 2020*(1), 1–9.

Wangenge-Ouma, G., & Kupe, T. (2021). Seizing the COVID-19 conjuncture: Re-positioning higher education beyond the pandemic. In E. Mogaji, J. Varsha, F. Maringe, & E. Hinson (Eds.), *Re-imagining educational futures in developing countries: Lessons from global health crises*. Palgrave.

Watermeyer, R., Crick, T., Knight, C., & Goodall, J. (2021). COVID-19 and digital disruption in UK universities: Afflictions and affordances of emergency online migration. *Higher Education, 81*, 623–641.

Zhang, J., Hayashi, Y., & Frank, L. (2021). COVID-19 and transport: Findings from a world-wide expert survey. *Transport Policy, 103*, 68–85.

Theme II

Technology Adoption

6

Influence of Technology on Student's Integrated Learning for Effective Well-Being in Developing Countries

Damini Goyal Gupta and Varsha Jain

Introduction

The outbreak of coronavirus disease (COVID-19) has had a significant impact on people's lives globally, particularly after the declaration of a global pandemic by the World Health Organization (World Health Organization, 2020) the second week of March 2020. The government's subsequent measures across the developing countries regarding imposing lockdown and urging everyone to stay at homes to curb infection rates led to the closure of all higher education institutes (El Said, 2021).

The pandemic had significantly affected the higher education students' lifestyles regarding (1) academic work and college life—switching to online learning mode, communication, library closures, adapting to new ways of assessment, and dealing with different workloads and performance levels (Jasmine, 2020); (2) social life—college closures, returning home, remaining confined within four walls with no access to social gatherings with friends, college colleagues, relatives, no celebrations, and even no travels; (3) financial situation—the loss of a part-time job or an internship, and concerns about placements, potential education, and career opportunities (De, 2020); and (4) emotional health—fears, frustrations, anxiety, anger, boredom (Coman et al., 2020). Thus, leading to a paradigm shift in the entire learning

D. G. Gupta • V. Jain (✉)
Marketing, MICA, Ahmedabad, India
e-mail: daminigupta.fpm20@micamail.in; varsha.jain@micamail.in

E. Mogaji et al. (eds.), *Re-imagining Educational Futures in Developing Countries*,
https://doi.org/10.1007/978-3-030-88234-1_6

environment and moving to online learning using different gadgets and applications over the Internet (Tam & El-Azar, 2020). However, Hodges et al. (2020) identified a difference between well-planned online learning and ad hoc online learning. This ad hoc and steep learning is seen in the crisis, as the speed of transition from offline and on-campus learning pedagogy to online learning may come as a shock to students and faculty members. In developing countries, the lower penetration of the Internet (44.4%) (Johnson, 2021) and underdeveloped digital infrastructure (Koomson, 2020) made the transition to an online learning environment challenging. However, the proactive nature of all the shareholders facilitated the process of bringing a change (Mogaji & Jain, 2020). As a result, the online learning environment was co-created, leading to students' enhanced learning experience and overall well-being.

In the emerging markets, the learning environment is different from that of the developed nations. For instance, the teacher-to-student ratio in developing countries is higher than in developed nations (Roser, 2017). Also, the lack of training and professional development to integrate technology into the learning ecosystem makes the transition to online education quite challenging (Sharma et al., 2020). The review of previous literature mentions that no significant work illustrates where technology usage of the students in developing countries connects with students' learning and well-being. Thus, this is the first attempt to understand the influence of technology adaption and usage on student's integrated learning for practical well-being in developing countries.

The approaches and processes in higher education, primarily for learning effectively, are distinctive in every country. The difference in learning takes place due to the unique adaption and usage of technology. After the onset of the global pandemic, the students have shifted to an online learning model, which has significantly affected their education and well-being. Therefore, this chapter aims to understand the influence of technology on students' integrated learning well-being in developing countries during the COVID-19 crisis. Thus, contributing to the existing knowledge by introducing a framework that connects technology usage with students' well-being in integrated learning (Fig. 6.1). The chapter also contributes to society by identifying the role played by students in reshaping the higher education system. Hence, this chapter will provide a direction to stakeholders—the top management and the faculties—to address the immediate concerns of students. In addition, the chapter will further facilitate the policymakers in identifying the gaps in the system and managing them to develop an integrated learning system in developing countries. Therefore, this chapter will be of great interest to students, future researchers, stakeholders, and policymakers for higher education in developing countries.

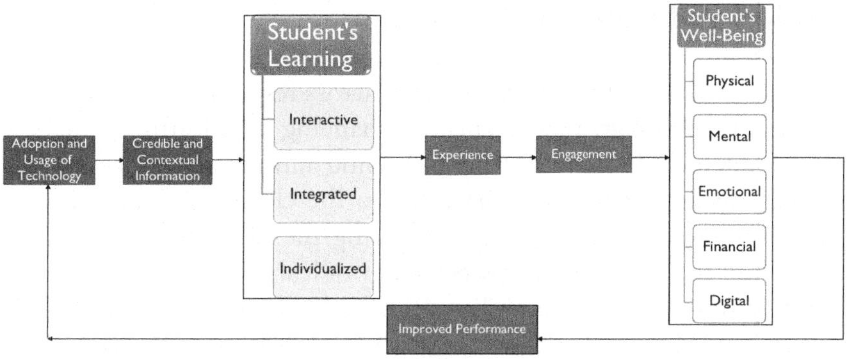

Fig. 6.1 Influence of technology on student's integrated learning for effective well-being in developing countries

The chapter consists of five sections that present a holistic view of the influence of technology on students' well-being. Section "Introduction" of the chapter introduces the readers to the aim of the chapter. Section "Influence of Technology on Student's Integrated Learning for Effective Well-Being in Developing Countries Framework" explains the framework that connects technology usage with students' well-being in an integrated learning environment. Subsequently, section "Opportunities" focuses on the opportunities posed by advancements in technology in higher education in developing countries. Further, section "Challenges" discusses the challenges faced by students in developing countries to adapt to the new learning pedagogy. Finally, section "Implications and Conclusion" discusses the implications for higher education stakeholders while shifting to online learning. Section "Implications and Conclusion" also presents authors' thoughts for future research opportunities in the education sector in developing countries.

Influence of Technology on Student's Integrated Learning for Effective Well-Being in Developing Countries Framework

This section will discuss how adaption and usage of technology have affected students' learning and how the paradigm shift in education pedagogy has affected their overall well-being positively and effectively.

Adoption and Usage of Technology

In this section, we will be discussing the factors responsible for the adaption and usage of technology by students in enhancing their learning process during the pandemic. The onset of the pandemic and the subsequent lockdown and social distancing measures have led to the closure of higher education institutions across most of the world during the 2020 academic year. This change led to the adaption of new pedagogy of learning and teaching through online mediums. Universities and students in developing countries were taken by surprise by the sudden transition to online learning. Nonetheless, they attempted to create strategies to rapidly adopt and use online learning technologies (Coman et al., 2020).

According to the Technology Acceptance Model (TAM), the actual use of a platform is influenced by the perceived ease of use of the instruments provided by the forum and by the perceived usefulness of those instruments (Venkatesh & Bala, 2008). In developing countries, the stakeholders use TAM to implement and integrate E-learning systems to make the learning process easy and straightforward. The shift towards e-learning modules using TAM further improved students' independence, self-discipline, and awareness (Almaiah et al., 2020) regarding different subject matters. Online learning facilitated the students to interact more with the faculties, thereby improving students' motivation to learn and increase participation in discussions (Coman et al., 2020). The students further claimed that they could comprehend information and navigate and view documents with ease (Pokhrel & Chhetri, 2021), making e-learning enjoyable (Vitoria et al., 2018). For instance, the students in Ecuador could navigate and access course-related content using social media and use a dedicated email address and phone number to connect with faculty to solve problems (The World Bank, 2020). This process eased the difficulty in adopting technology as an official tool for learning.

However, to maximize the benefits of online learning, good infrastructure concerning stable access to electricity and critical digital infrastructure—including universal Internet access, faster connections, and access to relevant content and enhanced digital skills—is a must for developing countries (Armbrecht, 2016; Scheerder et al., 2017; Sharma et al., 2020). Hence, the initiatives taken by stakeholders in developing countries during the pandemic have brought a drastic change. Many developing countries have adopted technology over the past decade and have modified it to local conditions in response to the pandemic. The Rwanda Education Board (REB), for example, has taken several measures to assist students with online learning through the use of a local intranet and web-based learning. Local telecommunication companies provide valuable help by waiving package charges to expand the use of multi-format online learning modules. As a result, students can have online access to books, watch course-related videos on REB's YouTube page, and communicate with faculty at any time using the REB platform (Rwanda Basic Education Board—REB, 2020). Hence, higher education stakeholders in developing countries have used the opportunity to enhance the penetration of online learning pedagogy. Stakeholders have made significant efforts to help the students adapt to the new technology using all the available resources and creating new provisions wherever possible. Thus, enhancing the learning process and paving the way for access to credible and contextual information facilitates students' integrated learning in developing countries.

Credible and Contextual Information

The online learning process becomes effective and efficient through the use of credible and contextual information. In developing countries, credible information can be accessed from sources such as government documents, scholarly articles, and databases, making them valuable sources of information for students (Benson, 1994; Lubans, 1998; Ryan, 1994). However, the Internet also includes millions of websites run by individuals, corporations, activist groups, clubs, and other organizations that can provide misleading or biased information. Students who use the Internet need assistance to deal with this. To assist students in seeking credible and contextual information, university reference librarians in developing countries have become expert web users (Lubans, 1998). The higher education institutes' libraries have access to scholarly databases, making them the most credible sources of information for students (University of the People, 2020).

Additionally, credible information needs to be in context with the students' learning objectives. Thereby, students can use cognition and connotation to extract knowledge from or apply knowledge to online information to enhance the learning process (Shackleton-Jones, 2019). The online learning management systems of universities and colleges further facilitate consuming credible and contextual information by using recommendation and adaption methods resulting in suggesting content based on the students browsing information, hence, strengthening the contextual information. For instance, Indonesia's government-regulated online learning system program SPADA is freely available to the partner institutes of the government of Indonesia. The program is designed to adapt the browsing history of individual students, and recommendations are made about articles, research papers, and news articles. This process strengthens the search for contextual information using Edtech (including online learning, radio, television, and texting). Further, this facility and access are via remote learning during the COVID-19 pandemic. Thus, navigating the students to the right content motivates and engages them in the online learning processes (Rahman & Furqan, 2019).

Hence, online resources such as the institute's library play a key role in providing credible and contextual information to students in higher education. Also, the students rely on them to progress in their academic journey, thereby making learning more integrated and effective.

Student's Learning

The democratization of technology, increased use of the Internet, and credible and contextual information in online learning all affect students' learning. This section will discuss the changing paradigm of student learning using the 3I's model (Sheth, 2020). The onset of the COVID-19 and the sudden shift to online education has made tablets and mobile phones the new textbooks, leading to a change from hard copies to soft copies of course material and ease of access to content anytime, anywhere (Casselden & Pears, 2019). For instance, a study conducted in Islamabad, the capital city of Pakistan, reveals that the use of smartphones and tablets in online learning focuses more on using e-books, audio/video, pictorial, and graphical content for facilitating student's learning process (Iqbal & Bhatti, 2020). Thus, the adaption of smartphones and other gadgets empowers the students to refer to the content conveniently, connecting with peers and faculty in real time and exploring more about an area of interest through the information available on the Internet. Thus, making online learning interactive, integrated, and individualized (3I's).

Interactive

The first I of 3I's model of students' learning is interactivity. Technology has made the process of learning interactive and personalized. The gap between teachers and students has disappeared, increasing direct interaction between them and thereby enhancing learning. The use of video-conferencing apps such as Zoom and Google Classroom facilitates one-to-one interaction between the faculty and students (Koomson, 2020). As a result, a collaborative and interactive learning environment has been created to provide immediate feedback, ask questions, and engage in learning. In times of crisis, the anywhere-anytime function of e-learning is proving to be beneficial. In El Salvador, for example, a call center staffed by five people and assisted by six subject-area specialists (faculties) promotes contact between students and faculties, allowing students to obtain immediate answers to their questions. WhatsApp and email services further facilitate consultations (Ministerio de Educacion, 2021), thus, reducing the gap in communication and leading to an interactive and personalized learning experience for the students. The increased interactivity between faculties and students has further enhanced the learning process and paves the way for integrated learning opportunities for students in developing countries.

Integrated

The use of technology and the growing interactivity in the learning process have facilitated students to explore the connection between traditionally disconnected subjects, leading to an era of interdisciplinary studies. This technology used is highly beneficial in today's highly competitive economy that favors skilled people in multiple disciplines. Creativity, adaptability, analytical thinking, and teamwork are highly regarded abilities (Edutopia, 2008). The integrated study is a perfect way to improve such skills in the classroom. It allows students to gain multifaceted knowledge and understand the importance of interrelationships in the real world. For instance, Uganda's management institute used technology-enabled integrated learning systems to enhance the learning outcomes for the students. The integration of Moodle and social media platforms and other gadgets such as laptops and desktops facilitate better engagement between faculty and students to achieve better learning outcomes (Kamya & Otim, 2019).

Interdisciplinary studies, also known as integrated studies, bring several disciplines together comprehensively, enabling students to understand the dynamic relationships and influences within a topic. For example, Sunway College, Malaysia, uses problem-based learning platforms to provide real-time challenges. These students integrate domain knowledge with problem-solving abilities to solve live issues. Importantly, teamwork, independent learning, and critical thinking also combine to solve real-time problems (Narayanasamy & Seow, 2015). Thus, making the process of learning more exciting and efficient for students as well as teachers. Furthermore, integrated learning caters to the different learning process of each student, giving rise to individualized learning.

Individualized

Online learning has benefitted students individually as constant feedback is received and queries are sorted spontaneously. Online learning platforms also foster individualized learning based on their programs and courses. Students review the content based on their specific needs and requirements, resulting in saving time and effort. Furthermore, in individualized learning models, faculty members have the opportunity to collaborate with students one-on-one rather than approaching the entire class (Forest Trail Academy, 2020). This approach improves the effectiveness and efficiency of the learning process.

Additionally, individualized learning encourages students to dig deeper into their course materials and ask more open-ended questions. Students do not need to be concerned about making mistakes because the whole process focuses on one-on-one contact (Coman et al., 2020). As a result, students gain confidence and can progress in their chosen field effectively and efficiently. Also, the individualized learning pedagogy improves students' perspectives by encouraging them to learn more about their areas of interest.

Experience

Students' experience is acquired by 3I's—Interactive, Integrated, and Individualized learning models (Sheth, 2020), thereby facilitating personalized learning, paving the way for one-on-one communication. The online learning pedagogy makes it possible to engage with students, listen to their individual needs, monitor their progress, and provide motivation through (a) using automatic emails and Short Message Service (SMS) based on learning analytics of students such as their grades, portal login activity, assignment completion and submissions (Broadbent, 2020); (b) improving the quality of feedback and student satisfaction by recording audio feedback and using feed-forward strategies (Asarta & Schmidt, 2020); and (c) giving personalized support in real time using a Live Chat option within the subject's Learning Management System (LMS) site to address a student's specific issues privately (Broadbent, 2020). For example, universities in Indonesia adapted to a new learning management system that elevates the quality standards of higher education, systemizes the learning processes, and seamlessly executes all the learning approaches effectively (Rahman & Furqan, 2019). Hence, the online learning experience is enhanced by personalized communication channels, which allow for easy feedback and discretion in problem-solving, thus building trust and engagement in the learning process.

Engagement

The engagement has become very important in online learning as it aligns personalized and individualized experiences of the students. Also, the use of technology in higher education has connected the stakeholders across the globe through a click. The connection not only is limited to students and teachers but also extends access to renowned professors and experts worldwide, making communication easy and making non-reachable territories reachable (Head & Eisenberg, 2009). Also, multiple teaching methods such as audio, video, pictures, and games further became touchpoints to develop engagement. In a study conducted on research, students reported that technology increased attention as the classes are categorized into parts with proper break times missing in physical courses (Kamya & Otim, 2019). Also, the use of activities and quizzes by faculty created engagement in class.

Furthermore, the international support system and opportunities apply expertise for real-time analysis and provide a promising glimpse of online education's energizing possibilities to students. Thus, online learning has increased students' engagement by accelerating connection and communication among different stakeholders worldwide. Also, multimedia in learning pedagogy further enhanced students' attention, leading to happiness and satisfaction, resulting in overall well-being.

Students' Well-Being

The increased level of engagement created by the online learning process has played a significant role in maintaining the well-being of students during unprecedented times. This section will examine the meaning of well-being for students with a particular focus on digital well-being, which is at the primary stage of evolution and integrates all other forms of well-being. Student's well-being emphasizes overall satisfaction, such as happiness, fitness, and aptitude to endure. The well-being of students is also based on the best possible quality of life based on reasonable living standards, robust health, and a sustainable environment, but not inherently limited to them (Muhajarine et al., 2012).

Students further attain well-being through a balanced use of time and access to and participation in leisure and cultural activities (Sirgy & Lee, 2006). Overall, students' well-being includes both objective and subjective parameters. Objective well-being refers to a student's assessment of well-being regarding the quality of life gained from material resources (Alatartseva & Barysheva, 2015) such as food, housing, income, and social attributes like education, health, political voice, social networks, and connections (Diener, 2000). Subjective well-being refers to students' psychological and emotional assessment of their lives (Diener et al., 1985) being, such as physical, mental, and emotional. Physical well-being is related to a balanced state of body, mind, and spirit. Mental and emotional well-being refers to a sense of positive self-regard and creating satisfying relationships. Finally, financial well-being is a sense of satisfaction with personal financial situations. (Walker, 2020).

However, the changes in individuals' lifestyles and high dependence on technology lead to a difference in students' well-being. The fear of missing out (FOMO) and the fear of being offline (FOBO) in the absence of easy access to mobile phones, draining the battery, or unstable network coverage affect students' well-being. The use of technological devices further ignites the deepest fears, anxieties that did not exist two decades ago (Wiederhold, 2017). Therefore, the students of the digital age have new struggles regarding decision-making. This pressure also elevates with staying connected or choosing to disconnect, thereby adversely affecting the state of well-being and integrating physical, mental, financial, social, and emotional well-being with digital well-being (Jisc, 2020). Therefore, the role played by faculties in facilitating the learning process and designing the curriculum to provide time to students to disconnect has made the process of online learning enriching and promotes students' well-being. For example, the universities in India have designed the curriculum for exclusive online learning. In such a learning environment, the actual class content is segregated into two parts where the conceptual understanding is provided as a pre-read for students in the form of 30-minute recorded videos, and the online classes are conducted for not more than 45 minutes with a break of 10–15 minutes in between two sessions. This process helps to minimize fatigue for students. Also, a comprehensive assignment towards the end of the course was adapted instead of several in-course tasks to avoid over-burdening students with lessons and limiting their "screen time" (Lakshman Naik et al., 2021; Mathivanan et al., 2021). Through these various integrated learning systems designed to care for students' multi-layered well-being, students' health is promoted, which opens the road for their performance to improve.

Improved Performance

The increased well-being of students has a direct influence on their performance. According to the broaden-and-build theory, a student's momentary thought-action range widens the available array of possible actions and thoughts that come to mind. For instance, students in a good mood consider more options in any given situation than those in a bad mood (Celestine, 2021). As a result, these expanded mindsets will have indirect and long-term adaptive benefits because they will help a person "construct" physical, psychological, intellectual, and social capital. According to Wright et al. (2007), this state of mind would make students more proactive and less susceptible to stress. This process would not only impact their academic performance directly but also act as a moderator. These broadened mindsets would further enhance the already existing beneficial effects of other forms of well-being on performance. We investigated students' online integrated learning processes in developing countries, which aided in improving academic performance while also assisting students in maintaining their well-being. We discovered that many market opportunities have emerged due to students' usage and adaption to technology.

Opportunities

The pandemic has brought several unprecedented changes in the higher education system in developing countries. However, the advancement in technology has posed an opportunity for higher education students across developing countries to revolutionize the learning system.

The rural and underprivileged students in many developing countries have very little or no access to learning. Still, with the adaption of technology and shift to online learning pedagogy, such students can be reached and subsequently be helped in education. For instance, the South African government has collaborated with an organization called Learn Appeal from the UK to provide Internet access and remote learning facilities to students who have no access to stable Internet in Africa by developing a tool known as The Learn Appeal Capsule. The Raspberry Pi 3 battery in the capsule lasts for over 24 hours of continuous use and can be recharged using a USB cable. The capsule also comes with a Wi-Fi router that can handle up to 200 users.

Furthermore, the capsule can hold up to 1000 hours of interactive educational content, making it a convenient way for students to learn and access accurate and relevant information. Another feature of the capsule that makes it very useful in renewable energy sources is wind or solar power (Learn Appeal, 2020). This learning made it possible to overcome the hurdle of unstable electricity issues and provide smooth access to learning sources, thus, providing an opportunity for students to learn and develop skills.

Online learning also opens up possibilities for access to specialized learning opportunities for students in developing countries. For example, MBA students from top colleges in developing countries can opt for free courses with certificates on online learning sites such as Coursera. They enroll in these courses to build new skills and rejuvenate career opportunities during their free time (Coursera, 2021). Thus, providing an opportunity to students to excel in an area of interest and regular coursework.

Furthermore, the online learning module facilitates global peer learning opportunities for students from different countries to meet online and learn from each other. MagicBox, for instance, is an online platform enabling peer-to-peer learning across the globe. The platform is integrated with several LMS tools such as Moodle, Schoology, Sakai, and Blackboard, providing group discussion features for peer-to-peer learning (Ferreri, 2020). Online education has facilitated the connection between students across geographies and has posed an opportunity to learn about different subject matters from experts and students while sitting at home.

Challenges

While the shift to online learning has brought opportunities for higher education students globally, there are still challenges specific to the developing-country context that creates limitations in leveraging the opportunities. Some of these challenges include:

1. Access to the Internet and technological devices: One of the significant challenges students face in developing countries regarding online learning is uninterrupted access to the Internet and access to designated technological devices to attend online classes (Mogaji & Jain, 2020). For example, the Internet penetration rate in Zimbabwe in 2021 is reported to be only 33.4% (Kemp, 2021). This penetration means that more than half of the population is deprived of Internet accessibility. Thus, making it difficult for the students in those areas to continue their education using online mediums.

2. Home environment and students' focus: Since many families in developing countries live in compact houses with a lack of private space, students struggled for freedom and peace to attend online classes from home (Milosievski et al., 2020). Also, students associate home with a space for relaxation; hence it becomes further complicated for them to concentrate and learn (Aguilera-Hermida, 2020).
3. Lack of social interaction: The lockdown guidelines prevented students from stepping out of their homes, making them stuck in confined boundaries. This guideline led to a decline in social interaction with friends and other family members (Coman et al., 2020). As a result, students struggled to find new ways of recreation, which also hampered their learning processes.
4. Emotional challenges: The students reported a loss of motivation and increased stress, anxiety, concerns regarding the future, and fear of getting infected (Aguilera-Hermida, 2020). These factors affected students' mental and emotional health and learning outcomes.

Implications and Conclusion

The effect of transition from face-to-face learning pedagogy to online learning pedagogy on learning and students' overall well-being has critically been analyzed in this chapter. Also, we have identified specific opportunities and subsequent challenges faced by students in the adaption of the new learning module. This section discussed (1) the implications to stakeholders—the policymakers and upper management of the colleges and universities of higher education, and (2) the implications to faculty members—the knowledge facilitators.

Implications to Stakeholders

The policymakers should focus on building the needed infrastructure such as uninterrupted electricity supply and Internet access to remote locations to facilitate an enhanced learning process for students.

In developing countries, mobile Internet penetration is higher as compared to other Internet sources. Thus, leaders from universities and colleges must facilitate the development of content accessible on mobile phones. Also, attempts should be made to provide the content in local languages.

College libraries should provide access to more databases related to students' well-being to overcome students' mental and emotional challenges. Additionally, school programs, activities, and courses should be designed to enhance the students' well-being.

The policymakers can further analyze the use of advanced technology such as Augmented Reality (AR), Virtual Reality (VR), and Mixed Reality (MR) in enhancing the learning process through online mediums in higher education in developing countries.

Implications to Faculty Members

In higher education, the role of faculty is essential and cannot be replaced by technology. However, technology should be used as an enabler for the learning process. Efforts to develop human-technology interfaces for integrated learning for students and enhancing the overall well-being need focus and development.

Faculty members can integrate several visuals and engaging activities to facilitate the learning process and make it more enjoyable.

This chapter contributes to understanding the influence of technology on student's integrated learning for practical well-being in developing countries during the critical time of the pandemic. The onset of the pandemic has affected the learning process and overall well-being of higher education students in developing countries due to the quick transition to online learning and the lack of infrastructure to support such a system. However, all the policymakers' proactiveness and collaborative efforts, higher education leaders, faculties, and students facilitated bringing a change in the pedagogy. The shift to online learning reduced the adaption and usage of technology by students. This adaption of technology helps in the credible and contextual information. The use of relevant details further led to the transformation of the new model of online learning based on 3I's—Interactive—facilitating increased communication between the faculty and students, Integrated—paving the way for interdisciplinary learning system, and Individualized—empowering students to decide their place of learning and area of expertise individually. The integrated learning process helped enhance the students' learning experience that helped create more engagement in the online learning process. The technological adaption and integrated learning process effectively improved students' overall well-being, which further improved performance. Thus, paving the way for further up-gradation in technological adaptation and usage.

References

Aguilera-Hermida, A. P. (2020). College students' use and acceptance of emergency online learning due to COVID-19. *International Journal of Educational Research Open, 1*. https://doi.org/10.1016/j.ijedro.2020.100011

Alatartseva, E., & Barysheva, G. (2015). Well-being: Subjective and objective aspects. *Procedia—Social and Behavioral Sciences, 166*, 36–42. https://doi.org/10.1016/j.sbspro.2014.12.479

Almaiah, M. A., Al-Khasawneh, A., & Althunibat, A. (2020). Exploring the critical challenges and factors influencing the E-learning system usage during COVID-19 pandemic. *Education and Information Technologies, 25*(6), 5261–5280. https://doi.org/10.1007/s10639-020-10219-y

Armbrecht, A. (2016). 4 reasons 4 billion people are still offline. *World Economic Forum*. https://www.weforum.org/agenda/2016/02/4-reasons-4-billion-people-are-still-offline/

Asarta, C. J., & Schmidt, J. R. (2020). The effects of online and blended experience on outcomes in a blended learning environment. *Internet and Higher Education, 44*. https://doi.org/10.1016/j.iheduc.2019.100708

Benson, T. W. (1994). Electronic network resources for communication scholars. *Communication Education, 43*, 120.

Broadbent, J. (2020). Am I just another number? Using online education innovations to personalise and improve the student experience in online learning. *Tertiary Online Teaching and Learning*, 13–24. https://doi.org/10.1007/978-981-15-8928-7_2

Casselden, B., & Pears, R. (2019). Higher education student pathways to e-book usage and engagement, and understanding: Highways and cul de sacs. *Journal of Librarianship and Information Science, 52*(7). https://doi.org/10.1177/0961000619841429

Celestine, N. (2021, March 25). Broaden-and-build theory of positive emotions. *Positive Psychology*. https://positivepsychology.com/broaden-build-theory/

Coman, C., Țîru, L. G., Meseșan-Schmitz, L., Stanciu, C., & Bularca, M. C. (2020). Online teaching and learning in higher education during the coronavirus pandemic: Students' perspective. *Sustainability, 12*(24), 10367. https://doi.org/10.3390/su122410367

Coursera. (2021, April 20). *Enrollment is open for the University of Colorado Boulder's Master of Science in data science—No application required*. Coursera Blog. https://blog.coursera.org/enrollment-is-open-for-the-university-of-colorado-boulders-master-of-science-in-data-science/

De, S. (2020). *Impacts of the COVID-19 pandemic on global education*. In COVID-19 Pandemic update 2020 (84–94). Ayodhiyapatinam, Salem: Royal Book Publishing—International. https://doi.org/10.26524/royal.37.6

Diener, E. (2000). Subjective well-being: The science of happiness and a proposal for a national index. *American Psychologist, 55*(1), 34–43. https://doi.org/10.1037/0003-066x.55.1.34

Diener, E., Emmons, R. A., Larsen, R. J., & Griffin, S. (1985). The satisfaction with life scale. *Journal of Personality Assessment, 49*(1), 71–75. https://doi.org/10.1207/s15327752jpa4901_13

Edutopia. (2008, October 6). Why should schools embrace integrated studies?: It fosters a way of learning that mimics real life. *Edutopia*. https://www.edutopia.org/integrated-studies-introduction

El Said, G. R. (2021). How did the COVID-19 pandemic affect higher education learning experience? An empirical investigation of learners' academic performance at a University in a developing country. *Advances in Human–Computer Interaction, 2021*, 1–10. https://doi.org/10.1155/2021/6649524

Ferreri, A. (2020, July 30). How to foster peer learning in the digital classroom—Magic Box™ blog. *Magic Box*. https://www.getmagicbox.com/blog/peer-learning-online-education-digital-classroom

Forest Trail Academy. (2020). How online learning is encouraging individualized learning. *Forest Trail Academy*. https://www.foresttrailacademy.com/how-online-learning-is-helping-foster-individualized-learning.html, *K12*.

Head, A. J., & Eisenberg, M. B. (2009). Lessons learned: How college students seek information in the digital age. *SSRN Electronic Journal*. https://doi.org/10.2139/ssrn.2281478

Hodges, C., Moore, S., Lockee, B., Trust, T., & Bond, A. (2020, March 27). The difference between emergency remote teaching and online learning. *Educause Review*. https://er.educause.edu/articles/2020/3/the-difference-between-emergency-remote-teaching-and-online-learning

Iqbal, S., & Bhatti, Z. A. (2020). A qualitative exploration of teachers' perspective on smartphones usage in higher education in developing countries. *International Journal of Educational Technology in Higher Education, 17*(1). https://doi.org/10.1186/s41239-020-00203-4

Jasmine, A. (2020). The impact of COVID-19 pandemic in higher education on teachers and students—A parallel study. *Paripex Indian Journal of Research, 9*(12), 1–3. https://doi.org/10.36106/paripex/3506943

Jisc. (2020, May 19). Towards happy and healthy students: Digital well-being and COVID-19. *Jisc*. https://www.jisc.ac.uk/news/towards-happy-and-healthy-students-digital-wellbeing-and-covid-19-19-may-2020

Johnson, J. (2021, January 27). Global internet access rate 2005–2019. *Statista*. https://www.statista.com/statistics/209096/share-of-internet-users-in-the-total-world-population-since-2006/

Kamya, M., & Otim, S. (2019). *Integration of Technology-Enabled Learning at Higher education in developing countries: A case of Uganda Management Institute (UMI)* [Paper presentation]. Pan-Commonwealth Forum, Scotland.

Kemp, S. (2021, February 12). Digital 2021: Zimbabwe. *DataReportal.* https://datareportal.com/reports/digital-2021-zimbabwe

Koomson, W. (2020, June 7). Effective distance learning pedagogy in developing countries. *Elearning Industry.* https://elearningindustry.com/distance-learning-pedagogy-developing-countries

Lakshman Naik, G., Deshpande, M., Shivananda, D. C., Ajey, C. P., & Manjunath Patel, G. C. (2021). Online teaching and learning of higher education in India during COVID-19 emergency lockdown. *Pedagogical Research, 6*(1), em0090. https://doi.org/10.29333/pr/9665

Learn Appeal. (2020, February 7). *Learn appeal capsule—The magic box.* https://www.learnappeal.org.uk/learn-appeal-capsule/

Lubans, J. (1998, April). How first-year university students use and regard Internet resources. www.lib.duke.edu/staff/orgnztn/lubans/docs/1styear/firstyear.html

Mathivanan, S. K., Jayagopal, P., Ahmed, S., Manivannan, S. S., Kumar, P. J., Raja, K. T., & Prasad, R. G. (2021). Adoption of e-learning during lockdown in India. *International Journal of System Assurance Engineering and Management.* https://doi.org/10.1007/s13198-021-01072-4

Milosievski, M., Zemon, D., Stojkovska, J. & Popovski, K. (2020, May 19). Learning online: Problems and solutions. *Unicef.* https://www.unicef.org/northmacedonia/stories/learning-online-problems-and-solutions. United Nations Children's Fund.

Ministerio de Educacion. (2021). La Educacion Sigue. *Ministerio de Educación.* https://www.mined.gob.sv/continuidadeducativa/

Mogaji, E., & Jain, V. (2020). Impact of the pandemic on higher education in emerging countries: Emerging opportunities, challenges and research agenda. *SSRN Electronic Journal.* https://doi.org/10.2139/ssrn.3622592

Muhajarine, N., Labonte, R., & Winquist, B. D. (2012). Undefined. *Canadian Journal of Public Health, 103*(5), e342–e347. https://doi.org/10.1007/bf03404438

Narayanasamy, P., & Seow, E. (2015). The challenges with problem-based learning: A case study on Mufy students studying economics and information and communication technology (ICT) [Conference session].

Pokhrel, S., & Chhetri, R. (2021). A literature review on impact of COVID-19 pandemic on teaching and learning. *Higher Education for the Future, 8*(1), 133–141. https://doi.org/10.1177/2347631120983481

Rahman, A., & Furqan, M. (2019). Adopting learning management system in Indonesian Higher Education: The encountering challenges to the transformation. *Asian EFL Journal, 23*(3.4), 83–97.

Roser, M. (2017). Teachers and professors. *Our World in Data.* https://ourworldindata.org/teachers-and-professors

Rwanda Basic Education Board—REB. (2020). *Facebook.* https://www.facebook.com/1994415110879008/posts/2567514926902354/?d=n

Ryan, S. M. (1994). Uncle Sam online: Government information on the Internet. *Communication Education, 43*, 151–158.

Scheerder, A., Van Deursen, A., & Van Dijk, J. (2017). Determinants of internet skills, uses and outcomes. A systematic review of the second- and third-level digital divide. *Telematics and Informatics, 34*(8), 1607–1624. https://doi.org/10.1016/j.tele.2017.07.007

Shackleton-Jones, N. (2019). *How people learn: Designing education and training that works to improve performance.* Kogan Page Publishers.

Sharma, H., Jain, V., & Mogaji, E. (2020). Defining developing countries in higher education context. *Research Agenda Working Papers.* 2021(No), pp. 1–9. https://ssrn.com/abstract=3774632

Sheth, J. (2020, December 18). The three I's of learning in the digital age. *Jagdish Sheth.* https://www.jagsheth.com/information-technology/the-three-is-of-learning-in-the-digital-age/

Sirgy, M. J., & Lee, D. (2006). Macro measures of consumer well-being (CWB): A critical analysis and a research agenda. *Journal of Macromarketing, 26*(1), 27–44. https://doi.org/10.1177/0276146705285669

Tam, G., & El-Azar, D. (2020, March 13). 3 ways the coronavirus pandemic could reshape education. *World Economic Forum.* https://www.weforum.org/agenda/2020/03/3-ways-coronavirus-is-reshaping-education-and-what-changes-might-be-here-to-stay/

The World Bank. (2020). How countries are using edtech (including online learning, radio, television, texting) to support access to remote learning during the COVID-19 pandemic. *World Bank.* https://www.worldbank.org/en/topic/edutech/brief/how-countries-are-using-edtech-to-support-remote-learning-during-the-covid-19-pandemic

University of the People. (2020, January 1). Tips to find credible sources for research: A guide for students. https://www.uopeople.edu/blog/ultimate-student-guide-to-finding-credible-sources/

Venkatesh, V., & Bala, H. (2008). Technology acceptance model 3 and a research agenda on interventions. *Decision Sciences, 39*(2), 273–315. https://doi.org/10.1111/j.1540-5915.2008.00192.x Model 3.

Vitoria, L., Mislinawati, M., & Nurmasyitah, N. (2018). Students' perceptions on the implementation of e-learning: Helpful or unhelpful? *Journal of Physics: Conference Series, 1088*, 012058. https://doi.org/10.1088/1742-6596/1088/1/012058

Walker, H. (2020, March 18). Holistic well-being: A more expansive consumer understanding of health. *The Grocer.* https://www.thegrocer.co.uk/consumer-trends/holistic-wellbeing-a-more-expansive-consumer-understanding-of-health/602995.article

Wiederhold, B. K. (2017). How digital anxieties are shaping the next generation's mental health. *Cyberpsychology, Behavior, and Social Networking, 20*(11), 661–661. https://doi.org/10.1089/cyber.2017.29089.bkw

World Health Organization. (2020). *Coronavirus disease (COVID-19) pandemic*. https://www.who.int/emergencies/diseases/novel-coronavirus-2019?adgroupsurvey

Wright, T. A., Cropanzano, R., & Bonett, D. G. (2007). The moderating role of employee positive well being on the relation between job satisfaction and job performance. *Journal of Occupational Health Psychology, 12*(2), 93–104. https://doi.org/10.1037/1076-8998.12.2.93

7

Mapping the Global EdTech Revolution during the Pandemic: From 'Determinism' to 'Solutionism'

Himani Sharma

Introduction

Universities worldwide are increasingly digitizing their operations to pace ahead in the global economy. However, they do not digitize alone but seek collaborations and partnerships from various tech-based service providers and creators. Educational technology (EdTech) companies have been one of the key benefactors for higher education owing to such partnerships. EdTech companies are not limited to online tutorial teaching and learning but include a whole suite of software, hardware, and digital tools and services that support knowledge dissemination.

In the past few years, EdTech companies worldwide have leveraged upon their digital readiness and advancements for partnering with various higher education institutions. In the past few months, the EdTech space has evolved significantly due to the pressing need for digitization because of the pandemic. This has paved way for rapid, radical, and fundamental changes in higher education. The changes have subsequently affected the operations, functions, and administration in higher education leading to a paradigmatic shift worldwide. Furthermore, the ongoing changes have created unified grounds of teaching and learning in higher education globally through digital

H. Sharma (✉)
MICA, Ahmedabad, India

University of Innsbruck, Innsbruck, Austria
e-mail: Himani_fpm18@micamail.in

E. Mogaji et al. (eds.), *Re-imagining Educational Futures in Developing Countries*,
https://doi.org/10.1007/978-3-030-88234-1_7

mediums. As a result, the world is witnessing a new revolution in the practices and processes of higher education. This new revolution in higher education has a distributed audiences who have both receptive and resistant views. There is a segment of stakeholders who believe that technology is the forebear of the future of higher education. They are the ones who orient themselves as determinists. While the determinists' segment advocates the significant role of technology in reshaping the system of society. They also further expound on the idea of technology as the solution to the problems in society. This chapter presents an overview of the global discourse around the prospects, promises, and penetration of technology in higher education in the twenty-first century with EdTech as the core. It outlines the changing landscape of higher education globally with specific reference to the pandemic and its effects. However, to add another layer of granularity it builds upon the phenomenon of technological determinism and technological solutionism and their consideration in the landscape of higher education.

Review of Literature

Technological Determinism

Technological determinism is a claim that technology alone determines the changes in the social and cultural structure. From a philosophical viewpoint, Dusek (2006) relates technological determinism to technology's autonomous and social-shaping tendencies leading to change. Further, Dafoe (2015) restates this claim by presenting four perspectives around technological determinism and argues that technological momentum and human choice are critical for shaping the socio-cultural systems. Veblen (1857) who originally coined the term 'technological determinism' explained how determinism is a causative link between technology and society. The theory assumes that technology has the potential to carve new avenues in society as it is the principal initiator of social change (Hodgson, 1998). This philosophical explanation of technological determinism has been used across various disciplines to discuss technological determinism in the context of new media (Hauer, 2017), new literacies and future learning (Mardiana & Daniels, 2019), digital skills in the twenty-first century (Laar et al., 2017), and robotics and artificial intelligence (Boyd & Holton, 2018). Some recent studies that have explored technological determinism in educational contexts are understanding ICT metaphors (Bardakcı & Kocadağ Ünver, 2020), educational theory in technology-enhanced learning (Maria, 2020), and learning of medium (Dai, 2020). However, limited studies have focused on unraveling the technological determinism in higher education specifically in the era of the EdTech revolution. In developed nations where EdTech is currently a rising phenomenon, it is critical to extend a philosophical and practical understanding of technological determinism and also explore the shift towards solutionism.

Technological Solutionism

There are firm believers and advocates of the notion that the world's problems can be fixed with technology and that the world will be a fundamentally better place to live with the adoption of their tech solutions. They tend to often overlook that the most pressing problems that society faces are deeply social, cultural, economic, and political. Technology may be support but cannot fix a problem on its own. Technological solutionism as a phenomenon claims that technology can solve any problem. However, this claim is often criticized for its over-ambitious assumptions. Milan (2020) argues that technology is often quantified for the wealthy which causes global uncertainties and disruptions. Developing nations as compared to the developed ones are not always privileged to have their social, economic, legal, and political issues resolved through technology. As a result, many a time the solution itself becomes a problem.

However, in the current scenario, when the pandemic came with challenges of its own, it also brought in a new wave of solutionism amidst the people, policymakers, and other stakeholders. The solutionist optimism this time was driven by the extensive use of technology that helped to operate while the whole world was under an indefinite lockdown. However, time and again there is a realization that despite the unwavering support from various technological tools the ultimate power lies with the human minds. Humans determine the future of society (Richard, 2013). Therefore, the support from technology is momentary yet not fundamental (Salvo, 2020).

With solutionism, there are other issues as well. There have been constant debates around the issue of big data, privacy, surveillance, and digital citizenship. On the one hand, technologists claim to carve personalized zones for each individual, whilst on the other hand, there is a breach of personal and private data. This is not just confined to industries but is present in all the segments of society. In 2010, Oliver explained that even the research around learning and technology is technologically determinist and has soft 'solutionism'. This is one of the major issues that Selwyn (2010) points out while discussing the issue of power and morality in the context of technology. Therefore, it can be argued that solutionism is an oversimplified concept that needs an inquiry for better understanding and critical explanation. This becomes even more important as the EdTech phenomenon (discussed in the segment below) revolutionizes the ecosystem of higher education.

Educational Technology (EdTech)

EdTech Imperative in Higher Education

In the year 2002 Ladytron released the song 'Startup Chime' with the lyrics 'technology is there to cure yourself'. Little did anyone know back then that technology would become an immediate cure to the challenges posed by the pandemic in 2020. The year 2002 was precisely when open educational resources (OERs) became popular, laying the foundation for modern EdTech; 18 years and there has been no looking back. With a series of advancements and disruptions EdTech has grown uninterruptedly. The EdTech industry has expanded its boundaries and covered all spheres of education. Teaching and learning at higher education have specifically been the center of the system with peripheral operations. Within the last two decades, the system of higher education has moved to many new stages of advancements. Wikipedia, blogs, open textbooks, MOOCs, learning analytics, blockchain, artificial intelligence, machine learning have all been a part of this ongoing journey. However, amidst this slugfest, EdTech companies have successfully managed to become a significant part of a putative domain of higher education. They have helped learners in maintaining learning continuity and deal with the urgency created by the pandemic. 'EdTech' is not a new buzzword in higher education. Its existence dates back to the time when teaching and learning were given an outsiders' objectivity. However, in the current scenario, it has regained momentum globally. Due to the pandemic, EdTech companies have managed to expand their business globally. By revamping the architecture of teaching and learning these companies have carved an extended space for EdTech in higher education.

The United States (US) dominates the EdTech market followed by India, Brazil, the UK (United Kingdom), and China. In the US, within the EdTech sector, higher education accounts for 54 percent. Despite some of the major concerns like data privacy, access, and mobility, EdTech in the US is scaling new heights. According to a report by Austrade, some of the highest valued EdTech in the higher education sector in the US are: Udacity, HotChalk,

Coursera, Age of Learning, PluralSight, Knewton, General Assembly, and Duolingo. India is another hub for nurturing the EdTech space in higher education. The Indian EdTech industry is expected to rise to 1.96 billion dollars in 2021, as per a report by KPMG and Google. This is a turning point for the Indian higher education system as the focus now could be on sustaining innovation and inclusivity (Kumar et al., 2019). By addressing issues like lack of job opportunities, limited industrial exposure, and creating affordable technological infrastructure, EdTech companies in India are on the way to redefining the norms of higher education. Similarly in other countries like Brazil, the UK, and China, the EdTech exposure is rising and so is its adoption for teaching and learning. Africa, which is also becoming a new spot for EdTech development, has hailed some new initiatives in this arena. 'Disrupt tutoring', a South African EdTech platform, is becoming quite popular along with the use of mobile technology for teaching and learning. Apart from that, other learning platforms like Obami, Siyavula, Pass.ng, and SmartED are on their way to create a promising future for learners in Africa.

Human Capital Theory

In the context of developing economies like India, Africa, and China, human capital is critical to higher education (Oliver, 2004). Economists Adam Smith and Gary Becker who initiated and popularized the theory of human capital argued that human capital is the stock of embodied attributes that have an economic value (Almendarez, 2016). These attributes include knowledge, experiences, sociability, creativity, and personal skills. Several other scholars have discussed the association between these attributes forming human capital and productivity. Novikov et al. (2020) explained that ever since the digital economy has been on the rise, the focus on human capital has increased. It is considered a determining factor for the development of the economy. The theory has also been used to discuss lateral mobility and promotions in the workplace (Jin & Waldman, 2019) where it is examined how task-specific human capital plays a role in enhancing employee productivity. Another extension of the theory is towards understanding factors of health and their role as a human capital at work (Hatak & Zhou, 2019).

However, in the given context of this chapter, human capital theory bridges the gap between higher education, EdTech, and employability. As manifested by the global education and industry leaders, higher education has a deep relationship with employability which is oriented from the development of human capital. Therefore, as defined by Goldin (2016), human capital is the skills possessed by an individual which has an economic value. These skills are part of an individual's fortune in return for which the industry pays a cost (Smith, 2003). This can be further understood by the following imperative of EdTech in higher education.

EdTech Narrative in Retrofitting Higher Education for Building Human Capital

In modern societies where digitization is a rage, higher education is widely recognized as an integral part of society at a macro level. Thus there is a renewed focus on expanding the system of higher education with the help of technology as the state of the art to boost the human capital of the nation. Figure 7.1 presents the relationship between higher education, technology, and growth from the lens of the human capital theory. According to the theory of human capital, higher education is the key to a nation's growth and development (Olaniyan & Okemakinde, 2008). It rests on the global benchmarks, community norms, and policies to channelize productivity for the growth of an individual, society, and nation as a whole. In the context of the modern-day education system, the theory implies an understanding that to amplify the potential of higher education a collaborative memorandum with technology is critical. Therefore, with the ability to provide on-demand and personalized sources of learning and creating an alternative avenue for the growth of higher education, EdTech companies apportion higher instrumentality for building human capital. The societies from all ideological spectrums are thus bound to adopt EdTech in higher education as a part of the planned economic system.

As showcased in the figure above, the process of learning in higher education is subjugated by global standards of education, education policies, aligned ecosystems, and society as a whole. As a result, the economies worldwide are not just focused on adopting technology but also registering the evolution of a new system of higher education. EdTech companies are monumental in creating a lackluster alternative for empowering higher education. Thus

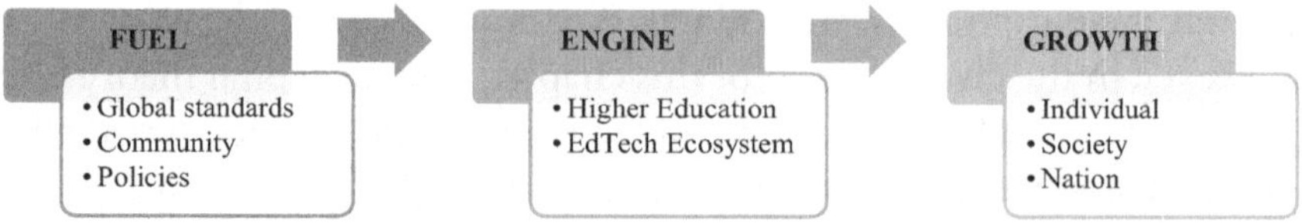

Fig. 7.1 Application of human capital theory in higher education. (Source: Adapted from Olaniyan and Okemakinde (2008))

contributing towards building a strong economic and social structure for an advanced future of things. However, this leap of faith needs backing from the policymakers, education analysts, visionary leaders, and other stakeholders to ensure that there is a designated balance between the force of human intellect and technology. For this, it is critical to outline the perils and promises of EdTech and keep a check on their integrity against predefined societal and human values.

Methodology

While exploring the phenomenon of technological determinism in the context of EdTech in higher education, a preliminary literature review was conducted to develop a baseline knowledge of the area and its aligned concepts. Applying the theory of human capital formation, a second-level semi-systematic review of the literature was conducted to conceptualize the phenomenon. The semi-systematic review helped in reporting the studies done so far and also unveiled key insights across different disciplines (Wong et al., 2013). This method also supported tracking down the evolution of the phenomenon from determinism to solutionism over time. However, the process of reviewing the literature was divided into four phases as suggested by Snyder (2019). Phase 1 included designing the review which focused on outlining the need and relevance of getting the literature. By carefully analyzing the current changes in higher education and body of knowledge, so far this phase addressed the critical question of whether the research is relevant and interesting for the stakeholders. Phase 2 was the actual phase where the review was conducted. Google Scholar, Summon, Scopus, and EBSCO were the four search engines used to explore the literature. Broadly 70 articles both academic and grey were identified for the purpose. In phase 3, out of the 70 articles, only 30 were retained as they helped in abstracting the required information and were rigorous in their approach. Finally, in phase 4, the literature review was written for the study. The literature review in the context of this study resulted in getting the evidence of an effect created by the EdTech revolution in the academic space of higher education in developing nations (Verlegh & Steenkamp, 1999). Therefore, the following research questions were addressed

RQ 1: What is the philosophical implication of technological determinism and solutionism in the context of EdTech and the current system of higher education?

RQ 2: How are EdTech companies changing the ecosystem of higher education? What are their promises and perils?
RQ 3: What leads to human capital formation? How does it contribute to the future of higher education?

Analysis and Discussion

An in-depth analysis of the literature unraveled some key insights which have potential implications for the triple helices of higher education, industry, and nation. Based on the analysis following key areas have been identified for discussion.

EdTech Companies and the Renewed Focus on Digitization: Perils and Promises

The year 2020 brought a mammoth of changes in the education industry. One of them being the rise in EdTech adoption in higher education. The pandemic gave EdTech a quantum leap in taking higher education towards a hybrid model of teaching and learning. The remarkable shift has carved a new optimism towards digital acceptance for education. Benefiting from this attitude change, EdTech companies have launched a new palimpsest for outweighing the traditional system of higher education. Table 7.1 below gives a snapshot of the transitions that are affecting the cogs of higher education by focusing on the promises and perils of the contemporary EdTech approaches.

EdTech companies have been around for more than a decade but had failed to deliver to the best of their potential. Until today when the pandemic sailed in and redefined the norms. The renewed functionality of EdTech has created a new systemic relationship between the service providers and stakeholders in higher education. However, not all promises made are promises fulfilled. Some of the critical promises made by EdTech companies need to be scrutinized. The potential claims raise several primary concerns demanding immediate attention.

Interestingly the leaders and business enablers in higher education do realize and acknowledge these pitfalls which obfuscate the fundamental notion of education for all. The idea of democratized education as discussed by Dewey (1916/1985) is challenged due to the limitations of EdTech ideology and practices. When education that is offered limits its reach to certain segments of the societies, then it does not qualify as equitable education. Therefore, it

Table 7.1 Disruptions in teaching and learning in higher education

Traditional approaches	EdTech approaches		
	Dimensions	Promises	Perils
Teacher-centered learning	Innovative services 'on demand'	The flexibility to learn from resources around the globe is instrumental for embarking on global standards in higher education.	Personalized learning is symbolic of privileged learning. It comes with a cost that may create a divide.
Curriculum management	Tech-driven digital content	The new content design imbibes sophisticated tools and updated knowledge on critical issues. It offers diverse learning.	Indigenous knowledge and practices suffer the cost of tech embodiment in higher education.
Textbooks	Systems and tools	Digitization has led to reduced cost, labor, and better scalability.	Substitution is not sufficient. Increased digital dependency is not the ultimate solution. It devalues the foundations of knowledge building.
Classroom-based learning	Advanced delivery mechanism	The online delivery mechanism enhances the accessibility and opportunity for learning.	Algorithm-driven learning in respective spaces hurts personal relationships and peer networks.
Grading and credentials	Skill-based assessment	The focus is on building meta-skills and enhancing employability.	Experiential learning is adversely affected in a software-driven simulated environment.

becomes crucial for the leaders, policymakers, and incumbents to carefully examine the growth of EdTech and regulate their profit ideologies. Even though regulation is important, one still needs to cautiously understand that unwarranted control is also perilous for creating an open culture of learning. A balanced stake curating a win-win space for all is the need of the hour and demand of the future.

Retrospections on the Success of EdTech in the Context of 3 C's: Creativity, Cost, and Crisis Management

Creativity

Creativity cuts across various cultures, industries, and disciplines as a quality of the human cognitive mind (Van Laar et al., 2019). As an essential element of the twenty-first century, creativity has become central to the processes in society. With rapid technological advancements, the phenomenon of creativity has become an indispensable part of higher education as well. The modern system of higher education imbibes and endorses creativity as a unique component for success and growth. This has been brought to light by the various unicorns in the EdTech business who have channeled their business models through creative execution and planning.

Realizing the need and potential for upskilling and lifelong learning, EdTech companies have harnessed their resources in offering services that are designed to their creative best. This has been successfully implemented by two of the leading EdTech companies, Examity and Coursera. Examity, which is one of the fastest-growing EdTech companies in North America, founded in 2013, envisions creating high-quality educational experiences for the learners. It is an innovative artificial intelligence (AI) based proctoring and monitoring service which offers creative measures to detect any signs of cheating or misconduct during online tests. Along with Amazon and Coursera, Examity's clientele includes Texas A&M, Penn State, Northeastern University, and Yale University. On similar lines of offering easy solutions, Coursera, a leading EdTech company in higher education since 2012, has managed to create a new vertical business model for fostering collaborative learning. By offering courses accredited by some of the top universities around the world, it is rewriting the palimpsest for modern higher education. Thus carving a linear path for admissions worldwide. Therefore, by contributing to the burgeoning grand narrative around the role of EdTech companies in disrupting and redefining higher education, Examity and Coursera are creatively taking the lead. Ceteris paribus, if the market continues to grow in a similar fashion and digitization is expanded further, these EdTech companies along with many others will soon transform the system of higher education. However, to do so the companies must not diverge from Clayton Christenson's disruption theory principles, which are discussed below in the context of the second C, i.e., cost.

Cost

Disruptive innovation posits innovations that make the product or service more accessible, viable, and affordable for the users. In the 1990s Clayton Christensen coined the term 'disruptive innovation' which has now become a rage in today's technology-driven era. His theory fits the definition of the new markets that have emerged in higher education. With their low-cost payment models, EdTech firms are optimizing disruption in higher education. To capture the state of the art, it is critical to explore how the theory of disruptive innovation applies to the cost-logic of EdTech companies. Initially, the revenue model for a majority of EdTech companies was an outcome of experimentation rather than strategic decision-making. The content was bundled and pre-packaged for selling to the users. However, on learning the complexity of the education market the EdTech leaders shifted to focus on gaining economies of scale and standardizing the services offered. As a result, four revenue models were devised which are illustrated in Fig. 7.2 below (Agarwal, 2020).

The cost-logic of EdTech companies has largely benefited them in appealing to users from diverse socio-economic and educational backgrounds. In

Most Popular Revenue Models In Edtech

Types of Revenue Models	Preferred Sectors	Advantages	Disadvantages
Freemium-Pay as you go	▪ Test preparation ▪ Skill development	▪ High traction ▪ Wider engagement ▪ Increased popularity	Eventually, a large proportion of users don't turn out to be buyers
Only pay as you go	▪ Online certification ▪ Test preparation	▪ Cost advantage in product offerings Wider options range for customers ▪ Quality user base	Relatively lower traction due to unavailability of free trials
Subscription	▪ Skill development Online certification	▪ Recurring revenue ▪ Substantial customer engagement ▪ Stability in revenue inflow	Difficult to maintain the value creation in customers mind if the USP of the offering is not prioritised
Enterprise Sales	▪ STEAM kit ▪ Performance assessment providers ▪ ERP solutions	▪ The higher ticket size of revenue ▪ Post sales revenue ▪ The purchasing power of the buyer is high	Higher dependency on traditional education enterprises & Unwillingness of the buyer to adopt new-age technology

Fig. 7.2 Revenue models in EdTech

developing nations like India, the freemium model has managed to garner good ROI (returns on investments) in terms of high enrollments. It offers higher flexibility and freedom to access the content and pay accordingly. Thus creating a win-win situation for the stakeholders involved at the delivery and consumption ends. Interestingly, like other industries, the cost-logic in the EdTech industry also gets affected by real-time situations. This gives us the understanding that during different economic phases the revenue models may gain or lose their significance. In such situations, strategic planning and clear vision help in dealing with market fluctuations. The fluctuations may be connotative of both positive and negative experiences. To deal with the changes and cope up with the challenges the companies need to be prepared on optimizing the opportunity or if needed use effective crisis management mechanisms.

Crisis Management

Crisis is defined as a downturn that might lead to deterioration. The year 2020 redefined the crisis which affected all the spheres of human living. The global health crisis COVID-19 not just caused physical and mental disturbances but also disturbed the socio-economic system of the world. If ever written, the history of the year 2020 will not just be the testimony of endless prophecies, the reflection of philosophies, but also a landmark of positivity for the EdTech industry. The pandemic sailed in with many challenges but also created space for digitization to expand now more than ever. The education sector which was once dominated by books and blackboards is becoming an open pool of opportunity driven by tech-based companies. Higher education specifically has witnessed a major drift towards the adoption and acceptance of EdTech. EdTech players optimized this momentum by offering services and content that was relevant, timely, and contributed towards lifelong learning. They focused on strengthening user engagement, scalability, and access. As a result, EdTech garnered investments worth 1.1 billion dollars in the year 2020. With their explosive growth, EdTech companies have now become an integral part of the higher education system.

In the words of Robert Hsiung, CEO emeritus, China, 'The same chaos that the virus is causing in countless industries is also making us focus on the possibilities of the online world for everyone from graduate students to my three-year-old daughter, who could begin her online education. There is currently a massive demand for high-quality online experiences; all businesses at all levels are working to create new solutions for online lessons. This is opening the way for the creation of new companies with the potential to become leaders in online education, especially when extraordinary circumstances, such as a health crisis, demand it' (Hsiung, 2020).

Outlook on a New Landscape: The Evolution from 'Determinism' to 'Solutionism'

To march ahead towards a new landscape in higher education, it is important to delineate the relationship between technology, society, and learning. The intrinsic and extrinsic connections between them frame technological experiences that are based on the learnings and lead to societal actions. In the era of modernity, dexterity, and flexibility, a new system of higher education is crucial for unpacking the convergence of new ideas and practices. This brand of system demands a mutual shift from a deterministic view to a solutionist view taking into consideration that technology alone is not sufficient. There, the following framework is suggested to design the ecosystem of higher education for the future (Fig. 7.3).

Implications

Policy and Societal Implications

Existing literature on technological determinism posits the idea of a society or culture driven by technology. The present trail of events falls under methodological determinism which takes into account the momentum, technologies available, and technologies in use. The argument that determinism builds upon the momentum can be better supported by what Roy Amara, an American futurologist had quoted in the 1970s, 'we tend to overestimate the impact of a new technology in the short run, but we underestimate it in the long run' (Ratcliffe, 2016). The current situation is substantive in the fact that technological interventions that were considered as an optional route for teaching and learning are now an essential part of the higher education system. The current circumstances where teaching and learning have been switched to a hybrid model fosters the need of the time. It brings a realization of the power, scope, and impact of technology in the future. Thus, there is an urgent need to draw ideas around the radius of determinism and yet be preventive of a complete solutionist approach while designing educational policies for higher education. In developing economies, it is critical to embody

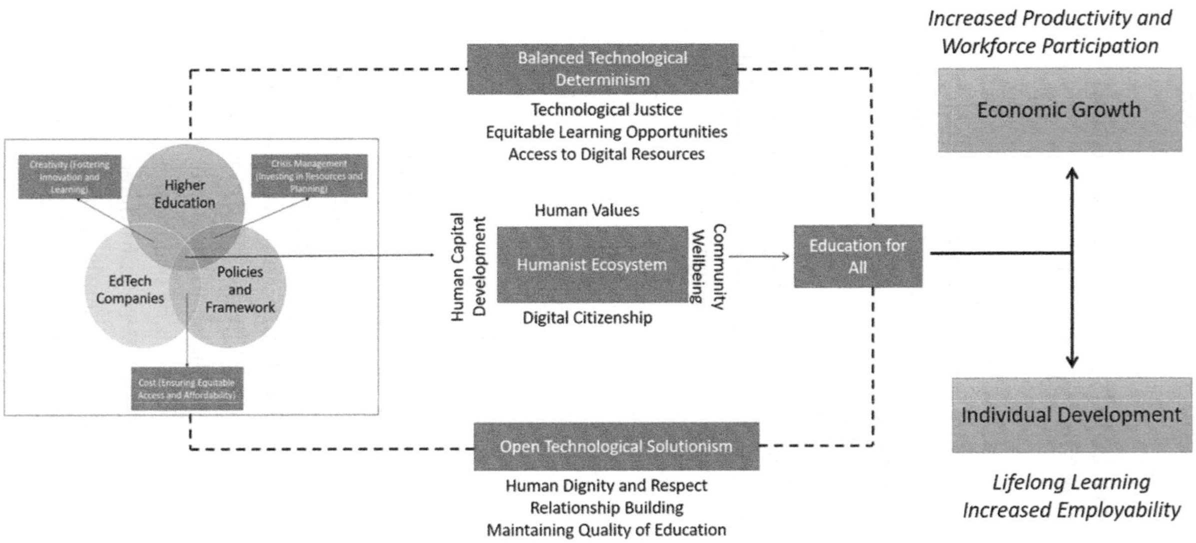

Fig. 7.3 Proposed framework for a humanist ecosystem of higher education

the philosophical ideas from the past and design the future with contemporary objectives (Hallström, 2020). The folly of solutionism needs to be outweighed by the right intellect, investment, and innovation. A society with imperfections is the one that has the scope to grow and seek alternatives because a solutionist mindset stigmatizes the notions of technological dependence and is instrumental in reinforcing capitalism. In nations where education is still a privilege, a balanced deterministic mindset is critical for the people to understand the importance of learning and sharing knowledge.

Academic Implications

Post-pandemic universities need a roadmap to amalgamate EdTech and other educational technology tools without compromising the dignity of an academic entity. In this course of the journey, cautious attention towards digital issues is crucial. Therefore, the landscape of higher education needs to take the road less traveled hitherto and ensure high stakeholder engagement in the long run. To overcome the impact of the COVID-19 health catastrophe, higher education needs to focus on three dimensions: collaborations (academic communities, partnerships, peer networks), conventionality (value-driven holistic learning), and inclusivity (hybrid learning, equity). However, above all, an academic entity is supposed to alibi quality. Quality in higher education is possible through three modes of teaching and learning. The first strategy involves nurturing the potential talent who can be trained to build up their skills and develop human capital. Another strategy is rigorous evaluation for credentials. To create a force of capable human beings who can contribute to the growth of the nations, the evaluations must be taken up seriously to award the right credentials. A balance between the entry and exit strategies can help the universities create a culture of quality education without a complete dependency on technology. The third and most important strategy for building a sustainable system of higher education is adopting a humanist approach (Thierer, 2018). Having firm control over technology and offering people-based solutions is key to maintain an equilibrium.

Here are seven possibilities inviting debate and action from the stakeholders in higher education for the future:

- Addressing the surge in demand for online adoption with contemporary strategies
- Partnering with technology for fluid and engaging learning experience
- Radical transformations in terms of value-driven teaching and learning

- Increase in investments in hybrid infrastructure and technology support
- Enhancing creative freedom and mobility by migrating to an elastic workforce
- Outlining the scope of EdTech interventions to hearten human intellect over technology

The recommendations above hint towards embracing the ideological changes that will help higher education become more sustainable in the future. The pandemic has given a realization of the changes that are bound to happen, but shaping them into an advantage is what higher education incumbents need to think of. There are no acceptable readymade solutions for any situation. Therefore, building upon the experiences and acting accordingly is the key. The solutions will differ, but the strategies should underpin a humanistic vision for higher education globally.

Conclusion

Higher education across the globe is determined to become hybrid, multimodal, customized, and flexible post the pandemic. With a keen focus on enhancing the meta-skills of the individuals, this new model of higher education is pacing ahead towards curating a future-ready system. Therefore, it can be arguably put forward that the partnership between EdTech and higher education is inevitable. Higher education now more than ever needs to lean upon technology to build a sustainable system propelling lifelong learning. However, as an integral part of the fabric of economies worldwide, a lot still needs to be done to retrofit the system of higher education. New possibilities ranging from technological advancements to pedagogical innovations, to cross-cultural collaborations, to entrepreneurial growth need to be acknowledged and optimized for building strong human capital. Furthermore, visionary leadership in higher education is critical to address the challenges of the digital divide at all levels. To address these challenges it is important to outline the existing lines of the relationship between EdTech companies, their services, and higher education. It is only possible with a collaborative restructuring of the norms in higher education and the market.

With an understanding that the pandemic has accelerated EdTech intervention in higher education, the academic community is heading towards critical transformations to empower the system. In this course of the transition, only the future can decide whether EdTech companies will retain their promises or not. Nevertheless, what is certain is that there is a deliberate shift towards better approaches to teaching and learning considering the uncertainties in the digital era.

References

Agarwal, M. (2020). *EdTech startups on cracking the revenue model formula in India* [online]. Retrieved March 30, 2020, from https://inc42.com/datalab/edtech-startups-on-cracking-the-revenue-model-formula-in-india/

Almendarez, L. (2016). Human capital theory: Implications for educational development in Belize and the Caribbean. *A Journal of Caribbean Culture, 59*(4), 21–33.

Bardakcı, S., & Kocadağ Ünver, T. (2020). Preservice ICT teachers' technology metaphors in the margin of technological determinism. *Education and Information Technologies, 25*, 905–925. https://doi.org/10.1007/s10639-019-09997-x

Boyd, R., & Holton, R. (2018). Technology, innovation, employment, and power: Does robotics and artificial intelligence really mean social transformation? *Journal of Sociology, 54*(3), 31–45.

Dafoe, A. (2015). On technological determinism: A typology, scope conditions, and a mechanism. *Science, Technology and Human Values, 40*(6), 1047–1076.

Dai, R. (2020). The argument of technologic determinism and the learning of medium. *International Journal of Social Science and Education Research, 3*(9), 122–128.

Dewey, J. (1985). Democracy and education. In *The middle works* (Vol. 9, pp. 1899–1924). Southern Illinois University Press.

Dusek, V. (2006). *The philosophy of technology: An introduction*. US: Blackwell Publishing.

Goldin, C. (2016). Human capital. In C. Diebolt & M. Haupert (Eds.), *Handbook of cliometrics* (pp. 55–86). Springer-Verlag.

Hallström, J. (2020). Embodying the past, designing the future: Technological determinism reconsidered in technology education. *International Journal of Technology and Design Education*, 1–15. https://doi.org/10.1007/s10798-020-09600-2

Hatak, I., & Zhou, H. (2019). Health as human capital in entrepreneurship: Individual, extension, and substitution effects on entrepreneurial success. *Entrepreneurship Theory and Practice, 45*(1), 18–42.

Hauer, T. (2017). Technological determinism and new media. *International Journal of English, Literature and Social Science, 2*(2), 1–4.

Hodgson, G. M. (1998). On the evolution of Thorstein Veblen's evolutionary economics. *Cambridge Journal of Economics, 22*(4), 415–431.

Hsiung, R. (2020). *Growing online management training in China* [online]. Retrieved September 10, 2020, from https://www.linkedin.com/pulse/growing-online-management-training-china-robert-hsiung/

Jin, X., & Waldman, M. (2019). Lateral moves, promotions, and task-specific human capital: Theory and evidence. *Journal of Law Economics and Organization, 36*(1), 1–46.

Kumar, A., Gupta, A., & Khetan, A. (2019). *EdTech in India—An Omidyar Network India & RedSeer Report* [online]. Retrieved December 12, 2020, from https://redseer.com/reports/edtech-in-india-an-omidyar-network-india-redseer-report-2019-20/

Laar, E., Deursen, A., Dijk, V., & Haan, J. (2017). The relation between 21st-century skills and digital skills: A systematic literature review. *Computers in Human Behavior, 72*, 577–588.

Mardiana, H., & Daniels, H. (2019). Technological determinism, new literacies, and learning process and the impact towards future learning. *Journal of Educational Science and Technology, 5*(3), 219–229.

Maria, Z. (2020). Educational theory in technology-enhanced learning revisited: A model for simulation-based learning in higher education. *Studies in Technology Enhanced Learning, 1*(1). https://doi.org/10.21428/8c225f6e.1cf4dde8

Milan, S. (2020). Techno-solutionism and the standard human in the making of the COVID-19 pandemic. *Big Data & Society*, 1–7. https://doi.org/10.1177/2053951720966781

Novikov, V., Klochko, E., Brizhak, O., & Digtyar, O. (2020). Digital economy: Human capital, technology, communications. *Proceedings of the 5th International Conference on Economics, Management, Law, and Education*. https://doi.org/10.2991/aebmr.k.191225.035

Olaniyan, D. A., & Okemakinde, T. (2008). Human capital theory: Implications for educational development. *Pakistan Journal of Social Sciences, 5*(5), 479–483.

Oliver, D. E. (2004). Human capital theory and higher education in developing countries. *Journal of Thought, 39*(1), 119–30.

Ratcliffe, S. (2016). *Amara's law*. Oxford Essential Quotations [online]. Retrieved December 11, 2020, from https://www.oxfordreference.com/view/10.1093/acref/9780191826719.001.0001/q-oro-ed4-00018679

Richard. (2013). *Robots aren't the problem: It's us*. Chronicle of Higher Education [online]. Retrieved May 10, 2020, from https://eric.ed.gov/?id=EJ999692

Salvo, D. P. (2020). *Solutionism, surveillance, borders, and infrastructures in the "Datafied Pandemic"*. Datactive—The Politics of Data According to Civil Society [Online]. https://Data-Activism.Net/2020/12/Bigdatasur-Covid-Solutionism-Surveillance-Borders-And-Infrastructures-In-The-Datafied-Pandemic/

Selwyn, N. (2010). Looking beyond learning: Notes towards the critical study of educational technology. *Journal of Computer Assisted Learning, 26*(1), 65–73.

Snyder, H. (2019). Literature review as a research methodology: An overview and guidelines. *Journal of Business Research, 104*, 333–339.

Thierer, A. (2018). *Is it "Techno-Chauvinist" & "Anti-Humanist" to believe in the transformative potential of technology?* [Online]. https://medium.com/@AdamThierer/is-it-techno-chauvinist-anti-humanist-to-believe-in-the-transformative-potential-of-14aa4e87a124

Van Laar, E., Van Deursen, A. J., Van Dijk, J. A., & De Haan, J. (2019). Determinants of 21st-century digital skills: A large-scale survey among working professionals. *Computers in Human Behavior, 100*, 93–104.

Verlegh, P. W. J., & Steenkamp, J. B. E. M. (1999). A review and meta-analysis of country-of-origin research. *Journal of Economic Psychology, 20*, 521–546. https://doi.org/10.1016/S0167-4870(99)00023-9

Wong, G., Greenhalgh, T., Westhorp, G., Buckingham, J., & Pawson, R. (2013). Rameses publication standards: Meta-narrative reviews. *BMC Medicine, 11*(20). https://doi.org/10.1186/1741-7015-11-20

8

Zoom-ing Past "the New Normal"? Understanding Students' Engagement with Online Learning in Higher Education during the COVID-19 Pandemic

Sooraj Namboodiri

Introduction

COVID-19 was declared a pandemic by the World Health Organization (WHO) in March 2020. What followed was a series of global shutdown of numerous businesses and economic activities, including the education sector. Amidst the chaos, confusion and uncertainty, governments, businesses and educational institutes were equally struggling with several challenges presented by the unexpected global shutdown. Countries around the world faced unprecedented challenges, especially the emerging economies, where these challenges were magnified. The economic losses faced by businesses across industries during this pandemic have been well documented (Jones et al., 2021), but the education sector has been comparatively neglected (Mogaji & Jain, 2020). Although the severity and infection rates of COVID-19 differ globally, approximately 990 million students across 130 countries were affected by the school closures due to the pandemic (UNESCO, 2020). The closure of educational institutions carries a substantial economic and social cost for individuals across various sections of the society, especially for the vulnerable and marginalized (Chen et al., 2021). The consequences of the disruptions and challenges presented by the pandemic not only aggravated

S. Namboodiri (✉)
MICA, Ahmedabad, India
e-mail: soorajnamboodiri.fpm19@micamail.in

E. Mogaji et al. (eds.), *Re-imagining Educational Futures in Developing Countries*,
https://doi.org/10.1007/978-3-030-88234-1_8

the existing disparities within the education system but also highlighted these disparities in other aspects of our lives.

Although there have been significant discussion surrounding successful or positive transitions towards the online mode of learning, these have primarily catered to the educated, urban or elite section of the population (García & Weiss, 2020; 'Online learning cannot just be for those who can afford its technology', 2020). Hence, issues caused by the digital divide is prominent when it comes to emerging economies where many students lack access to technology and infrastructure, stable internet connectivity or a conducive learning environment at home. To address various concerns stemming from social exclusion and access divide, countries across the world adopted online learning amidst healthcare and economic emergencies where ministries of education implemented policies to support students' remote learning during the pandemic. With educational institutions shut down—as part of the many protocols in place, such as social distancing, wearing masks, ensuring personal hygiene by routinely washing and sanitizing our hands—the education sector has been badly hit and the conventional model of education has taken a back seat. With the commercial viability in mind, institutes have swiftly embraced the work-from-home culture and online learning during the pandemic's early phase.

The transition from the "offline" or the traditional classroom experience to the online mode has been challenging for many. However, as time progressed during this lockdown period, it got worse, and it came with its own set of challenges. The idea of spaces has been removed from our learning experiences, and now classrooms exist wherever we carry, and sit with, our devices such as laptops, tablets or even smartphones. The students and the faculty now interact within the confines of their homes and small windows on their screen which may be similar to the online-distance learning model albeit with a curriculum designed for the conventional classroom model. Although the online learning phenomenon during the COVID-19 pandemic has received mixed responses, one of its merits was the opportunity to connect with one's colleagues and faculties, hearing their voices, ability to see their facial expressions and sharing a laugh with them. Whilst this does not make up for not being in the classroom physically, it is comforting on a certain level for many. The comfort of familiarity, connectedness has now faded away due to the extended lockdowns and restricted movements during the pandemic. The phenomena of teleco-presence and disembodiment have altered our existing social rituals, practices and norms of how we interact with each other (Zhao, 2005), and higher education is no exception. Similar to many modern-day institutions, educational institutions too function in a state of constant connectivity electronically.

Gradually, educational institutions across the world adapted to the "new normal" thrust upon them. This transition presented its own set of challenges which further aggravated the existing conditions such as internet connectivity issues, juggling between tech support, lack of educational infrastructure and the equality gaps amongst the students. Additionally, teachers who were new to the online mode of teaching were also struggling to keep up with various demands of the medium. Both the scale and the pace of change ushered in by the pandemic presented unprecedented challenges to online learning, both technical and human. As time progressed, the excitement and "newness" of the online mode of learning wore off, and there were rising concerns surrounding issues such as teachers struggling with lack of the whole in-class interactions and experience, unable to get through to the students and constantly trying to find ways to keep them engaged. Similarly, as students adjusted to the realities of remote learning, the majority are struggling to stay focused on the coursework, lack of privacy at home, loss of internship opportunities, mental health issues and uncertainty in the job market (Parry, 2021).

Presently, most educational institutions have extended this online mode of learning and anticipated the continuity of certain practices adopted amidst the pandemic during the gradual or staggered re-opening of institutes. Higher education is witnessing an inflection point where return to the old classroom model of teaching without incorporating some aspects of online learning is difficult to imagine. In continuing to deliver seamless learning, technology is playing an essential role nowadays. This raises the central question of how we engage the learners when they are not physically present in the classroom or the seminar halls. This is a complex question even in the cases of regular online learning programs. However, the pandemic has magnified this concern and presented both opportunities and challenges for online learning, highlighting the relevance of understanding student engagement. The stakeholders involved in educational institutions will have to devise and facilitate quality learning through the online medium collectively (Ndofirepi et al., 2020). There are no back seats in online education; all the learners are in the front row. This presents the need to have a certain level of intimacy in the form of interaction, engagement and active participation from the learners. Effective online learning requires detailed planning and increased effort as compared to traditional classrooms. This entails the collaboration of all the stakeholders—administration, top management or leaders of the institution, government or policymakers, teachers, tech support, student coordinators and support staff to provide a seamless learning experience to the students. Certain roles within institutions that were primarily considered as support functions such as tech support have received more attention during the pandemic. They have demonstrated that IT is a crucial part of education, from everyday operations to academic success in the classroom.

The present chapter aims to provide a holistic view of student engagement with online learning from a stakeholders' perspective. The framework offers practical and actionable insights into the key stakeholders in offering quality education during and post pandemic periods. The implications of the findings presented in the chapter are threefold. First, the chapter would benefit instructors seeking to enhance their online lectures through implementable engagement strategies. Second, it would assist course designers, administration and support staff within institutions to better facilitate and develop online courses. Third, it would provide the management in understanding challenges and opportunities with online learning to implement better institution-wide practices and policies.

The chapter is organized as follows. The first section establishes the context of the pandemic, online learning and higher education. The second section introduces and details the crucial role of students' engagement in online learning. The third section presents the triad of student engagement from a stakeholders' perspective—the role of institution, instructor and peer engagement. The fourth section discusses the residual legacy of the COVID-19 pandemic on higher education. This is followed by the conclusion section.

The Pandemic, Remote Learning and Zoom

The impact of the COVID-19 pandemic on higher education has been more than that of any other event in modern history, with institutions still coping with the challenges and struggling to restructure existing pedagogy to adapt to online learning. To avoid a complete shutdown of the education system and the learning process, institutions have moved to online platforms in their effort to continue some form of teaching. With respect to emerging economies where technology, opportunities and income are disproportionally distributed, certain groups of students might be prone to dropping out of the course. Challenges with technology, limited data plans, switching between devices for better connectivity, lack of motivation, distractions, time management, adapting to new technology and uncertainty about the future are a few of the common challenges students face. Two of focus areas essential for effective dropout prevention measures are academic and socio-emotional support. For students who struggle academically, credit recovery programs, instructional support, setting short-term goals and incentives can help improve their grades. Whereas socio-emotional aspects involve having a human connection, creating a sense of belonging, reaching out, being supportive and encouraging can prevent students from dropping out. There exists an additional challenge with online learning where the learners need to have the discipline and motivation to work in isolation. With a lack of accountability due to no face-to-face interaction, it is easier for learners to give up or completely disengage from the class without anyone noticing.

Online classes during the pandemic have also resulted in increased screen time amongst the learners where they are constantly glued to their mobiles, laptops or tablets, be it for work or leisure. In addition, video-conferencing applications such as Zoom have now become an integral part of our (work) lives—meetings, classes, presentations, interviews or even birthday celebrations. At least some aspects of our lives now involve this online form of interaction, staring at each other through the screen in front of us. Recently, the phenomenon of Zoom fatigue or Zoom gloom has received growing attention (Fosslien & Duffy, 2020; Jiang, 2020). It results from various factors such as the need to focus more intently for absorbing information, politely asking our loved ones not to disturb us, mental fatigue due to increased screen time and all the work-from-home situations one encounters. This becomes a lot more difficult for the learners who do not have a private space to work.

Another challenging aspect of remote learning is the issue of distractions. This can significantly affect the level of motivation to engage with the sessions. Amidst a variety of distractions, to have undivided attention and engagement with students during the limited time of the class is an imperative and challenging task for a quality learning experience. Due to a lack of communication between the instructors and learners in online learning environments, it is difficult for instructors to determine the degree of student engagement clearly. Delivering online courses which solely presents information is no different from lifelong learning or distance education programs. However, the critical challenge was adopting the online learning mode with a curriculum primarily designed for the conventional classroom model. Hence, online learning in higher education has to differentiate itself in the innovative pedagogical practices that connect, engage and transform students while achieving positive outcomes for all the stakeholders involved. Success with the program and positive learning outcomes are achieved only when the learners are actively engaged with the class (Kahu & Nelson, 2018). Therefore, the following section focuses on the fundamental role of understanding what encompasses student engagement and its key takeaways for stakeholders involved in online learning.

Online Learning and the Critical Role of Student Engagement

One of the most crucial aspects of one's learning, overall achievement and personal development is students' engagement, which refers to the effort or quality students commit towards purposeful educational activities which contribute towards certain desired outcomes (Hu & Kuh, 2002). Due to the complex and multidimensional nature of engagement, there exist various approaches in understanding engagement, such as the behavioral perspective, psychological perspective, socio-cultural perspective and the holistic perspective (Kahu, 2013). These focus on practicing effective teaching, engagement as an individual process, the role of social and cultural context and a comprehensive view of engagement, respectively. There exist three core elements present across all the definitions of students' engagement—cognitive, behavioral and affective (Handelsman et al., 2005). The cognitive aspect involves the extent to which students are investing mental effort and attending to the tasks involved in the learning process; the behavioral aspect refers to the extent students are actively involved and respond to the tasks presented; and the affective aspect refers to the extent the student is emotionally involved and invested and how they react to the tasks presented in the learning. The level of students' engagement is also highly affected by the relationships established with the instructor which fosters a sense of belonging leading to affective engagement. This instructor-learner relationship could also lead to behavioral and cognitive engagement. Furthermore, notable academic achievement is unobtainable without sustained, substantive engagement which goes beyond procedural engagement, which refers to engagement only being limited to the task at hand, at a certain point of time (Nystrand & Gamoran, 1991). Hence, ensuring situations that provide opportunities to the learners in pursuing their interests, expressing themselves freely and motivating them would result in greater engagement, autonomy and their overall well-being.

Student engagement is often used as a proxy for the quality of learning and teaching (Kuh, 2009) and is a widely accepted key metric for evaluating classroom success. It is an all-encompassing construct that acts as a general accountability measure to understand, explain and predict student behavior and involvement with the learning environments (Axelson & Flick, 2010). Learners' engagement is influenced by their cognitive capacities, ability to focus, level of motivation, the course design and how instructors facilitate the session. However, students' engagement is not limited to their own internal experience, it is also embedded in the socio-cultural context, shaped by the characteristics of the institution, the learners and the immediate stakeholders (Kahu, 2013). The interaction of these elements determines the varying levels of student engagement. The highest level of engagement is fostered where the social conditions of the learner facilitate competence, autonomy and relatedness. Engagement has been described as an all-encompassing construct that includes students' academic performance, achievement and classroom behavior; their motivational, cognitive, affective, social and contextual aspects of learning; and interaction with the instructors and the instructional materials (Azevedo, 2015). Therefore, it is imperative to understand that online engagement is not the result of one of these aforementioned factors; rather, it involves the interplay of all of them.

It has been observed that the students who are more engaged often exhibit more chances of successfully completing the course, higher satisfaction with the learning experience and overall a higher level of achievement with the course (Rice & Kipp, 2020). The factors that influence engagement and its consequences are cyclical and bi-directional in nature; i.e., having access to essential resources leads to increased self-efficacy of the learner, leading to engagement, which in turns increases the learner's self-belief. Likewise, establishing a positive relationship leads to better engagement, fosters good relationships and leads to higher chances of good grades, which in turn motivate students to be more engaged (Llorens et al., 2007). Although instructors and learners agree that synchronous learning was more engaging due to its similarity with the traditional classroom, many found the asynchronous variety to be more equitable since it presented certain students—who faced certain challenges such as bandwidth issues, difficulty to engage with the entire class or other factors beyond their control—the opportunity to participate in the class. The deepest engagements are formed in environments that promote emotional and social development, engaging instructional content and fostering certain relationships among the participants (Kahu & Nelson, 2018). However, with no face-to-face interactions, lack of familiarity with the whole online learning programs and little or no hands-on experience or opportunity to collaborate, many students might feel disconnected and isolated from the entire learning experience with remote or online learning. In addition, access to infrastructure and resources is unevenly distributed among students, highlighting inequality which may further aggravate the challenges faced by learners. These would result in a few learners who might end up dropping out of the programs. Such concerns are magnified with the COVID-19 pandemic, raising concerns about their academic progress and quality of education during this period.

How to Keep Students Engaged

One of the key problems associated with online learning is not only creating a space that promotes social interaction but also making a social presence felt in the online environment. Employing interactive and innovative ways of using technology coupled with thoughtful instructional design can help promote in-class discussions and positively improve overall student outcomes. In addition to the issues surrounding engagement and learning in the online environment, the chapter presents the three pillars of students' engagement, with a stakeholder's perspective (see Fig. 8.1), which depicts the shared role of educational institution, instructor and peer engagement in moving towards a successful online learning experience. Figure 8.1 is an adaption of the Adolescent Community of Engagement (ACE) framework (Borup et al., 2014), which addresses the unique student and environmental characteristics of the online learning environment. The chapter incorporates the role of higher educational institutions and presents a holistic view of student

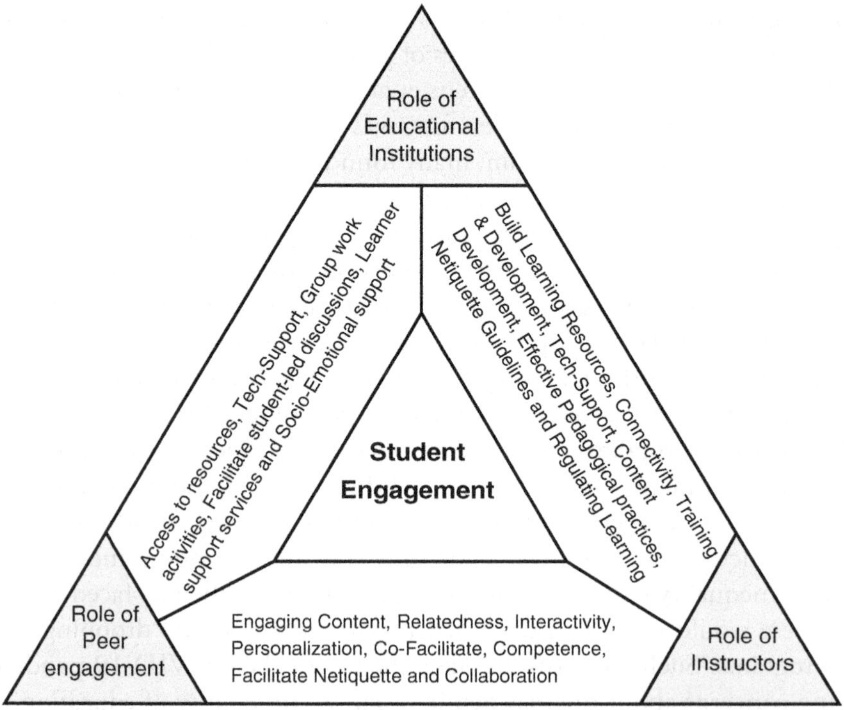

Fig. 8.1 Student engagement—a stakeholder's perspective, adapted from Borup et al.'s (2014) ACE framework

engagement, highlighting the role of key stakeholders involved in higher education—institutes, instructors and peers. The elements depicted between the three stakeholders represent their combined efforts which contribute towards student's engagement.

Role of Educational Institutions

The role of administration in educational institutions have evolved with time; now they are entrusted with adapting their leadership and administration practices in a dynamic environment driven by digital technologies, remote communication and collaboration. Although this is not an easy task, it does present institutions with an opportunity to create a stronger sense of community and encourage innovative teaching and learning methods. The first pillar of student engagement with online learning is the role of higher educational institutions. To achieve success with online learning requires cultivation of student engagement which is an indication of quality teaching practices and learning environments. Educational institutes and instructors play a vital role in ensuring student's success with online learning. Due to the challenges posed by the medium, students may feel isolated and disconnected; here the role of the instructor is key to foster a sense of community and encourage participation amongst the learners. Technology usage should provide instructors with improved access to content, data and expertise to improve the overall teaching-learning experience.

Regarding the course structure, content and delivery, it has been observed that presenting "bite-sized", spaced learning allows learners to process the information offered in chunks which increases the likelihood of learner retaining the information (Kang, 2016; Kondratjew & Kahrens, 2019). This presents an opportunity for the learner to review and recall information, thereby contributing towards their long-term memory. In addition, maintaining a healthy screen time is one of the challenges with remote learning, which requires effective curriculum planning, scheduling and customized teaching-learning material for online classes. Hence, educational institutions can assist instructors to understand and implement such practices in the class. It is essential to expose learners to, and engage them with, industry practices and professionals in higher education. Designing innovative pedagogical practices and introducing courses with contemporary and relevant content is crucial even during remote learning. These can be in the form of case studies, live projects, webinars, recorded interviews, capstone projects and inviting distinguished speakers to share their experiences.

Institutes should ensure that all the students, teachers and support staff have the minimal infrastructure and technology required to participate in, engage with or facilitate online learning (Farinloye et al., 2020; Simone, 2020). These may include tech support for internet connectivity issues, remote access to the library for academic resources and acclimatizing learners with various features of the application or the software that would promote interaction and engagement during the remote learning experience. They also need to ensure that instructors are provided with appropriate technology training sessions that are not limited to the usage of online conferencing applications such as Zoom or Google Meet (Carey, 2020). These should also be supplemented with sessions that empower teachers with the skills required in smooth functioning of online classes, supporting and establishing a positive rapport with the students, especially during this mode of "disembodied communication", apt use of technology in the classroom and strategies to make the most out of the blended learning approach.

To maximize benefits derived from online learning requires a concerted effort in providing a structure that moves beyond mere replication of offline classrooms. This can be achieved by introducing various engagement and collaboration tools which promote personalization, inclusion and active learning. Educational institutions would benefit from embracing a holistic, multi-stakeholder approach both within and outside the organization. Another significant aspect that is often overlooked while discussing engagement with online learning is taking care of one's mental health. It is important to take into account that achieving the right work (or learning)—life balance might be difficult for many during these times of uncertainty. With a unique environment presenting varied forms of stress and demanding work environments, institutes can provide platforms for students, teachers and support staff to freely interact online and share mental health and wellness resources to cope with any challenges they may experience.

Role of Instructors

Determining how to effectively engage learners has always been a challenging issue for instructors or educators. The second pillar of student engagement with online learning is the role of instructors. Although education technologies are at the center of online learning, they cannot replace instructors; they can only augment teaching. This involves recognizing ways to motivate learners, maximizing their takeaway or learning from the class, assisting them in focusing on the content or task assigned, and making the most out of the learning environment. These act as challenges even in the offline classes, but now remote learning has magnified them. Due to the nature of the medium, the content delivered via technology tends to be less interactive and compelling and makes student interaction more challenging. Online teaching requires thoughtful, intentional perspective in crafting the right instructional approach. Presently, these concerns are heightened due to the pandemic, forcing students to transition onto the online mode. Knowing that these students did not necessarily sign up for the online learning experience, achieving meaningful results is challenging for many instructors, especially in times of such uncertainty. Hence, they must "keep the class alive" or provide a stimulating remote classroom experience. The instructor's thoughtful approach in enabling the balance between learner's autonomy and instructor's control would determine the level of engagement with online learning. In letting go of some control, instructors can allow learners to form connections by themselves and encourage in-class discussions, which makes the experience more interesting while keeping students engaged with the arguments being presented by their peers.

One of the key issues with student engagement is its widely espoused narrow definition which attributes student engagement to instructor's competence and the lack thereof being some problems with the student (Zyngier, 2008). This outlook reduces engagement to a phenomenon in control with the instructors and espouses a myopic view ignoring other stakeholders' role in education. At the same time, substantial research in the area of engagement has shown that instructors significantly impact the learner's experiences, which influences their motivation, self-efficacy and perceived learning (Darling-Hammond et al., 2020). Whether the mode of online learning be synchronous (when both the learner and instructor are present at the same time) or asynchronous (both parties are not present at the same time), the instructor's role is to provide an opportunity to the learner in thoughtful engagement with the subject and promote peer-to-peer interaction virtually. There exist certain teaching behaviors that engage students such as challenging the learner to think, presenting the subject matter in an interesting way, showing enthusiasm towards their subject, encouraging students to question or challenge them, providing feedback to enhance student's learning, being available to reach out in case of queries, embracing the pedagogy which enables the students to apply their knowledge in addition to learning and genuinely caring about the students (Zepke et al., 2014).

An engaged instructor represents someone who is visible on the screen, addressing students actively in the class or through the text discussions, checking on student's progress of the tasks assigned and providing feedback, among others. There are ways where the instructors can increase their visibility and promote overall engagement with the class. These include, but are not limited to, posting regular announcements, using audio-visual tools like showing funny or informative videos during the class, timely response to learner's queries and requests, developing relatable activities, reaching out to learners using various communication tools that they are comfortable with, providing personalized feedback to establish a good rapport and also introducing the concept of virtual office hours where the learners can reach out to them. Another approach that has demonstrated success with student learning and engagement is gamification, which uses technology to introduce "game-like elements" into the sessions. These would involve achievement badges, introducing points system and competitive leaderboards. All these help break some of the invisible barriers and help the learners relax and be at ease with the remote classroom, leading to being more immersed and engaged with the class. A sagacious instructor might employ various strategies to build a rapport with the class and enhance overall engagement. Educators can successfully advance towards deeper engagement with online learning by understanding the crucial role of facilitating and promoting in-class interactions, engaging learners, promoting peer interaction through group-based activities and devising teaching strategies based on contextual and situational factors.

The Role of Peer Engagement

The third significant pillar of what contributes to overall student engagement, which is not emphasized much in online or remote learning, is the crucial role of peer-to-peer interaction and peer learning. There are different forms of peer learning, such as peer support groups, peer tutoring, peer-assisted learning and supplemental instruction. The opportunity to collaborate and work together on the assigned tasks, provide a platform of forums to share ideas and have one-on-one interaction with the instructor helps foster peer engagement. When learners are presented with course-related tasks that help them express themselves and their vulnerability, they appear more relatable and visible to their peers. Learner-to-learner interaction is a valuable component of remote classrooms. In order for information to develop into knowledge, learners must engage in tasks that assist them to make sense of the content they have been presented with. A sense of online learning community might help learners place the information in the context, thereby making the "sense-making" journey more engaging. A collaborative and supportive learning community also aids learners to retain and acquire knowledge. Online learning is considered most effective when learners have a social presence, cognitive presence and teaching presence during the discussions (Garrison et al., 1999). Establishing social presence aids pedagogical practices, which enables learners to work together and establish a bond.

Viewing education as a collaborative reconstruction of experience, knowledge and higher-order outcomes are achieved when institutions embrace a community-based inquiry with teachers and learners (Kolb & Kolb, 2005). This involves active class participation, interacting and being engaged with other peers. When learners interact with each other in the remote classroom, it creates a new dynamic potential of deeper learning and engagement. As an alternative to the traditional teaching method, the flipped classroom approach has demonstrated higher student engagement (Smallhorn, 2017; Steen-Utheim & Foldnes, 2018). The blend of synchronous and asynchronous modes of instruction allows students to take the lead, present their arguments and listen to their peers after viewing the recorded content. In addition, starting the sessions by dividing students into smaller groups ensures a level of fellowship or rapport with each other where no one is left behind or neglected. During online learning, these can take the form of discussion forums, online group projects and features such as "breakout rooms" on the video-conferencing application Zoom, allowing students to interact as a class and then continue discussions as separate groups for more focused and personalized learning.

The ecologies of learning and development spaces have been described as nested arrangements of structures consisting of microsystem, mesosystem, exosystem and macrosystem (Bronfenbrenner, 1977, 1979). Microsystem refers to the learners' immediate settings such as classrooms; mesosystem involves other concurrent settings such as courses, hostels or dorms and family; exosystem includes the formal and informal social structures such as institutional policies and campus culture; and macrosystem refers to the overarching wider cultural and institutional values which influence the learners' microsystem and mesosystem. Therefore, social system factors and learning spaces greatly influence the overall learning experiences (Kolb & Kolb, 2005). Remote learning and teaching during the pandemic have invited individuals (virtually) into their homes, and many families, staff members or students may not be comfortable with this. To address this, spatial reconfigurations can be tweaked to encourage engagement using virtual backgrounds, for instance, pictures of campus classrooms or the library. This can help simulate the classroom experience and recreate spaces that learners are otherwise distant from. This may help participants and instructors feel more connected and engaged with the virtual class. These highlight the role of peer engagement and the importance of learning spaces in virtual classrooms when learners work together in groups that foster peer learning and discussions. Through peer discussions, moderating arguments and self-regulation, learners carve their own path of inquiry while engaging in some form of teaching presence themselves. Although purportedly counterintuitive, in encouraging learners to act as moderators or lead discussions, the instructor witnesses substantially higher engagement (Baran & Correia, 2009).

The Residual Legacy of the Pandemic for Higher Education

Although the pandemic unleashed an innumerable set of challenges across industries, it also offered learning opportunities to re-evaluate and re-invent existing practices across educational institutions. This includes investing in advanced online platforms and innovative teaching methods and developing interactive and virtual learning content, among others. COVID-19 pandemic worked as a catalyst in academia's typically slow-paced world where educational institutions globally were now scurrying in search of innovative solutions within a limited period. This would also help institutes prepare for any unpredictable situations in the future (Mogaji & Jain, 2020). Many of the practices adopted during the shift might continue to persist post-pandemic and how it might disrupt the global education sector generally, and higher education in particular. Universities and institutes that are more innovative in creating and implementing online courses have swiftly adapted to the transition to online format. With the restrictions and lockdowns still in place, universities are now completely re-thinking higher education, with discussions ranging from moving towards hybrid campuses to location-agnostic campuses, from virtual campus tours to substantial changes in the recruitment process.

The drastic shifts in higher education induced by the COVID-19 pandemic have also resulted in an exponential growth of online education platforms, Ed-Tech start-ups, video-conferencing applications, online learning software and mobile learning applications (Terrisse, 2020). Even during the pre-pandemic period, there was increasing demand, growth and adoption of technology in education. Due to the flexibility, affordability, convenience and choices afforded by online learning, it is gaining popularity among students, and enrolment in courses are witnessing exponential growth (Quilantan, 2021). With rising opportunities, several universities and institutions are now entering the competitive market of e-learning. If institutions can leverage resources and technology through a strategic partnership with Ed-Tech firms, it could reduce the financial load on the learner and the institute while simultaneously creating the cycle of collaborative knowledge-sharing partnership benefiting all the stakeholders.

Another integral aspect of the pandemic's residual legacy that should elicit the education institute's attention involves identifying, diagnosing and treating the learning gaps that might have emerged during the pandemic. Likewise, building on the experience and knowledge gained from the abrupt shift to online learning may help government, policymakers and leaders of academic institutions take an informed decision in the future and introduce significant positive changes in the education sector. These include, but are not limited to, better student-faculty interaction, adapting to changes, standardization on common technology, faculty training, quality standards and curriculum design (Kieu et al., 2020). Although lack of experience and learning skills within an online environment may affect students' overall satisfaction with remote learning, when it comes to student learning outcomes, courses with high-quality and relevant content are proven to be equally effective as compared to the traditional ones (Busteed, 2019). Developing online courses helps institutions minimize their costs, concurrently maximizing student enrollments due to the flexible learning opportunities. Even during remote learning, student engagement plays a vital role in the learners' enrollment and retention, thereby contributing to the program's overall success.

Conclusion

As educational systems cope with the crisis, they have to chart plans for recovery with a renewed sense of collective responsibility to address the gaps in opportunity to ensure that learners have an equal chance of quality education. Given the crucial role of student engagement in learning, understanding the challenges and what keeps the students engaged with the online mode of learning, especially during the pandemic, can present numerous opportunities to educational institutions. While meeting the motivational needs is essential, engagement is also shaped by students' broader learning environment and the contextual factors that can diminish or enhance their overall engagement (Kahu & Nelson, 2018). The swift and fortuitous move to online learning during the pandemic will lead to the emergence of a hybrid model of education in the post-COVID-19 period where the role of technology will continue to accelerate, eventually making online learning an integral component in higher education. Similar to the physical classroom setting, online learning requires effective pedagogical practices and a well-designed curriculum. With an understanding of learners' needs, challenges faced during remote learning and empowering them with skills required for future employment, instructors can design pedagogical strategies to enhance learners' engagement. The distinct rapport and engagement formed online are not limited to enhancing the student experience; they also enhance the overall teaching experience.

Although there is no single panacea for improving student engagement during online learning, it requires the teamwork of all the major stakeholders, inter-departmental coordination and, most importantly, the need to be more flexible, to adapt and to overcome any challenges that emerge. Online learning requires the instructor to employ multiple strategies to strengthen the relationship with the learners, reach out to them and connect them with their peers. By providing students access to resources, necessary infrastructure and student learning support services, educational institutions can ensure that online learning would be a seamless experience for students as well as teachers and support staff. Engagement, support and ease of use with technology are a few of the challenges concerning learning online. Building opportunities for learners to engage with each other, instructors, other key stakeholders of the institution and ensuring a seamless execution process could help overcome challenges and achieve success with online learning.

Building on the ACE framework (Borup et al., 2014) and considering the unique characteristics of students and their learning environments, we incorporated the role of educational institutions as a dimension in our integrated framework. The insights and implications provided by the chapter would help policymakers, government, institutions and other stakeholders get an empathic understanding of what promotes and impedes students' engagement with online learning. Implications for educators and the management involve moving beyond simply creating behavioral interactions with students online to creating cognitively engaging, richer experiences by carefully considering learning design, study materials, tasks and assessments. In addition, the contemporary models of learning also emphasize the students' exploring, discovering and inquiring among themselves. Hence, incorporating inquiry-based and peer-based learning models can make a crucial difference in online learning. The stakeholder perspective presented in the chapter considers the complex system where institutions have to align and optimize value creation for all the stakeholders. Hence, engagement is a shared responsibility of stakeholders, requiring moving beyond merely replicating the "offline" or physical settings towards a combination of being learning-centered and learner-centered concurrently in achieving successful online learning.

References

Axelson, R. D., & Flick, A. (2010). Defining student engagement. *Change: The Magazine of Higher Learning, 43*(1), 38–43. https://doi.org/10.1080/00091383.2011.533096

Azevedo, R. (2015). Defining and measuring engagement and learning in science: Conceptual, theoretical, methodological, and analytical issues. *Educational Psychologist, 50*(1), 84–94. https://doi.org/10.1080/00461520.2015.1004069

Baran, E., & Correia, A.-P. (2009). Student-led facilitation strategies in online discussions. *Distance Education, 30*(3), 339–361. https://doi.org/10.1080/01587910903236510

Borup, J., et al. (2014). The adolescent community of engagement framework: A lens for research in K-12 online learning environments. *Journal of Technology and Teacher Education, 22*(1), 107–129.

Bronfenbrenner, U. (1977). Toward an experimental ecology of human development. *American Psychologist, 32*(7), 513.

Bronfenbrenner, U. (1979). *The ecology of human development: Experiments by nature and design*. Harvard University Press.

Busteed, B. (2019). *Online education: From good to better to best? Forbes*. Retrieved April 16, 2021, from https://www.forbes.com/sites/brandonbusteed/2019/03/05/online-education-from-good-to-better-to-best/

Carey, K. (2020, March 13). Everybody ready for the big migration to online college? Actually, No. *The New York Times*. Retrieved January 26, 2021, from https://www.nytimes.com/2020/03/13/upshot/coronavirus-online-college-classes-unprepared.html

Chen, L.-K., et al. (2021). *Teacher survey: Learning loss is global and significant. McKinsey & Company*. Retrieved April 4, 2021, from https://www.mckinsey.com/industries/public-and-social-sector/our-insights/teacher-survey-learning-loss-is-global-and-significant

Darling-Hammond, L., et al. (2020). Implications for educational practice of the science of learning and development. *Applied Developmental Science, 24*(2), 97–140. https://doi.org/10.1080/10888691.2018.1537791

Farinloye, T., Adeola, O., & Mogaji, E. (2020). Typology of Nigerian universities: A strategic marketing and branding implication. In E. Mogaji, F. Maringe, & R. E. Hinson (Eds.), *Understanding the Higher Education Market in Africa* (pp. 168–198). Routledge.

Fosslien, L., & Duffy, M. W. (2020, April 29). How to combat Zoom fatigue. *Harvard Business Review*. Retrieved October 21, 2020, from https://hbr.org/2020/04/how-to-combat-zoom-fatigue

García, E., & Weiss, E. (2020). *COVID-19 and student performance, equity, and U.S. education policy: Lessons from pre-pandemic research to inform relief, recovery, and rebuilding. Economic Policy Institute*. Retrieved April 11, 2021, from https://www.epi.org/publication/the-consequences-of-the-covid-19-pandemic-for-education-performance-and-equity-in-the-united-states-what-can-we-learn-from-pre-pandemic-research-to-inform-relief-recovery-and-rebuilding/

Garrison, D. R., Anderson, T., & Archer, W. (1999). Critical inquiry in a text-based environment: Computer conferencing in higher education. *The Internet and Higher Education, 2*(2), 87–105. https://doi.org/10.1016/S1096-7516(00)00016-6

Handelsman, M. M., et al. (2005). A measure of college student course engagement. *The Journal of Educational Research, 98*(3), 184–191. Retrieved January 23, 2021, from https://www.jstor.org/stable/27548076

Hu, S., & Kuh, G. D. (2002). Being (dis)engaged in educationally purposeful activities: The influences of student and institutional characteristics. *Research in Higher Education, 43*(5), 555–575. https://doi.org/10.1023/A:1020114231387

Jiang, M. (2020). *The reason Zoom calls drain your energy. BBC Worklife*. Retrieved January 24, 2021, from https://www.bbc.com/worklife/article/20200421-why-zoom-video-chats-are-so-exhausting

Jones, L., Palumbo, D., & Brown, D. (2021, January 24). Coronavirus: How the pandemic has changed the world economy. *BBC News*. Retrieved April 4, 2021, from https://www.bbc.com/news/business-51706225

Kahu, E. R. (2013). Framing student engagement in higher education. *Studies in Higher Education, 38*(5), 758–773. https://doi.org/10.1080/03075079.2011.598505

Kahu, E. R., & Nelson, K. (2018). Student engagement in the educational interface: Understanding the mechanisms of student success. *Higher Education Research & Development, 37*(1), 58–71. https://doi.org/10.1080/07294360.2017.1344197

Kang, S. H. K. (2016). Spaced repetition promotes efficient and effective learning: Policy implications for instruction. *Policy Insights from the Behavioral and Brain Sciences, 3*(1), 12–19. https://doi.org/10.1177/2372732215624708

Kieu, T., Mogaji, E., Mwebesa, C., Sarofim, S., Soetan, T., & Vululleh, S. P. (2020). Marketing higher education in Africa: Moving from research to practice. In E. Mogaji, F. Maringe, & R. E. Hinson (Eds.), *Strategic marketing of higher education in Africa* (pp. 221–237). Routledge.

Kolb, A. Y., & Kolb, D. A. (2005). Learning styles and learning spaces: Enhancing experiential learning in higher education. *Academy of Management Learning & Education, 4*(2), 193–212. https://doi.org/10.5465/amle.2005.17268566

Kondratjew, H., & Kahrens, M. (2019). Leveraging experiential learning training through spaced learning. *Journal of Work-Applied Management, 11*(1), 30–52. https://doi.org/10.1108/JWAM-05-2018-0011

Kuh, G. D. (2009). What student affairs professionals need to know about student engagement. *Journal of College Student Development, 50*(6), 683–706. https://doi.org/10.1353/csd.0.0099

Llorens, S., et al. (2007). Does a positive gain spiral of resources, efficacy beliefs and engagement exist? *Computers in Human Behavior, 23*(1), 825–841. https://doi.org/10.1016/j.chb.2004.11.012

Mogaji, E., & Jain, V. (2020). Impact of the pandemic on higher education in emerging countries: Emerging opportunities, challenges and research agenda. *SSRN Electronic Journal*. https://doi.org/10.2139/ssrn.3622592

Ndofirepi, E., Farinloye, T., & Mogaji, E. (2020). Marketing mix in a heterogenous higher education market: A case of Africa. In E. Mogaji, F. Maringe, & R. E. Hinson (Eds.), *Understanding the higher education market in Africa* (pp. 241–262). Routledge.

Nystrand, M., & Gamoran, A. (1991). Instructional discourse, student engagement, and literature achievement. *Research in the Teaching of English, 25*(3), 261–290. Retrieved January 23, 2021, from https://www.jstor.org/stable/40171413

'Online learning cannot just be for those who can afford its technology'. (2020). *Nature, 585*(7826), 482–482. https://doi.org/10.1038/d41586-020-02709-3

Parry, W. (2021). *Pandemic stress: The toll it's taking on students. Chemical & Engineering News*. Retrieved April 16, 2021, from https://cen.acs.org/education/undergraduate-education/Pandemic-stress-toll-s-taking/99/i2

Quilantan, B. (2021). *How the pandemic forever changed higher education. POLITICO*. Retrieved January 29, 2021, from https://politi.co/3okM5Um

Rice, K., & Kipp, K. (2020). *How can educators tap into research to increase engagement during remote learning?—EdSurge News. EdSurge*. Retrieved January 13, 2021, from https://www.edsurge.com/news/2020-05-06-how-can-educators-tap-into-research-to-increase-engagement-during-remote-learning

Simone, J. (2020). *How can school leaders support engaging remote education? EdTech Magazine*. Retrieved January 15, 2021, from https://edtechmagazine.com/k12/article/2020/09/how-can-school-leaders-support-engaging-remote-education

Smallhorn, M. (2017). The flipped classroom: A learning model to increase student engagement not academic achievement. *Student Success, 8*(2), 43–53. https://doi.org/10.5204/ssj.v8i2.381

Steen-Utheim, A. T., & Foldnes, N. (2018). A qualitative investigation of student engagement in a flipped classroom. *Teaching in Higher Education, 23*(3), 307–324. https://doi.org/10.1080/13562517.2017.1379481

Terrisse, A. (2020). *How has the pandemic changed the face of edtech? EU-Startups*. Retrieved April 5, 2021, from https://www.eu-startups.com/2020/09/how-has-the-pandemic-changed-the-face-of-edtech/

UNESCO. (2020). *Education: From disruption to recovery. UNESCO*. Retrieved December 8, 2020, from https://en.unesco.org/covid19/educationresponse

Zepke, N., Leach, L., & Butler, P. (2014). Student engagement: Students' and teachers' perceptions. *Higher Education Research & Development, 33*(2), 386–398. https://doi.org/10.1080/07294360.2013.832160

Zhao, S. (2005). The digital self: Through the looking glass of telecopresent others. *Symbolic Interaction, 28*(3), 387–405. https://doi.org/10.1525/si.2005.28.3.387

Zyngier, D. (2008). (Re)conceptualising student engagement: Doing education not doing time. *Teaching and Teacher Education, 24*(7), 1765–1776. https://doi.org/10.1016/j.tate.2007.09.004

9

AI Adoption in Universities in Emerging Economies: Prospects, Challenges and Recommendations

Himani Sharma, Taiwo Soetan, Temitope Farinloye, Emmanuel Mogaji, and Miguel De Freitas Noite

Introduction

The disparities between different countries around the world with regard to technology adoption is well evidenced (Azubike et al., 2021; Crawford et al., 2020). There is a digital divide, with these disparities often further enhanced by the poor socio-economic situation of individuals (Marinoni et al., 2020). The disparities are also evident in the quality of teaching and learning, especially when developing and developed countries are compared (Al-Ramahi & Odeh, 2020). The COVID-19 pandemic has now further exacerbated the existing inequalities in the global higher education community (Mogaji & Jain, 2020; Flynn, 2021). The pandemic has provided justification for humans to revisit how they engage in

H. Sharma
MICA, Ahmedabad, India

University of Innsbruck, Innsbruck, Austria
e-mail: himani_fpm18@micamail.in

T. Soetan
Red River College, Winnipeg, MB, Canada
e-mail: tsoetan@rrc.ca

T. Farinloye
Questbury Research Services, London, UK
e-mail: Temitope.farinloye@questbury.com

E. Mogaji et al. (eds.), *Re-imagining Educational Futures in Developing Countries*,
https://doi.org/10.1007/978-3-030-88234-1_9

different activities (Mogaji, 2020), including teaching and learning, but concerns remain about the growing inequality in education (Reich, 2020; Black et al., 2021).

In higher education, the pandemic has further intensified the need to adopt technology to engage with students and other stakeholders (Madsen & Strulik, 2020; Flynn, 2021). As a result, universities are now gearing up for the arrival of new technological tools to deliver the desired outcomes (Crawford et al., 2020; Teräs et al., 2020). In this ongoing disruption, artificial intelligence (AI) has specifically caught the attention of higher education managers (Krishnamurthy, 2020), whose possible intention is to reduce inequality and give every student an opportunity to learn and be supported in acquiring knowledge. Baker et al. (2019) broadly defined AI as 'computers which perform cognitive tasks, usually associated with human minds, particularly learning and problem-solving'. Zawacki-Richter et al. (2019) further reiterated that AI is an umbrella term to describe a range of technologies and methods—such as machine learning, natural language processing, data mining, neural networks or an algorithm—that have been integrated into higher education in the form of artificial intelligence in education (AIED).

AIED is acknowledged as one of the most prominent developments in the field of higher education. AI adoption and application for educational purposes are constantly on the rise (Richter et al., 2019). Chen et al. (2020) presented evidence of the increasing interest in, and impact of, AIED. The urgent shift to digitised operations has swept aside traditional practices in higher education, creating space for the growth of AI-driven learning. Furthermore, the adoption of AIED is expected to rise (Qin et al., 2020), thereby encouraging universities and other institutions of higher education to invest in the training, resources and infrastructure required to support AI-driven systems (Hamilton, 2021). But how are universities in developing countries positioned to adopt and benefit from the growing prospect of AIED?

Drawing upon the urgent discussions around the adoption of AIED in emerging economies (Mogaji & Jain, 2020; Popenici & Kerr, 2017), this chapter identifies the educational implications of AI in emerging economies by examining the challenges therewith and provides recommendations for AI's adoption. This study builds upon the triple-helix framework (illustrated in Fig. 9.1) to integrate the perspectives of AI, higher education and economic activities towards a renewed

E. Mogaji (✉)
Department of Marketing, Events and Tourism, University of Greenwich, London, UK
e-mail: E.O.Mogaji@greenwich.ac.uk

M. D. F. Noite
University of Greenwich, London, UK
e-mail: M.Noite@greenwich.ac.uk

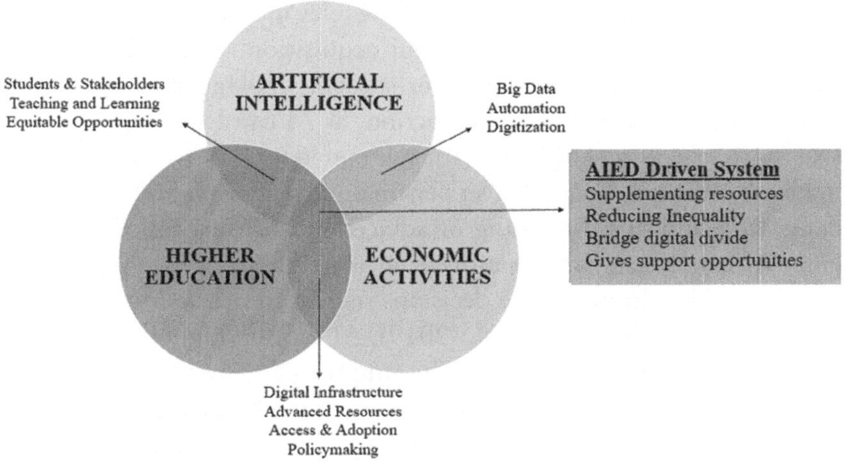

Fig. 9.1 AI adoption in higher education contextualised in emerging economies

understanding of contemporary education systems in emerging economies. This study makes a theoretical contribution to AIED (Krishnamurthy, 2020; Chen et al., 2020) by recognising the stakeholders, identifying the challenges and providing recommendations for the effective adoption of AIED in emerging economies. It moves beyond the usual need to transfer existing knowledge about AIED in developed countries to recognise that the inherent challenges of universities in emerging economies warrant a different approach to AIED.

The first section of the chapter focuses on discussing AIED. The section addresses the different typologies, benefits and implications of AIED issues. With a special emphasis on emerging economies, it theorises about the inherent challenges of features of AIED in developing countries. The latter segment of the chapter highlights the key recommendations of university managers and education technology developers as stakeholders. The concluding section discusses the relevant research agenda for, and opportunities for future research on, AIED.

AI in Higher Education

AI solutions are becoming more applicable in all sectors of the economy, and higher education is no exception (Wang et al., 2021). AI solutions open a new horizon of possibilities for teaching and learning in higher education, structurally changing university administration, student engagement and staff support (Popenici & Kerr, 2017). Luckin et al. (2016) presented three categories of AIED. They recognised that AI software applications in education can be used as (a) personal tutors, supporting and enhancing the student's ability to learn; (b) intelligent support for collaborative learning; and (c) intelligent virtual reality.

Wang et al. (2021) further recognised the relevance of AIED and identified four key benefits, which are (a) student acquisition, where AI can provide personalised support and assistance for students moving through the enrolment process; (b) learning and instruction, as AI can help instructors grade and support struggling students with relevant resources to succeed; (c) student affairs, in which AI can deliver personalised degree planning and support students with additional tutoring or advice; and (d) institutional efficiency, wherein AI can extract information from multiple campus systems and use the data to guide administrative decisions such as future course offerings.

In another study by Baker et al. (2019), AI tools in higher education were divided into three groups based on the support perspectives being provided. The groups are (a) learner-facing, helping the students engage with the subject matter and providing tools such as personalised learning management systems aligning with the learning and instruction strands of Wang et al. (2021); (b) teacher-facing, comprising tools used to enhance the teaching and facilitation of the courses and ensuring the teachers' workloads are reduced by automating tasks such as administration, assessment, feedback and plagiarism detection; and (c) system-facing, describing tools that support administrative duties at the instructional level, aligning with the institutional efficiency strands of Wang et al. (2021).

Zawacki-Richter et al. (2019) carried out a systematic review of research on AIED. Their iterative coding process led to four areas of AIED. The authors recognised (a) adaptive systems and personalisation, involving teaching course content, recommending personalised content, supporting teachers and learning design, using academic data to monitor and guide students and representing knowledge in concept maps; (b) assessment and evaluation, which involve automated grading, feedback, evaluation of student understanding, engagement, academic integrity and the evaluation of teaching; (c) profiling and prediction, which can be used for admission decisions and course scheduling, dropout and retention, student models and academic achievement; and (d) intelligent tutoring systems that aid in teaching course content, diagnosing strengths and automated feedback, curating learning materials and facilitating collaboration and the teacher's perspective.

AI in Higher Education in Developing Countries

With all these benefits, the concern of this chapter remains as to what the prospects of AIED in many of the developing countries are. While it can be agreed that AI in education has been around for many years, with a vast array of potential applications to support students, faculty members and administrators (Baker et al., 2019), there are inherent practical challenges in adopting AI in developing countries (Mogaji & Jain, 2020). From a theoretical perspective as well, there are limited studies emanating from these parts of the world. Popenici & Kerr (2017) found that the adoption of learning analytics services is still incipient in higher education institutions in Latin America. In a systematic review of research on artificial intelligence applications in higher education, Zawacki-Richter et al. (2019) revealed that 50 per cent of all the articles come from only four countries: the United States, China, Taiwan and Turkey, with no study from Africa.

It is important to contextualise developing countries beyond Africa regarding inherent characteristics that may present a challenge to AI adoption. What defines a developing country? Some may call developing countries emerging economies or the Global South. Using income classifications to group countries, the World Bank defines *developing countries* as the ones associated with low- and middle-threshold levels of gross national income (GNI) per capita (Sharma et al., 2020). However, the IMF classifies 37 countries as advanced economies against the remaining countries globally, categorised as emerging or developing economies (IMF, 2019). Statistically organised data support this classification. Nevertheless, the United Nations (UN) has no formal definition for developing countries, but it still characterises 159 countries across the world as 'developing'. These countries are categorised based on GNI, human capital and economic positioning (Sharma et al., 2020). According to the Economic Analysis and Policy Division (EAPD) of the United Nations (2020), the world is divided into three categories: developed economies, economies in transition and developing economies (UNDP, 2019).

Africa is not the only continent with countries that may be described as 'developing'. There are many developing countries in Asia and South America. As Chattopadhyay et al. (2022) noted, there are different names to describe these areas. While their education systems cannot be described solely within the context of emerging economies, they cannot be limited as developing countries, and moreover, they cannot be described as the Global South because there are countries in the region that are not considered developing countries. In all these classifications, developing countries are being measured on their economic capabilities, development prospects and social integration (Mogaji & Jain, 2020). Developing nations still face a dilemma about expanding higher education, quality trade-offs, equity and lifelong learning culture (Ndofirepi et al., 2020; Sharma et al., 2020).

From the technology and AI perspective, there are interesting challenges in many of these countries that need to be recognised in the push for integrating technology in higher education (Abdulquadri et al., 2021). Ungerer (2019) provided one of the earliest insights into AIED in an emerging-country context. By focusing on South Africa, the study recognised the challenges with manpower and suggested emerging countries should develop the necessary competencies to participate efficiently in a future AI-rich environment. Jaiswal et al. (2021) also explored the potential of AI for transformation of the education system in India. They conducted in-depth interviews with subject matter experts working on AI-related technologies and found that personalised learning, recommendation systems and adaptive assessments are helping students and supporting teachers. They acknowledged that education technology firms in an emerging country like India are deploying intelligent systems.

Access to data from universities poses a challenge for automation and artificial intelligence in higher education in developing countries (Mogaji & Jain, 2020). In the twenty-first century, data is the new coal (Raetzsch, 2016). As a result, data-related issues are probably the ones that have a high impact on the system of higher education. As per the given understanding, AI-driven systems rely heavily on the data that is fed into them. In a situation where data are not properly collected and processed at these universities, it becomes a challenge to properly integrate an AI-driven system for use in classroom teaching and learning (Dwivedi et al., 2019). Universities and other institutions of higher education have the heavy task of comparing the data they already have and the data required to run an AI-based system. This burden leads to the tedious tasks of cleaning and categorising the data sets required (Qin et al., 2020). Nevertheless, the actual bottleneck in the process is the procurement of data (Mogaji et al., 2020). The desired data sets are not always easily available and thus force the universities to seek synthetic data. Synthetic data is created artificially to suit the requirements of the system (Dilmegani, 2021).

The digital divide is also considered an issue quite peculiar to many universities in developing countries (Ndofirepi et al., 2020). Along with AI's potential to enhance the learning experience, the proliferation of smart devices and rapidly growing digitisation will further add to the growth of AI adoption in education (Zawacki-Richter et al., 2019). However, this anticipation for AI adoption may fail in economies and societies where a lack of digital exposure and access to resources are inherent (Mogaji & Jain, 2020). Many students in these developing countries do not have access to technology devices to use the AI systems (Azubike et al., 2021). The availability of the internet, digital devices like smartphones and laptops, and other technological tools is a major concern for students of diverse socio-economic and geographical backgrounds (Mogaji & Jain, 2020). Azubuike et al. (2021) found that more than half of the population in Nigeria does not have access to the internet; in addition, they found that socio-economic status contributes to the digital divide insofar as accessing remote learning, with disadvantaged populations having limited access to electricity and technological infrastructures.

In the current momentum of the pandemic, in which the world has embraced digitisation either wholeheartedly or by force, there has been a volcanic eruption of digital gaps exposed in different societies (Levander & Decherney, 2020). Caught on the two sides of the divide, higher education is challenged by the digital splits that barricade some students from receiving learning aids (Alexander, 2017). The concept of the digital divide is defined as the gap between individuals who have and those who do not have access to forms of information and communication technologies (Jan & Dijik, 2017). Tarman (2003) operationalises the digital divide to showcase the technological disparities and inequalities that exist in the system of higher education. The same can be visualised in the current situation, where universities and institutions of higher education are in a fix, having to handle the pre-existing challenges of the social, economic and cultural divide along with the digital gap.

AI has brought forth revolutionary changes and advancements in many vertical industries, one of them being higher education. With the increasing demand for personalised learning and a smart learning environment (Qin et al., 2020), AI-driven education has a huge scope in the learning industry worldwide (Chen et al., 2020). However, the demand for such an advanced education system depends on various factors, including the preparedness of the community, acceptance to change, adaptation, availability of resources and potential benefits (Wasilah et al., 2018). Since its very outset, AIED has had many challenges because education systems worldwide are averse to technological changes that go against their traditional systems. Even today, there is a certain degree of resistance from the faculty in accepting AI-driven media for the delivery of course content to the students (Rajecki, 2018). Faculty members still believe that AIED is at a very nascent stage and has a long way to go (Azubike et al., 2021). Initiatives towards the acculturation of AI-driven systems and higher education are critical to meeting the goals for AI adoption. Crafting new strategies and implementing them to accomplish the goals are the ways forward. According to Williamson (2019), for an entity such as higher education, public acceptance is important. In today's technology-driven era, there is a 'techlash' that affects the demand for big technologies in education. Techlash is a response from the stakeholders on whom the system is imposed. Universities and other institutions in higher education need a deep interrogation of their goals and value systems before implementing the cogs of AI-driven systems for higher education (Hamilton, 2021). Only then can these institutions sustain the expectations of the stakeholders.

This study presents the triple-helix framework (illustrated in Fig. 9.1) to integrate the perspectives of AI, higher education and economic activities towards a renewed understanding of contemporary education systems in emerging economies. It highlights the unique positioning of AI in context of universities in emerging economies (Ungerer, 2019; Jaiswal et al., 2021). This novel contribution recognised the intersection of AI and higher education which encompasses teaching, learning and equitable opportunities (Krishnamurthy, 2020; Chen et al., 2020). Importantly, we recognise the intersection between higher education and economic activities in the country which is reflected in deficit digital infrastructure, limited resources and digital divide (Mogaji & Jain, 2020, Azubike et al., 2021). The intersection of all three—AI, higher education and economic activities—present an AI-driven system that recognises the inherent challenges with data but still capable of meeting the basic needs of the University and presenting an opportunity to supplement teaching resources, reduce inequality, bridge the digital gap and give every student an opportunity to learn and to be supported in acquiring knowledge (Yang, 2019; Tanveer et al., 2020; AlAjmi et al., 2021).

Education at all levels is evolving at a pace faster than that of any other period in history. It is gratifying to witness the evolution and rise of new technologies, specifically in the field of higher education (Qin et al., 2020, Chen et al., 2020). Being the centre of the focus, AI is fostering more personalisation, real-time learning and improved outcomes, thus enhancing the system of higher education by providing an appropriate learning environment (Kashive et al., 2020). Even though AI is quickly gaining popularity, many institutions of higher education in developing countries still cannot find their way with this new advancement (Azubike et al., 2021). With the challenges having been highlighted, the subsequent section presents key recommendations relevant to stakeholders for integrating AIED in developing countries.

Recommendations for AI in Higher Education in Developing Countries

With the growing prospects of AIED, it is paramount to operationalise the scope and potential of AI and to put measures in place to support the process while still recognising the inherent challenges of universities in developing countries (Qin et al., 2020; Mogaji & Jain, 2020). The following recommendations are intended for university managers considering adopting an AI system and education technology developers anticipating a working relationship with universities. As Jaiswal et al. (2021) pointed out, these developers have a role to play in the proper integration of these AI systems.

Education technology developers and service providers have a mediating role to communicate with the right stakeholders (Ungerer, 2019). This mediating could be directly to the universities or directly to the students (Fitzharris & Kent, 2020). Education technology developers need to effectively present the services offered as solutions to the challenges in higher education in emerging economies (Garaika & Margahana, 2020). The instruction medium, methods and content need to be designed around aesthetics incorporating both human values and technological tools. These AI systems should be customised to contextualise the inherent challenges of the universities, should require less data, and should be easy to navigate and highly accessible (Abdulquadri et al., 2021). In addition, these systems should be developed taking into consideration in a way that requires less internet bandwidth, making it accessible.

Above all, universities need to create a supportive environment for adopting AIED. They need to recognise and acknowledge the importance of AI in delivering quality education (Qin et al., 2020). There should be some sense of awareness and recognition, a motivation to take action (Mogaji & Jain, 2020). This could come from the leadership of the university, who would gain a sufficient understanding of AI and other technology used in higher education and champion the idea of education technology developers proposing a solution (Hinson & Mogaji, 2020). AI can be considered a complex topic for discussion (Kankanhalli et al., 2019); therefore, the universities should have a team with the appropriate skills and expertise to oversee the discussion and select the company to work with.

Investing in AI systems is not a decision to be taken lightly (Mogaji et al., 2020), and therefore, universities need to be strategic in selecting the company to work with or the type of product to buy (Jaiswal et al., 2021). Alongside the issue of resistance, the demand for AIED is also affected by the cost involved in scaling up the deployment of advanced systems. Universities need to set aside dedicated funds cautiously for the availing of such technologies (Neelakantan, 2020). This is a challenge for many public universities where funding is very limited (Ndofirepi et al., 2020). The university needs to know what the company offers, how its systems can integrate with the existing infrastructure, what changes are involved and what adjustments the university may have to make to use the system, with education technology experts recommending different solutions that meet the financial, data and structural needs of the university.

Universities need to raise awareness about these tools and encourage their students to use them. Aoki (2020), experimenting with public trust in AI chatbots in the public sector, recognises that communicating the purposes of AI systems that would directly benefit citizens, such as achieving uniformity in response quality and timeliness in responding, would enhance public trust. Universities need to make the effort to communicate about their AI systems to build trust and encourage adoption. Communication could be achieved through the usual channels such as email and websites but could also be realised on social media and by working with tutors to reinforce the message (Farinloye et al., 2020).

The student also has a significant role to play in ensuring effective AI adoption in emerging economies (Phutela & Dwivedi, 2020). The number of youths in the population is growing. They are getting more conversant with technology, and mobile technology adoption is growing exponentially (Azubike et al., 2021). This situation offers students opportunities to engage with AI systems to enhance their learning experience. These opportunities could include using the learning analytics provided by the university to measure how the student is engaging with his or her studies or using the assistive technologies on the university website or mobile app (Knight et al., 2020). Student engagement with these touchpoints is important for improving the outcomes and results of the system.

Universities need to train their staff in the new revolution, the human–AI interaction and what to expect (Fontaine et al., 2019). This training can also offer a form of reassurance for those staff members thinking the machine is here to take their jobs. Alrashedi and Abbod (2020) explored the effect of using AI in the performance appraisal system at the University of Jeddah, Saudi Arabia, and reiterated the need to carry the staff along, keeping them informed and reassured about the benefits of AI. Muhaise et al. (2019) recognised that the staff in Uganda, another developing country, was reluctant to adopt an AI system because they were not properly consulted and reassured about the benefits and how their data would be processed.

No doubt, there are ethical implications that the universities and education technology developers should be aware of. Zawacki-Richter et al. (2019) recognised the emergence of new ethical implications and the risks with the development of AI applications in higher education. Russell and Norvig (2010) also warned in their work on AI that 'All AI researchers should be concerned with the ethical implications of their work'. In many countries with limited laws around privacy, ethics and data, laws such as the GDPR in

Europe (Mogaji & Jain, 2020), universities should demonstrate a high level of responsibility, developing quality and inclusive data systems and ethically calculating, processing, using and disseminating data in their control (Pedró et al., 2019). When these data are being shared with third parties such as the developers, data control measures must be put in place.

While we recognise the huge opportunities offered by education technology, the pedagogical, ethical, social, cultural and economic dimensions of AIED should be of concern for university management, staff, students and other stakeholders (Zawacki-Richter et al., 2019). It may be tempting to allow AI to do everything, replacing administrators and teachers, but universities should not get distracted from the real essence of teaching, the emotional connecting and support for students that a machine may not be able to provide. Selwyn (2016) warned that 'education is far too complex to be reduced solely to data analysis and algorithms. As with digital technologies in general, digital data do not offer a neat technical fix to education dilemmas—no matter how compelling the output might be'. It is therefore important to embrace an ethics of care (Hagendorff, 2020) and see the AIED as a support statement for complete teaching and learning.

Conclusion

This chapter recognises the COVID-19 pandemic as a great digital accelerant. Many universities have acknowledged the need to accelerate their adoption of technology to meet the changing style of teaching and learning as we adapt to this pandemic. Beyond the usual Zoom and Microsoft Teams, this acknowledgement has also further necessitated considering the adoption of AIED. AI is considered a subset of education technology within the ecosystem. While many start-ups are developing education technology, we acknowledge that AI offers a unique feature and may be of a considerable challenge for many of the universities in emerging economies.

There are potential benefits for AIED in developing countries; it could provide additional teaching support in situations where teaching resources are already stretched (Azubike et al., 2021, Qin et al., 2020). It gives the university an opportunity to best understand their students and how to meet their needs. AIED provides quantification and autonomous systems, which can track and quantify activities (Mogaji et al., 2021), creating value for the student and the university through a co-creation of knowledge (Hinson & Mogaji, 2020). Pedagogically, the students and staff get additional support with the evaluation of knowledge, assessment and feedback (Salama & Maclean, 2017).

This chapter makes a considerable theoretical contribution to AI adoption, technologies in higher education and higher education in emerging economies. Moving beyond the existing body of work on Western, educated, industrialised, rich and democratic (WEIRD) groups (Blanchard, 2015), this study recognises the socio-cultural imbalances in AIED research and highlights the challenges with the application and theory gaps during the rise of artificial intelligence in education (Chen et al., 2020). The study presents a theoretical framework that recognises the unique integration of AIED in emerging economies. Key recommendations are also presented, with managerial implications relevant to university managers and education technology developers.

Though this is a conceptual chapter, certain limitations need to be considered, thus creating scope for future research. This chapter has not been contextualised to a particular country, and therefore, the unique features of many of the emerging economies may not have been properly captured. Future studies should endeavour to understand AI adoption in higher education by the key stakeholders especially. First, research should endeavour to engage with the education technology developers and start-ups to understand their challenges in developing AI systems that can be used by universities in emerging economies, possibly extending the work of Jaiswal et al. (2021) on the transformation of the education system. Second, research should aim to uncover the universities' reluctance in adopting AI as part of their system. Third, the students' and staffs' attitudes and intentions towards AI can also be a subject of future research. Fourth, the role of policymakers in supporting universities to adopt AI is also worth exploring, at least to understand the role of ministries of education and technology in providing an enabling ecosystem for innovations in AI in education. Last, the ethical implications of data collection and data processing on the AI system should be theoretically examined.

References

Abdulquadri, A., Mogaji, E., Kieu, T. A., & Nguyen, N. P. (2021). Digital transformation in financial services provision: A Nigerian perspective to the adoption of chatbot. *Journal of Enterprising Communities: People and Places in the Global Economy*.

AlAjmi, Q., Arshah, R. A., Kamaludin, A., & Al-Sharafi, M. A. (2021). Developing an instrument for cloud-based e-learning adoption: Higher education institutions perspective. In *Advances in computer, communication and computational sciences* (pp. 671–681). Springer.

Alexander, B. (2017, October 23). Higher education, digital divides, and a balkanized Internet. https://er.educause.edu/articles/2017/10/higher-education-digital-divides-and-a-balkanized-internet

Alrashedi, A., & Abbod, M. (2020, September). The effect of using artificial intelligence on performance of appraisal system: A case study for university of Jeddah Staff in Saudi Arabia. In *Proceedings of SAI Intelligent Systems Conference* (pp. 145–154). Springer, Cham.

Al-Ramahi, N., & Odeh, M. (2020). The impact of innovative technology on the quality assurance at higher education institutions in developing countries: A case study of Jordan. *International Journal of Information and Education Technology, 10*(11).

Aoki, N. (2020). An experimental study of public trust in AI chatbots in the public sector. *Government Information Quarterly, 37*(4), 101490.

Azubuike, O. B., Adegboye, O., & Quadri, H. (2021). Who gets to learn in a pandemic? Exploring the digital divide in remote learning during the COVID-19 pandemic in Nigeria. *International Journal of Educational Research Open, 2*, 100022.

Baker, T., Smith, L., & Anissa, N. (2019). Educ-AI-tion rebooted. Exploring the future of artificial intelligence in schools and colleges. Retrieved from Nesta Foundation website: https://media.nesta.org.uk/documents/Future_of_AI_and_education_v5_WEB.pdf

Black, S. E., Muller, C., Spitz-Oener, A., He, Z., Hung, K., & Warren, J. R. (2021). The importance of STEM: High school knowledge, skills and occupations in an era of growing inequality. *Research Policy, 104249.*

Blanchard, E. G. (2015). Socio-cultural imbalances in AIED research: Investigations, implications and opportunities. *International Journal of Artificial Intelligence in Education, 25*(2), 204–228.

Chattopadhyay, A., Kupe, T., Schatzer, N. F., & Mogaji, E. (2022). Fireside chat with three Vice Chancellors from three continents: Re-imagining higher education in emerging economies. In E. Mogaji, V. Jain, F. Maringe & R. Hinson (Eds.), *Re-imagining educational futures in developing countries.* Cham: Palgrave.

Chen, X., Xie, H., Zou, D., & Hwang, G. J. (2020). Application and theory gaps during the rise of Artificial Intelligence in Education. *Computers and Education: Artificial Intelligence, 1*, 100002.

Crawford, J., Butler-Henderson, K., Rudolph, J., Malkawi, B., Glowatz, M., Burton, R., … & Lam, S. (2020). COVID-19: 20 countries' higher education intra-period digital pedagogy responses. *Journal of Applied Learning &Teaching, 3*(1), 1–20.

Dilmegani, C. (2021, February 2). The ultimate guide to synthetic data in 2021. https://research.aimultiple.com/synthetic-data/

Dwivedi, Y. K., Hughes, L., Ismagilova, E., Aarts, G., Coombs, C., Crick, T., … Williams, M. D. (2019). Artificial Intelligence (AI): Multidisciplinary perspectives on emerging challenges, opportunities, and agenda for research, practice and policy. *International Journal of Information Management, 101994.*

Farinloye, T., Adeola, O., & Mogaji, E. (2020). Typology of Nigerian universities: A strategic marketing and branding implication. In *Understanding the higher education market in Africa* (pp. 168–198). Routledge.

Fitzharris, R., & Kent, S. (2020). Adoption of bring-your-own-device examinations and data analytics. In *Adoption of data analytics in higher education learning and teaching* (pp. 327–348). Springer.

Flynn, S. (2021). Education, digital natives, and inequality. *Irish Journal of Sociology*.

Fontaine, G., Cossette, S., Maheu-Cadotte, M. A., Mailhot, T., Heppell, S., Roussy, C., … & Dubé, V. (2019). Behavior change counseling training programs for nurses and nursing students: A systematic descriptive review. *Nurse Education Today, 82*, 37–50.

Garaika, M., & Margahana, H. (2020). Adoption of educational technology: Study on higher education. *International Journal of Management (IJM), 11*(1), 61–71.

Hagendorff, T. (2020). The ethics of AI ethics: An evaluation of guidelines. *Minds and Machines, 30*(1), 99–120.

Hamilton, M. (2021). Envisioning education 4.0—A scenario planning approach to predicting the future. In *Future directions in digital information* (pp. 267–283). Chandos Publishing.

Hinson, R. E., & Mogaji, E. (2020). Co-creation of value by universities and prospective students: towards an informed decision-making process. In *Higher education marketing in Africa* (pp. 17–46). Palgrave Macmillan.

IMF. (2019). World Economic Outlook Database October 2019. https://www.imf.org/en/Publications/WEO/weo-database/2019/October

Jaiswal, A., Arun, C. J., & Varma, A. (2021). Rebooting employees: Upskilling for artificial intelligence in multinational corporations. *The International Journal of Human Resource Management*, 1–30.

Jan, A. G., & Dijik, V. (2017). *Digital divide: Impact of access*. John Wiley & Sons, Inc.

Kankanhalli, A., Yannis, C., & Sehl, M. (2019). IoT and AI for smart government: A research agenda, 304–309.

Kashive, N., Powale, L., & Kashive, K. (2020). Understanding user perception toward artificial intelligence (AI) enabled e-learning. *International Journal of Information and Learning Technology, 38*(1), 1–19.

Knight, S., Gibson, A., & Shibani, A. (2020). Implementing learning analytics for learning impact: Taking tools to task. *The Internet and Higher Education, 45*, 100729.

Krishnamurthy, S. (2020). The future of business education: A commentary in the shadow of the Covid-19 pandemic. *Journal of Business Research, 117*, 1–5.

Levander, C., & Decherney, P. (2020, June 10). The COVID-igital divide. https://www.insidehighered.com/digital-learning/blogs/education-time-corona/covid-igital-divide

Luckin, R., Holmes, W., Griffiths, M., & Forcier, L. B. (2016). *Intelligence Unleashed: An argument for AI in Education*. Pearson Education, London.

Madsen, J., & Strulik, H. (2020). Technological change and inequality in the very long run. *European Economic Review, 129*, 103532.

Marinoni, G., Van't Land, H., & Jensen, T. (2020). The impact of Covid-19 on higher education around the world. *IAU Global Survey Report*. https://www.iau-aiu.net/IMG/pdf/iau_covid19_and_he_survey_report_final_may_2020.pdf

Mogaji, E. (2020). Impact of COVID-19 on transportation in Lagos, Nigeria. *Transportation Research Interdisciplinary Perspectives, 6*, 100154. https://doi.org/10.1016/j.trip.2020.100154

Mogaji, E., & Jain, V. (2020). *Impact of the pandemic on higher education in emerging countries: Emerging opportunities, challenges and research agenda*. Research Agenda Working Papers. https://doi.org/10.2139/ssrn.3622592

Mogaji, E., Soetan, T. O., & Kieu, T. A. (2020). The implications of artificial intelligence on the digital marketing of financial services to vulnerable customers. *Australasian Marketing Journal; AMJ*.

Mogaji, E., Balakrishnan, J., Nwoba, A. C., & Nguyen, N. P. (2021). Emerging-market consumers' interactions with banking chatbots. *Telematics and Informatics, 65*, 101711.

Muhaise, H., Kareyo, M., & Muwanga-Zake, J. W. F. (2019). Factors influencing the adoption of electronic health record systems in developing countries: A case of Uganda. *American Scientific Research Journal for Engineering, Technology, and Sciences (ASRJETS), 61*(1), 160–166.

Ndofirepi, E., Farinloye, T., & Mogaji, E. (2020). Marketing mix in a heterogenous higher education market: A case of Africa. In *Understanding the higher education market in Africa* (pp. 241–262). Routledge.

Neelakantan, S. (2020, January 2). Successful AI examples in higher education that can inspire our future. https://edtechmagazine.com/higher/article/2020/01/successful-ai-examples-higher-education-can-inspire-our-future

Pedro, F., Subosa, M., Rivas, A., & Valverde, P. (2019). Artificial intelligence in education: Challenges and opportunities for sustainable development. http://repositorio.minedu.gob.pe/handle/20.500.12799/6533

Phutela, N., & Dwivedi, S. (2020). A qualitative study of students' perspective on e-learning adoption in India. *Journal of Applied Research in Higher Education*.

Popenici, S. A., & Kerr, S. (2017). Exploring the impact of artificial intelligence on teaching and learning in higher education. *Research and Practice in Technology Enhanced Learning, 12*(1), 1–13.

Qin, F., Li, K., & Yan, J. (2020). Understanding user trust in artificial intelligence-based educational systems: Evidence from China. *British Journal of Educational Technology, 51*(5), 1693–1710.

Raetzsch, C. (2016). Is data the new coal?—Four issues with Christian fuchs on social media. *Networking Knowledge Journal of the MeCCSA Postgraduate Network*, pp. 1–21.

Rajecki, K. (2018, December 28). AI in academia: Much potential, much resistance. https://www.forbes.com/sites/oracle/2018/12/28/ai-in-academia-much-potential-much-resistance/?sh=3bb32d265484

Reich, J. (2020). *Failure to disrupt: Why technology alone can't transform education.* Harvard University Press.

Richter, O. Z., Marín, V. I., Bond, M., & Gouverneur, F. (2019). Systematic review of research on artificial intelligence applications in higher education—Where are the educators? *International Journal of Educational Technology in Higher Education, 16*(39), 1–27.

Russell, S., & Norvig, P. (2010). *Artificial intelligence: A modern approach, 3rd Ed.* Prentice Hall: Upper Saddle River

Salama, A. M., & Maclean, L. (2017). Integrating Appreciative Inquiry (AI) into architectural pedagogy: An assessment experiment of three retrofitted buildings in the city of Glasgow. *Frontiers of Architectural Research, 6*(2), 169–182.

Selwyn, N. (2016). *Is technology good for education?* John Wiley & Sons.

Sharma, H., Jain, V., & Mogaji, E. (2020). Defining developing countries in higher education context. *Research Agenda Working Papers, 2021*(1), 1–9. Available at SSRN: https://ssrn.com/abstract=3774632

Tanveer, M., Hassan, S., & Bhaumik, A. (2020). Academic policy regarding sustainability and Artificial Intelligence (AI). *Sustainability, 12*(22), 9435.

Tarman, B. (2003). The digital divide in education. *International Conference for the History of Education, ISCHE, XXV*, 1–26.

Teräs, M., Suoranta, J., Teräs, H., & Curcher, M. (2020). Post-Covid-19 education and education technology 'solutionism': A seller's market. *Postdigital Science and Education, 2*(3), 863–878.

Ungerer, L. M. (2019). AI in higher education: Considering the ecosystem in an emerging-country context in Emerging education futures: Experiences and visions from the field. In Moravec, J. W. (Ed.), *Education Futures.* Minneapolis, Minnesota.

UNDP. (2019). *Human Development Report 2019.* New York: United Nations.

United Nations. (2020). Economic analysis and policy division | UN DESA | United Nations Department of Economic and Social Affairs. https://www.un.org/development/desa/en/about/desa-divisions/policy-analysis.html

Wang, Y., Liu, C., & Tu, Y. F. (2021). Factors Affecting the Adoption of AI-Based Applications in Higher Education. *Educational Technology & Society, 24*(3), 116–129.

Wasilah, W., Nugroho, L. E., & Santosa, P. I. (2018). IT-based change resistance in higher education. *International Journal of Engineering & Technology, 7*, 98–103.

Williamson, B. (2019, September 26). EdTech resistance. https://codeactsineducation.wordpress.com/2019/09/26/edtech-resistance/

Yang, X. (2019). Accelerated move for AI education in China. *ECNU Review of Education, 2*(3), 347–352.

Theme III

Staff Wellbeing

10

Physical Activity Among African Academics in a Post-COVID-19 Era: The Terrain for Action

Nestor Asiamah

Introduction

Occupational sitting is a global health risk associated with physical inactivity (PI), sedentary behaviour, and poor health (Chau et al., 2012; Marshall & Gyi, 2010). The risk of non-infectious diseases (e.g. diabetes, stroke, hypertension, and Alzheimer's disease) and mortality increases with occupational sitting (Marshall & Gyi, 2010; Simons et al., 2013; Picavet et al., 2016). There is a consensus among researchers that occupational sitting is a health risk in all employee groups but is more prevalent among administrative employees or individuals working in service organizations (Picavet et al., 2016). While employees in manufacturing firms are more likely to undertake work-related PA and avoid excessive occupational sitting, their counterparts in service organizations (e.g. banks and educational institutions) perform their core job tasks while sitting or working with the computer. Worse yet, full-time employees spend at least eight hours daily at work, which means that busy employees may spend most of their time in the week sitting. According to Hogan et al. (2016), prolonged sitting of at least one hour a day is associated with health risks, including the above non-communicable diseases.

N. Asiamah (✉)
University of Portsmouth, Portsmouth, UK

Africa Centre for Epidemiology, Accra, Ghana
e-mail: nestor.asiamah@myport.ac.uk

E. Mogaji et al. (eds.), *Re-imagining Educational Futures in Developing Countries*,
https://doi.org/10.1007/978-3-030-88234-1_10

Academic staff of universities are among the segments of the general population facing the highest risk of occupational sitting (Hogan et al., 2016). The core job tasks of teaching staff are teaching, research, and student assessment (Rapanta et al., 2020; Hogan et al., 2016). Of these three tasks, only onsite teaching (i.e. teaching in a physical classroom) involves walking and other physical activities on campus. Student assessment (e.g. design of quizzes and examinations, invigilation, and marking) and research (e.g. reading and literature review) are sedentary, except in situations where invigilation encourages walking, whereas research (i.e. data collection) involves physical activities in the field. It can, therefore, be inferred from the above that the work of teaching staff is more sedentary. This assertion is supported by studies (Hogan et al., 2016; Simons et al., 2013) that have reported an average occupational sitting time of about eight hours a day for academics. Non-teaching staff, who are university administrators, can be more inactive because their job tasks require several hours of sitting with screens (e.g. computers). More so, non-teaching staff have no or little opportunity to maintain PA in the way of onsite teaching. The incidence of PA insufficiency is, thus, likely to be higher in non-academic staff, compared with academics.

The outbreak of coronavirus disease 2019 (COVID-19) exacerbated occupational sitting among academics for a couple of reasons. First, academics became redundant after universities were temporarily closed down as part of COVID-19 containment strategy or social distancing measures. Therefore, academics lost the opportunity to keep active through onsite teaching. Other factors such as lack of access to community services, financial difficulties, and exposure to domestic violence made academics more vulnerable to PI and led to a decline in physical and mental health (Asiamah et al., 2020a; Varea & González-Calvo, 2020). Compounding this problem is the resolve of universities to move classes online (Adarkwah, 2020), which necessitated online teaching and student assessment. Recent studies (Asiamah et al., 2020a; Varea & González-Calvo, 2020) have shown that these changes among academics have dire implications for public health and the quality of university services. From a public health point of view, these changes do not only worsen occupational sitting and PI, but also reduces work satisfaction, occupational health, and individual performance (Rosenkranz et al., 2020; Hendriksen et al., 2016; Bruce, 2010). If so, the quality of services provided by universities can be expected to fall.

The concern of many researchers (Adarkwah, 2020; Asiamah et al., 2020a; Varea & González-Calvo, 2020) is that occupational sitting and the incremental effect of COVID-19 containment measures on it are long-term risks. Asiamah et al. (2020a) observed that the adverse effect of COVID-19 on PA needs urgent public health interventions because similar or even more infectious pandemics may break out in future. True to this view are key developments in universities in Africa, including the adoption of blended (i.e. online and onsite) teaching approaches and the institutionalization of long-term social distancing measures by universities after they reopened in the final quarter of 2020 (Jacob, 2020; Lone & Ahmad, 2020). Some (Lone & Ahmad, 2020; Asiamah et al., 2020a) have reasoned that social distancing will eventually be incorporated into university management culture, or university staff will become accustomed to a work environment where social distancing or the use of sedentary modes of working is normative. That being so, adherence to social distancing measures in the long-term is necessary. A long-term decline in the health, work satisfaction, and individual productivity of university staff in a post-COVID-19 world is, thus, possible. This viewpoint is corroborated by studies (White et al., 2020; Bogaert et al., 2014) reporting a negative association between health status (e.g. PI and chronic conditions) and performance indicators. To maintain or improve the quality of educational services, interventions to occupational sitting and PI among university staff ought to be developed and rolled out.

The aim of this chapter is to draw on primary data to recommend ways in which African universities can reduce the risk of PI-associated new work patterns in a post-COVID-19 context. The specific objectives addressed are to: (1) provide implications of core job tasks for PA; (2) demonstrate the potential role of neighbourhood walkability in enhancing PA; and (3) analyse the role of campus residency in PA improvement among academics in a post-COVID-19 context. This chapter demonstrates PI as a potential risk associated with new work patterns necessitated by COVID-19 control measures in African universities in a post-COVID-19 era. It recommends ways to reduce PI and its potential adverse impacts on the health and productivity of university staff. Finally, recommendations in this chapter are expected to guide universities and ministries of education to provide policy-led interventions to PI and other related occupational health risks. University staff are also expected to gain an understanding of how they can avoid PI and its health risks in their effort to accomplish their job roles.

This chapter comprises an introductory section where the study's context and problem are clearly identified and defined. Subsequently, the focus of the study and its theoretical foundation are provided. The research methodology employed to gather and analyse data is then discussed and justified. Data are then analysed to address the specific research objectives presented above. A discussion of the findings follows data analysis and is aimed at analysing the relationship between findings, the theoretical foundation provided, and related empirical studies. Implications of the results for theory and practice are also discussed. Limitations of the study are also provided alongside relevant future research directions. Finally, conclusions are presented in line with the results relating to the specific objectives. The theoretical approach to the study is presented in the next section.

Study Focus and Theoretical Approach

Populations at the highest risk of PI are vulnerable to chronic conditions and mortality (Hinckson et al., 2017; Van Holle et al., 2016). For this reason, the maintenance of PA over the life course is a hallmark of ageing well, an idea that has encouraged the development of novel PA promotion programmes and interventions such as the 'smart cities' (Koohsari et al., 2018) and 'ageing in place' campaigns (Federmeier & Kutas, 2005). The smart cities campaign is a flagship of PA promotion that emphasizes the creation of cities and neighbourhoods that encourage walking, bicycling, skating, and other physical and social activities (Koohsari et al., 2018; Federmeier & Kutas, 2005). This initiative draws on bio-ecological models, particularly Lawton and Simon's (1968) Person-Environment (P-E) fit model. This model argues that behaviours such as PA are the results of the interplay between the environment and individual factors. The Bronfenbrenner's (1979) model, another popular bioecological model, similarly posits that behaviours are tied to a complex social system comprising the society, family, workmates, and neighbours. The foregoing two models suggest that human behaviours are dependent on ecosystem factors, namely social networks, the built environment (e.g. services, parks and gardens), and personal factors.

More recently, Wahl and Gerstorf (2018) drew on the above landmark models to develop the 'Context Dynamics in Aging' (CODA) framework. This framework promises to serve as an all-encompassing lens for seeing and understanding contextual factors that affect PA and health. The framework asserts that behaviours such as PA that contribute to health are affected by the built environment and social networks. The CODA is also prominent for including factors of neighbourhood walkability, defined as the extent to which the built environment or a community supports PA (Koohsari et al., 2018, 2020). Research to date has shown that neighbourhood walkability increases PA and health among residents of a community (Hosler et al., 2014; Oyeyemi et al., 2019; Koohsari et al., 2020). This evidence has encouraged the design of neighbourhoods in developed countries such as the UK, Singapore, Japan, and the US to support PA. Per the CODA, the risk of PI faced by academics can be avoided or reduced by maximizing neighbourhood walkability or designing university campuses to encourage PA among staff and students. The CODA and the foregoing models are particularly suited for this study because they assume that walkable neighbourhoods provide an opportunity for university staff to age well as they carry out job roles. This is to say that faculty members can 'age in place' or maintain PA and health as they age as individuals in their neighbourhoods.

Ageing in place or context is another prominent public health promotion paradigm that encapsulates interventions and recommendations for PA promotion for all segments of the population (Federmeier & Kutas, 2005; Wiles et al., 2011). Its programmes emphasize the need for people to age successfully in their homes and neighbourhoods where opportunities and resources for healthy behaviours such as social networks, social support, and walkable factors are more abundant (Koohsari et al., 2018), compared to long-term care facilities or any other place the individual is not familiar with. An underlying principle of ageing in place is that people who age in their homes and neighbourhoods utilize social capital (e.g. social networks and social support) and walkable attributes to maintain social engagement and PA (Wiles et al., 2011; Koohsari et al., 2018). From this perspective, ageing in place and the smart cities campaign overlap conceptually and share the goal of enabling individuals to maintain PA in the ageing process. Interestingly, research to date has provided compelling evidence on the positive effect of PA on health over the life course (Blom et al., 2020; Genin et al., 2018; Heiestad et al., 2020). Research has also evidenced that PA is higher among residents of smart or walkable cities (Koohsari et al., 2018) and those ageing in context (Federmeier & Kutas, 2005; Wiles et al., 2011). Therefore, one of the best ways to mitigate the high risk of PI faced by university staff is to understand PA promotion strategies applicable to universities from the perspectives of ageing in place and the smart cities campaign.

This study aims to use ageing in context and the smart cities campaign as a lens to identify key measures that can be taken to reduce PI among university staff. Since neighbourhood walkability enhancement is at the very core of ageing in context campaigns, the ideal way to guide stakeholders to reduce PI is to demonstrate how neighbourhood walkability moderates the relationship between academic job tasks and PA. Interventions implied by this relationship are, therefore, proffered for stakeholders' consideration and action. These interventions, which characterize key steps, actors, and collaborations, are hereby referred to as 'the terrain', which needs to be understood for PI among university staff to be curbed going forward. The post-COVID-19 context is operationally defined as the time after the reopening of universities in Africa when staff were required to resume work while observing more stringent social distancing measures. As indicated early on, working in this context is expected to be a long-term process because society is being compelled to take lasting countermeasures against COVID-19 or any future infectious disease, a reason why 'ageing in place' is an appropriate context for identifying interventions to PI among academics. The researcher's specification of the said terrain is an approach that draws on primary data collected in the foregoing post-COVID-19 context. The next section provides an overview of the methodology applied in collecting and analysing these data.

Methods

Design and Participants

This study adopted a cross-sectional design. The study participants were full-time academics working in African private and public universities. The study focused on African settings where COVID-19 restrictions had been lifted and universities were asked to reopen. The specific inclusion criteria used to select participants are: (a) having worked as a full-time academic for at least a year in the current university; (b) having a minimum of a diploma, which was used as an indicator of the ability to read and write in English; (c) active engagement in teaching or any other academic job task after reopening; (d) compliance with institutional or national social distancing protocols; and (e) willingness to participate in the study voluntarily. Since the study adopted an online survey method, a probability sampling method could not be adopted. To maximize the statistical power of the analysis, the researcher endeavoured to reach as many participants as possible using the snowball sampling method. A minimum sample size of 500 participants was deemed appropriate for this study as it had produced reliable findings in a related study conducted in Ghana (Asiamah et al., 2020a).

The four main constructs measured in this study are job components, neighbourhood walkability, campus residency, and PA. Demographic and personal characteristics were also measured as potential confounding variables. The researcher measured PA with the International Physical Activity Questionnaire (SF-IPAQ). Recommendations and a formula reported by Lee et al. (2011) were applied to generate an index from this questionnaire. To measure neighbourhood walkability, the 11-item Australian version of the Neighbourhood Walkability Scale adapted from Merom et al. (2015) was used. The five anchors of the scale are: strongly disagree—1, disagree—2, somewhat agree—3, agree—4, and strongly agree—5. In the current study, this measure produced a Cronbach's alpha value of 0.81. Appendix 1 shows how the job components, campus residency, and demographic attributes were measured whereas the following subsection discusses the structure of the survey used.

Survey Structure, Piloting, and Validation

An online self-reported questionnaire was employed in this study to gather data as social distancing protocols being observed did not support physical administration of questionnaires. Moreover, the use of an online survey was the only way to gather data from participants located in different African countries.

The procedure for piloting and validating the online survey has been reported by Asiamah et al. (2020a). The survey was constructed and hosted on Google Forms, which is free and was deemed the most convenient for the study. The survey was developed from scratch because no default template was applicable. The questionnaire had four parts; the first part presented the survey completion instructions and ethical statement whereas the second part presented seven measures of the job components. The third part presented measures of neighbourhood walkability while the final part captured personal and demographic attributes.

Data Collection Approach

This study received ethical clearance from an institutional ethics review committee (# 0022020ACE). The first question of the survey included the ethical statement of the study as well as survey completion instructions. The inclusion criteria were also presented to ensure that only those who were eligible could participate. The survey was published online on October 10, 2020, by sharing it on some WhatsApp platforms including or comprising academics. The collection of data was coordinated by Research Associates from the Africa Center for Epidemiology (ACE). ACE had four WhatsApp groups that contained about 360 academics and doctoral students. These platforms featured academics from 11 African countries and were therefore the ideal place to launch the survey. Members who met the inclusion criteria on these platforms were asked to complete the survey (posted as a short link) and share it with their colleagues. There was no need for participants to download the survey before completing it. Moreover, the survey could be completed with a relatively weak internet connection. The average survey completion time was about five minutes. To avoid multiple responses from the same participant, the survey was programmed appropriately in Google Forms. The survey was closed on November 15, 2020. After applying the selection criteria, 1064 completed surveys were incorporated into statistical data analysis. The next subsection presents the statistical analysis method employed.

Statistical Analysis Method

Data were analysed with version 26 of SPSS (i.e. Statistical Package for the Social Sciences). Data were summarized with descriptive statistics (frequencies, percentages, mean, standard deviation, skewness, and kurtosis) to identify potential outliers in the data. Estimates of kurtosis and skewness as well as stem-and-leaf plots met recommended rules of thumb (Garson, 2012) and, therefore, evidenced the absence of outliers in the data. A sensitivity analysis employed by Asiamah et al. (2020a) was applied to identify the ultimate covariates or confounding variables. This analysis was adopted to ensure that only relevant confounding variables were incorporated into the final analysis.

To address the research goal, three stages of analysis were conducted. In the first phase, the hierarchical linear regression (HLR) analysis was employed to assess the relationship between core job components and PA. In the second phase, the moderating role of neighbourhood walkability in the relationship between the job components and PA was evaluated using HLR. To test this relationship, the following four interaction terms were computed: NW*teaching-online (i.e. the interaction between neighbourhood walkability and online teaching), NW*teaching-onsite (i.e. the interaction between neighbourhood walkability and onsite teaching), NW*assessment (i.e. the interaction between neighbourhood walkability and assessment), and NW*research (i.e. the interaction between neighbourhood walkability and research). In the third phase, the moderating influence of neighbourhood walkability on the relationship between campus residency and PA was assessed. The interaction term created in this respect was NW*CR (i.e. the interaction between neighbourhood walkability and campus residency). The statistical significance of results was detected at $p < 0.05$. Findings of the study are presented in the next section.

Findings

In Appendix 2, 68% ($n = 720$) of the participants were men whereas 32% ($n = 344$) were women. About 35% ($n = 372$) of participants were resident in Ghana, 38% ($n = 400$) were resident in Nigeria, 26% ($n = 272$) were resident in Kenya, and 2% ($n = 20$) were resident in Tanzania. About 83% ($n = 880$) of participants lived off their university campus, whereas 17% ($n = 184$) lived on campus. Appendix 2 shows other relevant participant characteristics. In Table 10.1, there is a positive correlation between PA and neighbourhood walkability ($r = 0.205$, $p = 0.000$, two-tailed) and teaching onsite ($r = 0.064$, $p < 0.05$, two-tailed), suggesting that PA increases as onsite teaching and neighbourhood walkability increase. The table shows other key correlations on which the HLR analysis is based. Table 10.2 shows HLR coefficients on two regression models. In the first model, research has a positive association with PA ($\beta = 0.2$; $t = 2.42$; $p < 0.05$) whereas assessment has a negative association with PA ($\beta = -0.97$; $t = -11.49$; $p = 0.000$). This result confirms that PA reduces as student assessment increases but increases with research.

In the second model, the moderating effect of neighbourhood walkability rendered the relationship between online teaching ($\beta = 0.06$; $t = 2.28$; $p < 0.05$) and onsite teaching ($\beta = 0.17$; $t = 7.25$; $p = 0.000$) positively significant. This moderating effect also buffered the negative association between assessment and PA ($\beta = -0.65$; $t = -7.28$; $p = 0.000$). These results connote that neighbourhood walkability contributes to PA by reducing the negative influence of sedentary job tasks (i.e. online teaching and assessment) on PA. In the first model of Table 10.3, neighbourhood walkability has a positive association with PA, suggesting that PA increases with neighbourhood walkability. In the second model of the table, campus residency has a positive association with PA, which implies that academics who lived on campus had higher PA. In the third model, neighbourhood walkability moderates the relationship between campus residency and PA by further strengthening this relationship. Thus, the positive influence of campus residency on PA increases as neighbourhood walkability increases. The above findings are discussed in the next section.

Discussion

This study aimed to draw on findings of a cross-sectional analysis to specify interventions to PI among academics in a post-COVID-19 context where lessons from COVID-19 would cause changes in work patterns in universities. In this section, specifications of interventions and their actors are highlighted under the following subsections.

Table 10.1 The correlation between academic job components, neighbourhood walkability, and physical activity

Variable	Mean	SD	1	2	3	4	5	6	7	8	9	10	11	12
1. Teaching online	5.3	4.2	1	-0.231**	0.047	0.048	-0.095**	-0.048	-0.015	-0.137**	-0.006	-0.181**	-0.106**	-0.069*
2. Teaching onsite	6.0	4.9		1	-0.033	-0.055	0.093**	0.064*	-0.102**	-0.095**	-0.035	-0.014	0.025	-0.05
3. Research	2.3	1.1			1	0.972**	-0.208**	-0.748**	0.102**	0.067*	0.038	0.014	-0.073*	-0.069*
4. Assessment	7	3.2				1	-0.215**	-0.779**	0.094**	0.068*	0.054	-0.024	-0.057	-0.076*
5. Neighbourhood walkability	27.7	6.2					1	0.205**	0.011	-0.109**	-0.011	-0.04	0.209**	0.053
6. Physical activity	4475.3	2754.33						1	-0.127**	-0.140**	-0.067*	-0.03	0.111**	0.014
7. Gender (reference—male)	–	–							1	0.097**	-0.03	-0.062*	0.066*	0.012
8. Education	–	–								1	0.156**	0.589**	0.065*	0.432**
9. Income (USD)	–	–									1	0.172**	0.062*	0.192**
10. Rank	–	–										1	0.121**	0.628**
11. Campus residency	–	–											1	0.124**
12. Age (years)	44.25	9.632												1

– Not applicable; *SD* standard deviation; *USD* United States dollars

$^{**}p < 0.001$; $^{*}p < 0.05$

Table 10.2 The relationship between academic job components, neighbourhood walkability, and physical activity among academics

		Coefficients					Model fit				
Model	Independent variable	*B*	SE	β(*t*)	95% CI	Tolerance	R^2	Adjusted R^2	Change in R^2	Durbin-Watson	*F*-test
1	(Constant)	10542.99	404.78	(26.05)**	±1588.61		0.616	0.613	0.003	1.602	180.78**
	Teaching online	-10.29	13.28	-0.02(-0.78)	±52.12	0.91					
	Teaching onsite	-0.07	11.24	0.00(-0.01)	±44.10	0.91					
	Research	515.03	212.43	0.20(2.42)*	±833.71	0.05					
	Assessment	-836.87	72.86	-0.97(-11.49)**	±285.96	0.05					
	Covariates										
	Gender (reference—male)	-304.48	117.88	-0.05(-2.58)*	±462.63	0.95					
	Education	-251.09	108.28	-0.06(-2.32)*	±424.95	0.61					
	Income (USD)	-23.88	42.64	-0.01(-0.56)	±167.33	0.95					
	Rank	-53.39	52.16	-0.03(-1.31)	±204.70	0.46					
	Age	-5.55	7.44	-0.02(-0.75)	±29.18	0.58					
2	(Constant)	8558.31	473.82	(18.06)**	±1859.55		0.445	0.44	0.005	1.66	90.25**
	NW*Teaching online	130.67	57.33	0.06(2.28)*	±225.00	0.95					
	NW*Teaching onsite	249.92	34.47	0.17(7.25)**	±135.27	0.96					
	NW*Research	176.62	786.03	0.02(0.23)	±3084.85	0.07					
	NW*Assessment	-1943.31	267.12	-0.65(-7.28)**	±1048.33	0.07					
	Covariates										
	Gender (ref.—male)	-344.94	142.04	-0.06(-2.43)*	±557.44	0.94					
	Education	-366.87	130.21	-0.09(-2.82)*	±511.00	0.61					
	Income (USD)	-12.07	51.39	-0.01(-0.24)	±201.69	0.94					
	Rank	-7.39	62.33	0.00(-0.12)	±244.63	0.46					
	Age	11.32	8.91	0.04(1.27)	±34.98	0.59					

USD United States dollars; *NW* neighbourhood walkability; *SE* standard error (of B); *CI* confidence interval

$^{**}p < 0.001$; $^{*}p < 0.05$

[1]Model testing primary associations

[2]Model testing moderating relationships

Table 10.3 The association between neighbourhood walkability, physical activity, and campus residency

Model	Predictors	Coefficients			95% CI	VIF	Model fit				
		B	SE	*B*(*t*)			R^2	Adjusted R^2	Change in R^2	Durbin-Watson	*F*-test
1[a]	(Constant)	3831.57	676.45	(676.45)**	±2654.8		0.081	0.076	0.005	1.6	14.95**
	Neighbourhood walkability	85.51	13.45	0.19(6.36)**	±52.78	1.03					
	Gender[d]	-585.74	180.19	-0.10(-3.25)**	±707.16	1.04					
	Education	-645.18	165.89	-0.15(-3.89)**	±651.06	1.63					
	Income (USD)	-150.48	65.49	-0.07(-2.3)*	±257	1.05					
	Rank	52.22	77.7	0.03(0.67)	±304.95	2.04					
	Age	19.44	11.39	0.07(1.71)	±44.71	1.68					
2[b]	Campus residency[e]	1037.74	224.34	0.14(4.63)**	±880.44	1.03	0.064	0.059	0.005	1.57	11.63**
	Gender[d]	-644.99	182.37	-0.11(-3.54)**	±715.72	1.04					
	Education	-750.82	166.08	-0.17(-4.52)**	±651.78	1.6					
	Income (USD)	-165.95	66.15	-0.08(-2.51)*	±259.6	1.05					
	Rank	13.6	78.61	0.01(0.17)	±308.52	2.05					
	Age	24.54	11.44	0.08(2.15)*	±44.89	1.67					
3[c]	(Constant)	6360.19	554.55	(11.47)**	±2176.37		0.077	0.061	0.016	1.56	13.03**
	NW*CR	39.4	7.26	0.17(5.43)**	±28.5	1.04					
	Gender[d]	-688.43	182.22	-0.12(-3.78)**	±715.15	1.05					
	Education	-739.54	165.49	-0.17(-4.47)**	±649.46	1.6					
	Income (USD)	-170.85	65.92	-0.08(-2.59)*	±258.69	1.05					
	Rank	0.75	78.44	0.00(0.01)	±307.83	2.06					
	Age	24.04	11.39	0.08(2.11)*	±44.71	1.67					

USD United States dollars; *NW* neighbourhood walkability; *CI* confidence interval; *VIF* variance inflation factor; *CR* campus residency
$**p < 0.001$; $*p < 0.05$
[a]First model with neighbourhood walkability as predictor
[b]Second model with campus residency as main predictor
[c]Third model with NW*CR as main predictor
[d]Reference—male
[e]Reference—living on campus

Academic Job Tasks and Physical Activity

The study found that research is positively associated with PA, suggesting that PA increases as research work increases. In contrast, student assessment has a negative association with PA, which means that PA reduces as student assessment increases. What could be inferred from these findings is that research work in the post-COVID-19 context involved physical and social activities relating to field research work. Further to this, academics did less of desk research (i.e. literature review and reading) and were personally involved in physical activities relating to research, possibly because they had a backlog of field research tasks that could not be undertaken before schools reopened. The negative relationship between assessment and PA also suggests that academics, even in the post-COVID-19 era, did more of sedentary assessments. This assertion is congruent with the thought of some researchers (Asiamah et al., 2020a; Venkatesh & Edirappuli, 2020; Varea & González-Calvo, 2020) that academics would continue to observe social distancing even after schools reopen. Also consistent with this result is the hypothesis of Varea and González-Calvo (2020) that student assessment in the post-COVID-19 period would be carried out online. Deductively, at least one academic job task in the post-COVID-19 period is likely to discourage PA among academics, as a result of which interventions are needed from key actors.

Given the above results, the way forward is reducing the risk of sedentary job tasks in universities for PI and increasing work-related PA. Since sedentary job tasks are a risk factor for PI and chronic conditions, universities would have to adopt a policy emphasizing minimal online teaching and learning. Another reason why excessive online teaching and learning must be avoided by universities is the fact that most faculties are still learning to use online teaching resources whereas many students have been dissatisfied with online teaching and learning rolled out in response to COVID-19 (Upoalkpajor & Upoalkpajor, 2020; Varea & González-Calvo, 2020). Even so, online teaching and learning may become a routine in the post-COVID-19 world, as a result of which universities ought to adopt innovative approaches that tend to prevent prolonged sitting in online teaching. A feasible approach is educating staff members to remain active while teaching online. For instance, academics can be trained to stand and move slowly while teaching online. With a three-dimensional (3-D) online classroom view option, teachers can walk slowly while teaching online. A 3-D view can visualize both blackboard contents, the instructor, and relevant course materials concurrently. As to whether this method can function effectively in developing countries is, however, yet to be empirically established. Universities may have to invest in research investigating the feasibility and effectiveness of this method.

The fact that academic institutions operate under the government's watch should always be borne in mind by universities when developing occupational health policies for their employees. Involving governments and ministries of education in health programmes for university staff would encourage the government to provide a congenial environment for implementing interventions. From this point of view, governments can make PA-oriented teaching (both onsite and online) mandatory and a programme subject to routine surveillance and monitoring. This can be done through a legislative instrument that binds all universities to educate their staff to reduce occupational sitting, meet recommended PA levels, and avoid sedentary behaviour. What makes this and similar steps necessary is the high prevalence of chronic conditions among academics (Hogan et al., 2016), which is a recipe for underperformance. In the current study, 21% of academics had at least one chronic condition (see Appendix 2), which is far larger than ratios reported for even vulnerable groups such as older adults (Asiamah et al., 2020b, c). No doubt, failing to take radical measures against PI can have dire consequences for productivity and health in a post-COVID-19 world. Interestingly, neighbourhoods, including university campuses, can be designed to reduce the risk of PI among academics. The next subsection elaborates on this idea.

Neighbourhood Walkability and Physical Activity

Neighbourhood walkability positively moderates the association between the core academic tasks and PA, implying generally that neighbourhood walkability buffers the negative influences of sedentary job tasks on PA and increases the positive influences of PA-oriented job tasks on PA. This result backs the P-E fit theory of Lawton and Simon (1968) as well as Wahl and Gerstorf's (2018) CODA framework. Suffice it to say that neighbourhood walkability provides opportunities for PA and social activities even in sedentary work contexts where job tasks require prolonged sitting and reading. This outcome is also consistent with several empirical studies that have confirmed a positive association between neighbourhood walkability and PA in African and developed contexts. In Nigeria, for example, Oyeyemi et al. (2019) confirmed a positive association between neighbourhood walkability and PA. In Ghana, Asiamah et al. (2020c) confirmed that walkable contextual factors were negatively associated with sedentary behaviour, which means that walkability can buffer sedentariness in African populations. In Japan, neighbourhood walkability was found to have a positive association with PA (Koohsari et al., 2018, 2020). It is, thus, understandable that designing neighbourhoods to make them highly walkable is a general intervention to PI.

The foregoing evidence calls to mind the role of governments in providing healthy environments for all. According to findings of this study, most academics may not reside on their university campuses, which means that the walkability of neighbourhoods ought to be improved. The basis of improving neighbourhood design and walkability is sufficient political will; governments' commitment to public health would make programmes aimed at improving walkability more acceptable and meaningful to them. In line with developed countries such as the UK and Singapore, African governments would have to provide essential community services, safe roads and streets, and green spaces while enforcing neighbourhood peace and stability to maximize walkability, social engagement, and PA. This effort can be expected to have a ripple effect on university campuses and encourage PA in all segments of the population, including academics. Owing to the high rate of chronic conditions faced by academics, universities ought to take independent steps in the light of the said national legislative instrument to improve the mix of services available on their campuses. Universities are also encouraged to increase contextual resources for PA such as green spaces, sidewalks, wide streets, and spacious classrooms that can encourage academics to walk slowly while teaching. Interestingly, the provision of the above resources may not change behaviours in the right direction if university staff and possibly students are not well educated to understand the risk of PI they face, why they need to achieve recommended PA levels, and how they can use campus resources to maintain PA. Training and special health education programmes can be executed by universities to create awareness of PI risks and how to utilize campus resources to avoid or reduce these risks. As explained in the next subsection, the risk of PI can be reduced by revising or modifying campus residency policies in universities.

Campus Residency and Physical Activity

The study also reports a positive association between campus residency and PA, which suggests that academics who were living on campus reported higher PA time. More interestingly, the strength of this relationship was increased by neighbourhood walkability, which connotes that campus residency better supports PA in more walkable universities or campuses located in walkable neighbourhoods. This result reflects high walkability attributes seen on university campuses in African countries. To explain, campuses of the University of Ghana, the University of Cape Town in South Africa, and the University of Ibadan in Nigeria feature lots of green parks, lawns, services, and streets, which are the core of neighbourhood walkability relevant to social engagement and PA among students and university staff (Koohsari et al., 2018; Oyeyemi et al., 2019). Workers are more likely to use campus resources and services if these walkable attributes are available. More so, the availability of tarred streets and sidewalks would encourage walking, bicycling, or skating for a purpose or recreation. It is also worth indicating that this result affirms the positive moderating influence of neighbourhood walkability on the association between core job components and PA.

Considering the above evidence, universities may have to provide accommodation for all academics who are willing to live on campus. As the current study indicates, universities provide accommodation for a minor segment of its employees, possibly due to financial constraints. Universities can improve their capacity to build more staff flats in the light of the aforesaid national legislation for PA and health that is expected to increase the commitment of governments to the health of their labour force, particularly university staff. This legislation may call for beefing up the portion of national funds (e.g. Ghana Education Trust Fund) aimed at infrastructural development. Beyond the provision of more flats for university staff, campus walkability ought to be enhanced further as mentioned above, a step that is an appropriately urgent way to address the high prevalence of chronic conditions among academics. Last but not least, individual academics need to take extraordinary steps to reduce the health risks they face, bearing in mind the fact that their health does not only determine their productivity and career progress but also forms the basis of their happiness and general life satisfaction. This assertion is a way to emphasize the need for individuals to take personal steps to avoid occupational risks (e.g. prolonged sitting and PI) even in the absence of institutional and national interventions. Developing a personal plan in this direction would help every academic to invest in exercise and health education programmes while taking prophylactic steps to avoid key health risks such as high blood sugar and overweight. Regular PA and recommended nutritional practices must be observed simultaneously at the individual level (Asiamah et al., 2020b). The applicability of the above recommendations, however, would be enhanced if limitations of this study discussed in the next section are addressed in future research.

Study Limitations

This study adopted a cross-sectional design that is not robust against confounding influences. As such, future researchers are advised to replicate this study with experimental designs such as the randomized controlled trial.

Since data were collected using an online instrument, it was not possible to reach a probabilistic and powered sample. Similarly, the study was focused on academics or excluded non-academic staff. As such, this study's findings may not be generalizable to other contexts, especially non-African contexts. However, their implications and recommendations can apply to non-academic staff who work side by side with academics. Finally, recommendations provided in this study are only implications of the results and are, therefore, inconclusive. For this reason, more studies investigating the health risks faced by university staff as well as applicable interventions to these risks are needed. The next section presents conclusions based on the study's findings.

Conclusion

It is concluded that neighbourhood walkability plays an important role in buffering the potential negative influences of sedentary job tasks on PA in a post-COVID context. Academics living on more walkable campuses are more likely to maintain PA in the post-COVID-19 context, which suggests that walkability of campuses reduces the risks of PI associated with social distancing measures. These outcomes reinforce the need for neighbourhood walkability to be improved as an intervention to social distancing measures taken in response to the spread of a pandemic. Hence, stakeholders are obliged to take specific actions to reduce PI associated with academic posts. The specific stakeholders are universities, university staff, and governments. Universities are responsible for implementing health education programmes for staff, designing their campuses and classrooms (both physical and virtual) to encourage PA, and collaborating with the government and civil society to develop interventions to occupational sitting. University staff are expected to understand the risks of PI and sedentary behaviour, develop and maintain PA trajectories in compliance with global PA recommendations, support interventions rolled out by their universities and governments, and apply a scheme of routine self-evaluation to achieve recommended PA levels. Governments are expected to support universities by providing relevant legislations and funding for institutional health programmes, investing in walkable neighbourhoods, and keeping an open-door policy for collaborations with academic and research institutions. The foregoing measures can be an effective way to avoid significant increases in the risks of PI and their detrimental effects on health and productivity.

Appendices

Appendix 1: Operationalization and Coding of Job Components, Participant Characteristics, and Covariates

Variable	Indicator	Definition (operationalization)	Coding (values)	Dummy-coding
Participant characteristics	University classification*	Whether the individual's primary university was a public, private, or hybrid academic institution	Public (1), private (2), hybrid**** (3)	Applied
	Sex*	Reported gender of the participant	Male (0), female (1)	Applied
	Country*	The country where the participant was working as a faculty member	Nigeria (1), Ghana (2), Kenya (3), Tanzania (4)	Applied
	CDS*	Whether the participant had at least one clinically diagnosed chronic disease condition	None (0), ≥1 (1)	Applied
	Income (USD)**	The faculty's gross monthly income in United States dollars	0–500(1), 501–1000 (2), 1001–1500 (3), 1501–2000 (4), Above 2000 (5)	Not applied
	Rank[a**]	The academic rank of the participant	Teaching assistant (1), assistant lecturer (2), lecturer (3), senior lecturer (4), assistant professor (5), associate professor (6), full professor (7)	Not applied
	Residency*	Whether the faculty was resident on the campus of his or her primary academic institution	No (0), Yes (1)	Applied
	Job tenure***	The number of years the participant had served as an academic faculty	–	Not applied
	Alternative role(s)*	Whether the participant had other academic job roles outside his/her primary academic institution	No (0), Yes (1)	Applied
	Educational level**	The highest educational qualification acquired by the academic	Diploma (1), first degree (2), master's degree (3), PhD or equivalent (4)	Not applied
	Age (yrs)***	The age of the academic in years	–	Not applied

Research	Research***	The amount of time the academic had spent in the last seven days on research-related activities	–	Not applied
Teaching	Teaching online***	The time spent by the academic on online teaching over the last seven days	–	Not applied
	Teaching onsite***	The time spent by the academic on teaching in a physical classroom over the last week	–	Not applied
Student assessment	Marking***	The amount of time spent by the academic on marking of examination/test scripts over the last week	–	Not applied
	Marks organization***	The amount of time spent by the academic on organizing test/examination scores over the last week	–	Not applied
	Quizzes and exams***	The amount of time the academic spent on conducting quizzes and examinations over the last week	–	Not applied
	Project supervision***	The amount of time spent by the academic on student research project supervision over the last week	–	Not applied

– Not applicable; *CDS* chronic disease status
*Nominal variable; **Ordinal variable; ***Continuous variable; ****An institution with public and private ownership status
[a]Each category was associated with its research specialization

Appendix 2: Descriptive Statistics Summarizing Participant Characteristics

Variable	Group	*n*(%)
Income (USD)	0–500	192(18.0)
	501–1000	388(36.5)
	1001–1500	224(21.1)
	1501–2000	96(9.0)
	Above 2000	164(15.4)
	Total	1064(100)
Educational level	Diploma	16(1.5)
	First degree	76(7.1)
	Master's degree	480(45.1)
	PhD or equivalent	492(46.2)
	Total	1064(100)
Sex	Male	720(67.7)
	Female	344(32.3)
	Total	1064(100)
Alternative role(s)	No	624(58.6)
	Yes	440(41.6)
	Total	1064(100)
Campus residency	No	880(82.7)
	Yes	184(17.3)
	Total	1064(100)
Country	Ghana	372(35.0)
	Nigeria	400(37.6)
	Kenya	272(25.6)
	Tanzania	20(1.9)
	Total	1064(100)
Chronic disease status	None	836(78.6)
	≥1	228(21.4)
	Total	1064(100)
University classification	Public	760(71.4)
	Private	280(26.3)
	Hybrid (public and private)	24(2.3)
	Total	1064(100)
Rank[a]	Teaching assistant	96(9)
	Assistant lecturer	192(18)
	Lecturer	380(35.7)
	Senior lecturer	248(23.2)
	Associate professor	76(7.1)
	Professor (full)	72(6.8)
	Total	1064(100)

n frequency; *USD* United States dollars
[a]Each category was associated with its research specialization

References

Adarkwah, M. A. (2020). "I'm not against online teaching, but what about us?": ICT in Ghana post-Covid-19. *Education and Information Technologies, 16*(1), 1–21. https://doi.org/10.1007/s10639-020-10331-z

Asiamah, N., Opuni, N. F., Mends-Brew, E., Mensah, S. W., Mensah, H. K., & Quansah, F. (2020a). Short-term changes in behaviors resulting from COVID-19-related social isolation and their influences on mental health in Ghana. *Community Mental Health Journal, 57*(1), 1–14. https://doi.org/10.1007/s10597-020-00722-4

Asiamah, N., Petersen, C., Kyriakos, K., & Eduafo, R. (2020b). The association between physical activity and self-reported health in older adults: Lessons implied by lifestyle factors. *Advances in Gerontology, 33*(2), 289–298. https://doi.org/10.34922/AE.2020.33.2.010

Asiamah, N., Petersen, C., Kyriakos, K., & Eduafo, R. (2020c). The built environment and socio-demographic correlates of partial and absolute sedentary behaviours in community-dwelling older adults in Accra, Ghana. *Journal of Cross-Cultural Gerontology, 36*(1), 1–21. https://doi.org/10.1007/s10823-020-09417-5

Blom, E. E., Aadland, E., Skrove, G. K., Solbraa, A. K., & Oldervoll, L. M. (2020). Health-related quality of life and physical activity level after a behaviour change program at Norwegian healthy life centres: A 15-month follow-up. *Quality of Life Research, 29*(1), 1–11. https://doi.org/10.1007/s11136-020-02554-x

Bogaert, I., De Martelaer, K., Deforche, B., Clarys, P., & Zinzen, E. (2014). Associations between different types of physical activity and teachers' perceived mental, physical, and work-related health. *BMC Public Health, 14*(1), 1–9. https://doi.org/10.1186/1471-2458-14-534

Bronfenbrenner, U. (1979). *The ecology of human development: Experiments by nature and design*. Harvard University Press.

Bruce, E. (2010). Exercise as a factor in the job satisfaction of law enforcement officers. *Journal of Strength and Conditioning Research, 24*(1), 1. https://doi.org/10.1097/01.jsc.0000367076.30318.e5

Chau, J. Y., Van Der Ploeg, H. P., Dunn, S., Kurko, J., & Bauman, A. E. (2012). Validity of the occupational sitting and physical activity questionnaire. *Medicine and Science in Sports and Exercise, 44*(1), 118–125. https://doi.org/10.1249/MSS.0b013e3182251060

Federmeier, K. D., & Kutas, M. (2005). Ageing in context: Age-related changes in context use during language comprehension. *Psychophysiology, 42*(2), 133–141. https://doi.org/10.1111/j.1469-8986.2005.00274.x

Garson, D. (2012). *Testing statistical assumptions. Statistical Associates Publishing* (2012th ed., pp. 1–52). Blue Book Publishing.

Genin, P. M., Dessenne, P., Finaud, J., Pereira, B., Dutheil, F., Thivel, D., et al. (2018). Effect of work-related sedentary time on overall health profile in active vs. inactive office workers. *Frontiers in Public Health*, 1–8. https://doi.org/10.3389/fpubh.2018.00279

Heiestad, H., Gjestvang, C., & Haakstad, L. A. H. (2020). Investigating self-perceived health and quality of life: A longitudinal prospective study among beginner recreational exercisers in a fitness club setting. *BMJ Open, 10*(6), 1–8. https://doi.org/10.1136/bmjopen-2019-036250

Hendriksen, I. J. M., Bernaards, C. M., Steijn, W. M. P., & Hildebrandt, V. H. (2016). Longitudinal relationship between sitting time on a working day and vitality, work performance, presenteeism, and sickness absence. *Journal of Occupational and Environmental Medicine, 58*(8), 784–789. https://doi.org/10.1097/jom.0000000000000809

Hinckson, E., Cerin, E., Mavoa, S., Smith, M., Badland, H., Witten, K., et al. (2017). What are the associations between neighbourhood walkability and sedentary time in New Zealand adults? The URBAN cross-sectional study. *BMJ Open, 7*(10), 1–10. https://doi.org/10.1136/bmjopen-2017-016128

Hogan, V., Hogan, M., & Hodgins, M. (2016). A study of workaholism in Irish academics. *Occupational Medicine, 66*(6), 460–465. https://doi.org/10.1093/occmed/kqw032

Hosler, A. S., Gallant, M. P., Riley-Jacome, M., & Rajulu, D. T. (2014). Relationship between objectively measured walkability and exercise walking among adults with diabetes. *Journal of Environmental and Public Health, 2014*(1), 1–6. https://doi.org/10.1155/2014/542123

Jacob, O. N. (2020). Impact of COVID-19 pandemic school close down on the research programme of higher institutions. *International Journal of Advances in Data and Information Systems, 1*(1), 40–49. https://doi.org/10.25008/ijadis.v1i1.189

Koohsari, M. J., Nakaya, T., & Oka, K. (2018). Activity-friendly built environments in a super-aged society, Japan: Current challenges and toward a research agenda. *International Journal of Environmental Research and Public Health, 15*(9), 1–9. https://doi.org/10.3390/ijerph15092054

Koohsari, M. J., McCormack, G. R., Nakaya, T., Shibata, A., Ishii, K., Yasunaga, A., et al. (2020). Walking-friendly built environments and objectively measured physical function in older adults. *Journal of Sport and Health Science, 9*, 651–656. https://doi.org/10.1016/j.jshs.2020.02.002

Lawton, M. P., & Simon, B. (1968). The ecology of social relationships in housing for the elderly. *The Gerontologist, 8*(2), 108–115. https://doi.org/10.1093/geront/8.2.108

Lee, P. H., Macfarlane, D. J., Lam, T. H., & Stewart, S. M. (2011). Validity of the international physical activity questionnaire short form (IPAQ-SF): A systematic review. *International Journal of Behavioral Nutrition and Physical Activity, 8*(1), 1–11. https://doi.org/10.1186/1479-5868-8-115

Lone, S. A., & Ahmad, A. (2020). COVID-19 pandemic – An African perspective. *Emerging Microbes & Infections, 9*(1), 1–28. https://doi.org/10.1080/22221751.2020.1775132

Marshall, S., & Gyi, D. (2010). Evidence of health risks from occupational sitting where do we stand? *American Journal of Preventive Medicine, 39*(4), 389–391. https://doi.org/10.1016/j.amepre.2010.07.001

Merom, D., Gebel, K., Fahey, P., Astell-Burt, T., Voukelatos, A., Rissel, C., et al. (2015). Neighbourhood walkability, fear and risk of falling and response to walking promotion: The easy steps to health 12-month randomized controlled trial. *Preventive Medicine Reports, 13*(2), 704–710. https://doi.org/10.1016/j.pmedr.2015.08.011

Oyeyemi, A. L., Kolo, S. M., Rufai, A. A., Oyeyemi, A. Y., Omotara, B. A., & Sallis, J. F. (2019). Associations of neighborhood walkability with sedentary time in Nigerian older Adults. *International Journal of Environmental Research and Public Health, 16*(11), 1–12. https://doi.org/10.3390/ijerph16111879

Picavet, H. S. J., Pas, L. W., van Oostrom, S. H., van der Ploeg, H. P., Verschuren, W. M. M., & Proper, K. I. (2016). The relation between occupational sitting and mental, cardiometabolic, and musculoskeletal health over a period of 15 years – The Doetinchem Cohort Study. *PLoS ONE, 11*(1), 1–11. https://doi.org/10.1371/journal.pone.0146639

Rapanta, C., Botturi, L., Goodyear, P., Guàrdia, L., & Koole, M. (2020). Online university teaching during and after the Covid-19 crisis: Refocusing teacher presence and learning activity. *Postdigital Science and Education, 2*(1), 923–945. https://doi.org/10.1007/s42438-020-00155-y

Rosenkranz, S. K., Mailey, E. L., Umansky, E., Rosenkranz, R. R., & Ablah, E. (2020). Workplace sedentary behavior and productivity: A cross-sectional study. *International Journal of Environmental Research and Public Health, 17*(18), 1–14. https://doi.org/10.3390/ijerph17186535

Simons, C. C. J. M., Hughes, L. A. E., van Engeland, M., Goldbohm, R. A., van den Brandt, P. A., & Weijenberg, M. P. (2013). Physical activity, occupational sitting time, and colorectal cancer risk in the Netherlands cohort study. *American Journal of Epidemiology, 177*(6), 514–530. https://doi.org/10.1093/aje/kws280

Upoalkpajor, J. N., & Upoalkpajor, C. B. (2020). The impact of COVID-19 on education in Ghana. *Asian Journal of Education and Social Studies, 9*(1), 23–33. https://doi.org/10.9734/ajess/2020/v9i130238

Van Holle, V., Van Cauwenberg, J., De Bourdeaudhuij, I., Deforche, B., Van de Weghe, N., & Van Dyck, D. (2016). Interactions between neighborhood social environment and walkability to explain Belgian older adults' physical activity and sedentary time. *International Journal of Environmental Research and Public Health, 13*(6), 569. https://doi.org/10.3390/ijerph13060569

Varea, V., & González-Calvo, G. (2020). Touchless classes and absent bodies: Teaching physical education in times of Covid-19. *Sport, Education and Society*, 1–15. https://doi.org/10.1080/13573322.2020.1791814

Venkatesh, A., & Edirappuli, S. (2020). Social distancing in covid-19: What are the mental health implications? *British Medical Journal, 369*, 1. https://doi.org/10.1136/bmj.m1379

Wahl, H. W., & Gerstorf, D. (2018). A conceptual framework for studying context dynamics in aging (CODA). *Developmental Review, 50*(2), 155–176. https://doi.org/10.1016/j.dr.2018.09.003

White, R. L., Bennie, J., Abbott, G., & Teychenne, M. (2020). Work-related physical activity and psychological distress among women in different occupations: A cross-sectional study. *BMC Public Health, 20*(1), 1–9. https://doi.org/10.1186/s12889-020-09112-7

Wiles, J. L., Leibing, A., Guberman, N., Reeve, J., & Allen, R. E. S. (2011). The meaning of "aging in place" to older people. *The Gerontologist, 52*(3), 357–366. https://doi.org/10.1093/geront/gnr098

11

Covid-19: Study of Online Teaching, Availability and Use of Technological Resources

Ariana Daniela Del Pino Espinoza, Narce Dalia Ruiz Guzmán, Freddy Veloz de la Torre, Maria Nuria Lloret Romero, Ariana Andrea García León, Antonio Pérez, and Sylvia Arredondo

Introduction

The situation caused by the Covid-19 global crisis has led universities to make abrupt and immediate changes to continue training their students virtually (Bao, 2020). Universities have had to urgently adapt their strategies to respond to the crisis since the beginning of the epidemic to carry on with their daily tasks efficiently (Ali, 2020; Kieu et al., 2020). Time, however, was against the stakeholders as they had to plan to immediately adjust their teaching style and

A. D. Del Pino Espinoza (✉) • F. Veloz de la Torre • A. A. García León
Escuela Superior Politécnica del Litoral, Guayaquil, Ecuador
e-mail: ariddel@espol.edu.ec; fveloz@espol.edu.ec; aagarci@espol.edu.ec

N. D. Ruiz Guzmán
Tecnológico de Monterrey, Monterrey, Mexico
e-mail: narce.ruiz@tec.mx

M. N. Lloret Romero • A. Pérez
Universitat Politècnica de València, Valencia, Spain
e-mail: nlloret@upvnet.upv.es; aperez@upv.es

S. Arredondo
Universidad Nacional de Costa Rica Heredia, Heredia, Costa Rica
e-mail: sylvia.arredondo.guevara@una.cr

E. Mogaji et al. (eds.), *Re-imagining Educational Futures in Developing Countries*,
https://doi.org/10.1007/978-3-030-88234-1_11

pedagogical approach (García-Peñalvo et al., 2021). Considering the change in the paradigm of innovative teaching, learning materials and resources that have been planned for face-to-face teaching were being changed immediately to accommodate online teaching (Burki, 2020; Blankenberger & Williams, 2020). The lack of online development of the pre-pandemic curricula forced teachers to make a titanic effort to convert their predominant classroom teaching into the online model (Mishra et al., 2020). This lack of resources comes with a certain level of nervousness and uncertainty regarding the current situation (Hiremath et al., 2020). Additionally, this effort was aggravated by the small timeframe and the staff's inexperience in online teaching formats, resulting in models that had to be readapted constantly to meet the required educational standards (Rashid et al., 2020).

Undoubtedly, technologies play an active role in academic life and generate knowledge in "the training of participatory citizenship" (Erstad et al., 2021). However, in terms of technological infrastructure, each institution has had an unequal approach depending on how much they had previously invested in tools that would allow online teaching (van der Spoel et al., 2020). Many Universities in emerging economies were not funded enough and had limited technological infrastructure to cope with the change in pedagogical approach (Mogaji & Jain, 2020; Sharma et al., 2020). However, once the technological needs have been met and, in many cases, successfully resolved, the central problem has become how to deliver education in virtual environments (Salinas & De-Benito, 2020).

This technological challenge leads to other concerns around the preparedness of lectures in developing countries regarding teaching in the Covid-19 era (Akinde, 2021; Rahiem, 2020). Some teachers are unaided and lack the technological and methodological knowledge to carry out their lectures online (Mogaji et al., 2020). Virtual classes and online teaching pose challenges to teachers from the point of view of design. Studies such as Richardson et al.'s (2017) indicate the importance of social presence within the virtual learning environment: collaboration between students in different settings, diverse technological conditions and perhaps without prior knowledge of each other (Bishop-Monroe et al., 2021). Student-student and student-teacher interactions are critical in achieving successful learning experiences in virtual environments (Agormedah et al., 2020).

There are different requirements and new processes to designing online education, and they involve innovation and teaching practices in the development of training (Olaleye et al., 2020). With this innovation to virtual change in learning/training to improve learning outcomes, it is essential to recognise the difference between face-to-face teaching in the classroom and online teaching (González-Pérez et al., 2019). This difference presents a challenge for lecturers in adjusting their teaching content and pedagogical approach (Del Pino & Lloret, 2021). In addition, the pandemic has led to a great deal of interest in the use of digital media and universities (Casero-Ripollés, 2020), and universities are being challenged to take up responsibilities and gear themselves up for technological innovations.

While Crawford et al. (2020) have provided insight through desktop analysis of university and government data to provide a timely map of the intra-period higher education responses to Covid-19 across 20 countries and Marinoni et al. (2020) surveyed universities to understand the impact of Covid-19 on higher education around the world, this present study offered a novel and different approach. The study surveyed university lecturers from other countries to understand their experience, level of preparedness and challenges as they switched from face-to-face teaching to online classes. The survey was conducted across multiple universities in Costa Rica, Ecuador, Mexico and Spain, to understand the experience the lecturers have gone through adapting to the digital environment. The study also sought to find out the scope of the measures implemented by lecturers and universities from these countries. Understanding their experience will allow the creation of better tools, implementing more strategic training plans and a better understanding of the infrastructure needed to maintain and elevate the current education level in this new virtual paradigm (Hassan et al., 2020).

The subsequent part of this chapter is presented in five sections. The following section offers relevant literature on virtual learning, new interactions and how universities have evolved in digital environments. The next two sections are about the methodology used and the results arrived at, respectively. A discussion of the results appears in the penultimate section. The final section concludes the chapter and highlight the limitations of the study.

Literature Review

It is well known that the first online learning took place in 1892 at the University of Chicago (Marshall Crotty, 2012), and before that, in 1728, learning material was received by mail. In 1840 in the United Kingdom, Johns Hopkins developed the first educational material by correspondence, created through a typewriter in forensic medicine focused on autopsies (Maina, 2020). Now, in 2020, making these materials is mandatory, given the current situation during a pandemic. The problem is not the virtual classroom. For some time now, the classroom has been changing and evolving into new spaces of interaction (Karim et al., 2019) using different systems to teach in a classroom and at the same time online through social networks (Junco et al., 2011). The problem is the abrupt change; curricula had to be metamorphosed in a few weeks. According to Afshar (2020), a digital evangelist, "The best teachers are lifelong learners," which was proven true as faculty members had to adapt quickly and thrive in the new virtual environment.

As Maina (2020) from the UOC expresses in his webinar, we live an emergency non-face-to-face teaching situation rather than an online education, so we cannot expect results according to its principles, as it is not designed and planned for online education. At present, we will not eliminate the digital gap and the social and educational inequalities; do not confuse interaction with synchronous communication. Therefore, the change from the classroom format to virtual format prevails. There has been a boom in online tools and virtual communication platforms, which have been proven to be essential in enhancing the teaching-learning experience for both the teacher and the student and in enriching the interaction. Online platforms like Zoom, Microsoft Teams, Canvas and Remind, which are not new to the WebSphere and were not necessarily created for educational purposes, have become a must in the virtual classroom.

Interaction involves being connected with students through other channels such as WhatsApp and Facebook, which makes it so that we seek new resources or strategies (Escobar-Mamani & Gómez-Arteta, 2020) with the tools nearby so we can motivate or attract the student to the globalised world, avoiding the misuse of social networks and trying to compensate for the lack of technologies at home (Nie et al., 2019). This is an essential part of the online platform for professional learning (Charalambousa & Ioannou, 2008; Delgado et al., 2015; Kao et al., 2011), it directly influences how students stimulate the production of ideas (Stein et al., 2009), the exchange of opinions, the level of student satisfaction (Durrington et al., 2006), the objectives, the student's achievement and the learning outcomes that the teacher wants to achieve (Bernard et al., 2014). With the change of the teaching paradigm, we are no longer the ones who know the most. Now our millennial students will teach us about technological resources while transmitting knowledge about the subject (Wisniewski, 2019).

The university is expected to innovate in providing education (Zhang et al., 2004). There are new upcoming methods, such as the non-traditional classroom, where applied online learning with supervised learning is tested on students (Hao et al., 2018). According to Fisher et al. (2014), eventually, e-learning becomes part of most classrooms, either with formal or informal interaction. Some universities and institutes have invested in a learning platform such as a "learning management system or a learning content management system to offer high-quality online courses"—with the quarantine restriction system; classes must be registered for the student. Still, with this, there will be no interaction (Rosell, n.d.).

Despite the efforts of universities, teaching through applications is not online education. An attempt is made to adapt a traditional class to an online class model even though their structures and logic are different. We must not take as the fact that the current generation are professionals in technologies; the current generation was a "digital native" when they were "native to social networks" (Gökerik et al., 2018). Online classes are knowledge capsules that involve reading, videos, a short evaluation or quiz, a blog and a class at some point. We cannot assume that everyone has the internet, so classes must be adapted to a mobile phone format (Celedón, 2020).

Method

Quantitative data was collected through a survey consisting of 26 questions distributed in several blocks. The first block focuses on multiple-choice questions about generic issues regarding participants' origin, age, employment status and teaching time. The second block was made up of six questions based on their knowledge of the development of virtual classes, such as teaching, reception by the students, technical problems encountered by both teachers and students, tools used, experiences and challenges of online training. Finally, in the last block, six questions were asked about strategies, planning of teaching and the level of knowledge acquired in teaching; three questions were asked about active breaks, activities and class sessions; three questions were asked about evaluations, performance and participation; and finally, four questions were asked about the effort to prepare and manage online training and the increase in virtual classes, as well as the use of mixed models and the paradigm change.

This survey was shared online between April and May 2020, during the change from face-to-face to virtual class models during the Covid-19 pandemic. The survey was sent to university lecturers at several universities of Costa Rica, Ecuador, Mexico and Spain. These universities were selected due to the close relationship the research team has with them. Costa Rica faculty members are the most represented with 50% of the answered surveys, followed by Spain, Ecuador and Mexico. The universities participating in this survey in descending order in the 2020 Qs World University Rank are Tecnologico de Monterrey (158) from México, Universidad Politécnica de

Valencia (336) from Spain, Universidad Nacional de Costa Rica (801–1000) from Costa Rica and Escuela Superior Politécnica del Litoral—ESPOL (801–1000) from Ecuador. At the end of the data collection period, 625 valid responses were collected and descriptively analysed for the study. Costa Rica had the highest number of respondents with 51% (n = 319), Spain followed this at 33% (n = 206) and Ecuador at 10% (n = 62). The lowest number of participants was from Mexico, with 6% (n = 38).

Results

The highlights of the survey are:

- Only 49% of the professors had received training on online teaching pre-pandemic.
- 64% of the faculty members had not given an online class pre-pandemic.
- 65% of the teachers considered that the tools and methodology provided by the university were adequate.
- 86% of the professors reported they had to make an extra effort to prepare for an online class.
- 93% of the teachers consider post-pandemic online teaching as a positive experience.

Costa Rica

In the case of Costa Rica, 65% answered that it was the first time they taught an online course, 51% had received previous training online teaching, 71% find the tools and methodology implemented adequate, 90% say they had to make an extra effort preparing online classes and 98% see the online post-pandemic teaching as a positive experience.

Among the challenges encountered when moving from a face-to-face to a virtual class, 65% of the teachers indicated a lack of interaction with students. Regarding engagement, teachers agree that students participate 40% less, 32% the same and 28% more under the new virtual models for the courses. However, 90% of teachers consider that virtual classes require a more significant effort in planning and execution. To further engage the students, it was also found that 51% of the respondents use didactic tools during the entire online class to maintain student participation. When teaching the courses in the online format, the tools most often used by respondents were multimedia materials, videos and webinars to maintain immediate remote communication with students. In terms of platform use, teachers pointed to internet access and the joining of institutional platforms such as Zoom and Microsoft Teams as the most significant technical and technological drawbacks they have had when developing any course, given that they had not used it assiduously before.

When asked "what kinds of activities have you considered including during your next virtual class session?", participants indicated videos and presentations made by the students or dynamic exercises such as "Kahoot"—this is a free platform that allows the creation of evaluation questionnaires. Kahoot is a tool by which the teacher creates classroom competitions to learn or reinforce learning and where the students are the contestants—participation of experts through meetings in Zoom or other platforms. Concerning using the different technological tools, we posed the question: "Do you think that the virtual classroom allows the student to learn more and create more autonomous learning habits?" In response, 53% of the sample indicated that they do, encouraging responsible habits regarding work delivery, time management, being proactive through research and organising themselves to meet objectives.

In the case of active breaks for students, it was found that most of the respondents use relationship exercises, and they do them every hour according to the duration of the course. On the other hand, 44% do not provide breaks; however, this depends on the course model, if it is synchronous or asynchronous, since, in the latter, students choose when and how fast to complete the course contents according to their possibilities.

In Costa Rica, the average age range was 44, 75 ± 17 years, of which 61% are full-time professors and 49% part-time. Thus, we can observe that most respondents had been teachers for more than 20 years and were the oldest. This data is essential when understanding the following responses since age and seniority are necessary conditions for adaptation to virtual teaching methodologies.

Regarding the experience in offering online education before the Covid-19 context, if analysed by age group, it can be seen that 57% of the 36–45-year-old group have received some course in this area, and there is no significant difference with those who have not; however, in the 56–65-year-old group, 68%, i.e. more than half, indicating that they have not received online learning courses. From this point, we can see the importance of age in terms of knowledge of methodologies and technologies for virtual training: as we pointed out previously, the older the person, the less training in the field of virtual teaching. Now, it may be that conditions before Covid-19 allowed for classroom teaching in most universities. Still, it is striking that, on the one hand, Costa Rica (with professors with less than 10 years of service) and Spain (with professors with more than 20 years of experience) have not had the opportunity to use the technological tools that currently allow for the continuation of academic training processes.

Ecuador

In the case of Ecuador, 55% answered that it was the first time they taught an online course, 70% had received previous training about online teaching, 70% find the tools and methodology implemented adequate, 92% say they have to make an extra effort preparing online classes and 94% see the online post-pandemic teaching as a positive experience. Although, as in Costa Rica, the main challenge for 52% of Ecuadorian teachers is the lack of interaction with their students. For 30% of teachers, the biggest challenge is technical and connectivity problems.

This lack of interactivity also responds to the fact that 80% of the teachers, as answered in the survey, do not use any additional technological tools to teach their classes. They repeat the lecture mode in Zoom or Microsoft Teams and do not provide more interactive questions. However, 94% of the teachers use additional communication channels, such as chats. When asked about active breaks, 32% of the teachers answered that they do not take such breaks, 38% say they do relaxation exercises and 30% responded that they do other activities. 41% of teachers have had failures due to a lack of technological infrastructure at home, and 26% have had problems managing specialised tools. It should be noted that not all students have computers or tablets to work within their classes.

Other problems are evident in the research, such as frequent blackouts that occur more so than usual. Tools such as Kahoot are also used, and WhatsApp groups are introduced and so also the university platforms. The use of cameras and microphones is mandatory in most of the classes observed.

In Ecuador, it is common to have more than two, and low financial resources mean that having a computer—or more—is a luxury. Asynchronous courses offer the advantage of discrete-time management. Due to mobility restrictions, confident students and teachers are difficult to do all at once. Synchronous courses benefit from answering questions immediately, but it does not mean that they fulfil the same objective, despite using other tools such as WhatsApp or Facebook groups. Both have improvised in terms of study and workspaces.

Mexico

In the case of Mexico, 59% answered that it was the first time they taught an online course, 55% had received previous training in online teaching, 68% find the tools and methodology implemented adequate, 59% say they have to make an extra effort preparing online classes, and 100% see the online post-pandemic teaching as a positive experience. Also, in Mexico, the challenge faced by teachers is the lack of interactivity with their students. 63% respond that it is their greatest challenge.

All the teachers who answered the survey in Mexico responded that they use additional tools in their online sessions, including webinars and multimedia materials. 86% of teachers implement different communication strategies, such as chats. In a country like Mexico, the population's access to the internet is 70%. When asked about the connectivity situation to the teachers, 40% of the teachers answer that they have not had major technical or technological problems. 30% responded that the main problem of this type is internet connectivity.

Only 18% take active relaxation breaks in class. Moreover, 45% of teachers do not take this type of break. Although, in the case of Mexico, the high rates of inequality between public and private education become more evident; there was a digital divide in terms of access to technology and online resources. While those in private universities continued their studies almost immediately after the lockdown, the continuity for those in public universities was hampered by delays and more significant challenges.

Mexico, a young country, denotes in the responses that 60% of the teachers who answered the survey are in the age range of 36–45 years. While 22% are over 46 years old and 18% are teachers under 35 years old. 31% have more than 20 years of experience in education. 13% have 15 years of experience, 36% have 10 years teaching and 20% have only five years. Even when the teachers are young, the level of expertise is appropriate for their age. In the group interviewed in Mexico, 50% are full-time teachers and the other half are part-time teachers.

Spain

In the case of Spain, 67% answered that it was the first time they taught an online course, 35% had received previous training in online teaching, 54% find the tools and methodology implemented adequate, 85% say they have to make an extra effort preparing online classes and 85% see the online post-pandemic teaching as a positive experience.

As for the use of the platforms, it is worth noting that 55% had not found any problem in terms of the use of the platforms or infrastructure; the highest point being problems with internet access and the ambivalence between the use of tools external to the institution such as Zoom and Skype and the use of Microsoft Teams, a more official tool, among those surveyed. It is noteworthy that several teachers did not have computer equipment at home to provide quality teaching: many of them had equipment shared with their families, and, in other cases, their equipment was too obsolete to provide good quality teaching.

Regarding the tools used, it is noteworthy that 70% used resources in portable document formats (PDF) as material for online teaching, with webinars and audio-visual materials also being widely used. It is essential to understand that a PDF document itself is not an online learning tool. It can be considered a support material, but it is not an interactive resource that the student can work within a synchronous and active way. We believe that it has been necessary to use this type of material for an urgent situation, but as this type of training progresses officially, PDF materials should not be the basis for online teaching as they do not allow for genuine interaction between student and teacher.

This may explain why teachers have mostly replied that the most significant difficulty in their virtual experience has been interaction with students. Interacting with the students with eminently textual materials does not facilitate that interaction. Similarly, webinars, asynchronous recordings or streaming masterclasses do not help students interact with the teacher either. Therefore, there is a need for further development of teaching materials. In some cases, this is an effort on the part of the teacher, as it also requires support service at the university to transform contents into quality interactive materials.

This is an important fact to analyse since this faculty is mainly made up of career civil servants with fixed positions. Most have also said they have not had any previous relationship with virtual teaching. This complicates the adaptation to the new environment. If the teachers have more experience in virtual training, they will have more responsibility and degree of involvement in the university, whilst on the other hand, if they have neither knowledge nor sufficient experience in virtual training, we run into a severe problem at the time of applying the new models that virtual training requires with quality and efficiency.

We must also point out that retraining is voluntary at the Spanish university, so the institution is not to blame for teacher training. There are training courses in the teacher training programme, but there was a lack of interest on the part of teachers to enter these fields before the pandemic. If we were to carry out this study today, interest in teacher training would undoubtedly have increased exponentially, given that the shortcomings in teaching during the pandemic have made the need for advanced knowledge in these areas very plausible.

Discussion

This study sought to examine the level of preparedness of teachers teaching online class during the pandemic. While the notion that online classes have been operating with limited face-to-face engagement abounds, our study provides an international perspective on how the pandemic has changed online learning. We surveyed over 600 teachers across four countries. The results showed that teachers faced considerable difficulties adjusting to a different form of online learning due to the pandemic.

The most developed countries have managed to take advantage of technological advances for teaching-learning (Mogaji & Yoon, 2019). Still, Latin countries have not fully implemented online learning or have seen the need to transform or adapt in digital spaces with the resources available to students. It is clear that many Latino students do not have computers, but they do have mobile devices, so classes must adapt to small devices and teach quickly and effectively.

The economy of online classes benefits students and saves mobility and food, but easy-to-use platforms are still preferred. This allows coordination with other tasks at home. In specific courses where learning is entirely autonomous, the teacher becomes more of a guide or a supervisor to clarify doubts (Hinson & Mogaji, 2020). Self-regulation is essential for the student to succeed in this type of environment. The abrupt change for everyone, studying in person and interacting with others in a virtual space, where it is impossible to get technological equipment due to the surrounding circumstances due to the socio-economic situation. Latin American countries have a higher rate of poverty and corruption. Many students have not been able to study or have adapted with the few resources they can get.

Engaging the students with activities and planning for the classes during this testing time was challenging for the teachers. Across all teachers, 87% of respondents felt that virtual classes were more challenging to plan and implement, with no differences between countries of origin. Since a student cannot spend two hours listening to a teacher from a screen without disconnecting psychologically and given that the teacher in many cases cannot even see what students are doing, because many of them disconnect the camera, the teacher can't motivate or change the tone of the lecture as it could be done in person. Therefore, it is essential to design the synchronous teaching, thinking about much shorter lecture times if necessary, and with breaks for constant student interaction. Using chat became a convenient opportunity for teachers to engage with their students. 62% of respondents acknowledge that chat was the primary tool used for student interaction, which shows that, in general, teachers try to use the same tools for communicating with students as in a face-to-face class, with chat replacing a face-to-face classroom debate. This shows that teachers use the resources they know best, but these resources are not enough for students to interact correctly with the teacher when transferred to the virtual environment.

Our study also identified a relationship between age, level of preparedness and the ability to adopt technology for teaching and engagement. Universities with younger faculty members could quickly move to virtual teaching due to the more technological training and the smaller digital gap between their staffing team (Agbo et al., 2020). Spain and Ecuador are the only countries with teachers over 65 years old who work full time. In the other countries surveyed, ages were much lower. For example, most of the teachers in Costa Rica and Mexico are in the 36–44 age range, while in Spain, most teachers are in the 46–55 age range. Overall, 60% of the respondents were in the 46–65 age range, with the majority being full-time teachers with over 20 years of experience. However, in this age group—especially between 55 and 65 years of age—we find the most significant number of teachers who had not had any training before the pandemic in online learning methodologies or technologies, a much higher number than in other countries. Therefore, these teachers are more likely not to adopt any teaching technology, retain their teaching style and engage less with their students.

The evaluation method was also another important consideration in the wake of this pandemic, with lecturers taking more responsibility in developing ways to access their students (Prigoff et al., 2021). 53% of the sample indicate that they used—and are using—exercises designed by themselves and 67% did notice differences in student performance. In Spain, 45% of teachers think that students participate less than 40% in Costa Rica, 35% in Ecuador and 30% in Mexico. The stress of coping within the pandemic has contributed to how students are engaging and performing when accessing online learning. However, supporting students will become more critical than ever as it can be the differences between ranking position, long-term sustainability and reputation of these universities (Kiraka et al., 2020).

This study provides a theoretical contribution to the increasing body of works on how university lecturers cope during the pandemic and their plan in the post-Covid era (Crawford et al., 2020; Marinoni et al., 2020; Hassan et al., 2020). First, we provide a multinational insight from South America to Europe, understanding the precarious situation of the students and the changes lecturers are making, especially with the context of an emerging economy with limited resources and infrastructure (Mogaji & Jain, 2020). Second, we present a theoretical understanding of student engagement, lecturers' level of preparedness and student evaluation (Mishra et al., 2020; Rahiem, 2020; Rashid et al., 2020). These findings are relevant to academic researchers and practitioners interested in higher education and lecturers' training and support.

In addition, managerial implications are relevant for university managers, course administrators and programme leaders. The teaching staff has made a titanic effort in record time, even though they have neither the training nor the tools to teach. Current teaching methodologies are not helpful for online teaching and must be reviewed to ensure good continuity of student learning to meet curriculum and learning outcomes (Al-Ataby, 2020; Cavus et al., 2021). Universities should offer more training in pedagogical approaches and develop specific content for online training that is better suited to students and faculty (Ndofirepi et al., 2020; Adeyanju et al., 2020). The institutions must cover the technological needs of the teaching staff offering online learning—if the teacher needs a good connection from home or adequate equipment, it must be provided by the university itself (Bao, 2020; Blankenberger & Williams, 2020). In Spain, the new law on teleworking clarifies that entities should offer the means to the worker, so the institution itself must solve this issue. Incorporating advisory teams in creating multimedia and interactive content in universities should be a priority to help teachers develop materials with optimum quality (Gottlieb et al., 2020).

Conclusion

The preliminary study revealed that most teachers had not had infrastructure problems when teaching their classes, although they have had connectivity problems, a key aspect for online courses (Mogaji & Jain, 2020). Considering that the teachers have been very committed and that they have tried to adapt to the new circumstances quickly and with outstanding professionalism

(Rashid et al., 2020), we believe that there has been a very significant effort and the teachers themselves are aware of their gaps in knowledge about the tools for creating multimedia and interactive content (Mishra et al., 2020).

Universities have had to adapt even more than teachers and students. This study showed that not all universities were prepared for change, but they adapted (Mogaji & Jain, 2020). They started marathon training sessions and reused existing instruments until they met expectations (Agormedah et al., 2020). Universities will change teaching based on this, including a percentage of virtual education for life in their curricula. These data can give a clear idea of what education was like in Latin countries and how it could evolve.

The common denominator in many cases is that teachers do not only require infrastructure in their homes to do their work better (this is something that can be implemented quickly) (Ali, 2020); the major problem that has arisen in this pandemic is not the need for infrastructure, but rather the need to propose a change in the methodology for carrying out the work and in less-than-ideal conditions. We found that classroom flipping goes beyond speaking presence but requires a mix of learning tools for better engagement. Higher education providers are expected to keep working towards adaptive learning, making e-learning content mobile; likewise instructional design should encompass a variety of multimedia resources. Lecturers should create a supportive learning environment, providing ongoing feedback. Specific training is required in the development of these teaching methodologies for online training and the development of materials and content now in fully multimedia and interactive spaces. All this without knowing how to develop them and with what tools we can adapt to the content. Today's technologies play an essential role in active learning with connectivity (Ito et al., 2013).

Though effort has been made to provide a multinational insight from the study, we acknowledge some limitations. Therefore, the result should be interpreted in the context of the limitations. First, this is a descriptive study to give an overview of preparedness and teachers' effort. Future studies should aim to carry out other statistical analysis to understand better the differences across the countries and any different significant correlation. Second, the result only presents insights from the teachers. The opinion of the students on these online learning programmes has not been surveyed, and further study can examine the students' experiences about how their online learning has evolved in the wake of the pandemic. Third, in the future, we hope to conduct another survey to contrast the data collected so far and learn how the entire educational system in these Spanish-speaking universities changed during and after Covid-19.

References

Adeyanju, S., Mogaji, E., Olusola, J., & Oyinlola, M. (2020). Factors influencing students' choice of a federal university: A case study of a Nigerian federal university. In *Higher education marketing in Africa* (pp. 135–163). Palgrave Macmillan.

Afshar, V. (2020). https://twitter.com/ValaAfshar/status/1255166252395438080

Agbo, F. J., Olawumi, O., Oyelere, S. S., Kolog, E. A., Olaleye, S. A., Agjei, R. O., & Olawuni, A. (2020). Social media usage for computing education: The effect of tie strength and group communication on perceived learning outcome. *International Journal of Education and Development Using Information and Communication Technology, 16*(1), 5–26.

Agormedah, E. K., Henaku, E. A., Ayite, D. M. K., & Ansah, E. A. (2020). Online learning in higher education during COVID-19 pandemic: A case of Ghana. *Journal of Educational Technology and Online Learning, 3*(3), 183–210.

Akinde, T. A. (2021). Inhibitors to the electronic teaching and learning of library science in the Nigerian universities of the post-COVID-19 pandemic era and the way forward. *American Journal of Information Science and Technology, 5*(2), 30–39.

Al-Ataby, A. (2020). Technology-enhanced learning and teaching in COVID-19 era: Challenges and recommendations. *International Journal for Innovation Education and Research, 8*(10), 317–331.

Ali, W. (2020). Online and remote learning in higher education institutes: A necessity in light of COVID-19 pandemic. *Higher Education Studies, 10*(3), 16–25.

Bao, W. (2020). COVID-19 and online teaching in higher education: A case study of Peking University. *Human Behavior and Emerging Technologies, 2*(2), 113–115.

Bernard, R., Borokhovski, E., Schmid, R., Tamim, R., & Abrami, P. (2014). A meta-analysis of blended learning and technology use in higher education: From the general to the applied. *Journal of Computing in Higher Education, 26*(1), 87–122.

Bishop-Monroe, R., Di Paolo Harrison, B. M., Knight, M. E., Corritore, C., York, A. S., & Rybarczyk, B. (2021). Preparing doctoral students to teach in an increasingly virtual world: A response to COVID-19 and beyond. *Online Learning, 25*(1), 166–181.

Blankenberger, B., & Williams, A. M. (2020). COVID and the impact on higher education: The essential role of integrity and accountability. *Administrative Theory & Praxis, 42*(3), 404–423.

Burki, T. K. (2020). COVID-19: Consequences for higher education. *The Lancet Oncology, 21*(6), 758.

Casero-Ripollés, A. (2020). Impact of Covid-19 on the media system. Communicative and democratic consequences of news consumption during the outbreak. *El profesional de la información, 29*(2), e290223. https://doi.org/10.3145/epi.2020.mar.23

Cavus, N., Sani, A. S., Haruna, Y., & Lawan, A. A. (2021). Efficacy of social networking sites for sustainable education in the era of COVID-19: A systematic review. *Sustainability, 13*(2), 808.

Celedón, C. (09 de April de 2020). *Una clase por zoom no es una formación online*. Obtenido de Timeline. https://timeline.cl/2020/04/cristian-celedon-experto-en-educacion-una-clase-por-zoom-no-es-una-formacion-online/?fbclid=IwAR12wULOBEofs-RXoX3Ds0Tm41xwBH

Charalambousa, K., & Ioannou, I. (2008). The attitudes and opinions of Cypriot primary teachers about the use of the internet for their professional development and as an educational tool. *Learning, Media and Technology, 33*(1), 45–57. https://doi.org/10.1080/17439880701868879

Crawford, J., Butler-Henderson, K., Rudolph, J., Malkawi, B., Glowatz, M., Burton, R., Magni, P., & Lam, S. (2020). COVID-19: 20 countries' higher education intra-period digital pedagogy responses. *Journal of Applied Learning & Teaching, 3*(1), 1–20. https://doi.org/10.37074/jalt.2020.3.1.7

Del Pino-Espinoza, A., & Lloret-Romero, N. (2021). *Improving university reputation through academic digital branding*. IGI Global.

Delgado, A. J., Wardlow, L., McKnight, K., & O'Malley, K. (2015). Educational technology: A review of the integration, resources, and effectiveness of technology in K-12 classrooms. *Journal of Information Technology Education: Research, 14*, 397–416.

Durrington, V., Berryhill, A., & Swafford, J. (2006). Strategies for enhancing student interactivity in an online environment. *College Teaching, 1*(54), 190–193. https://doi.org/10.3200/CTCH.54.1.190-193

Erstad, O., Miño, R., & Rivera-Vargas, P. (2021). Educational practices to transform and connect schools and communities [Prácticas educativas para transformar y conectar escuelas y comunidades]. *Comunicar*, (66), 9–20. https://doi.org/10.3916/C66-2021-01

Escobar-Mamani, F., & Gómez-Arteta, I. (2020). WhatsApp for the development of oral and written communication skills in Peruvian adolescents [WhatsApp para el desarrollo de habilidades comunicativas orales y escritas en adolescentes peruanos]. *Comunicar*, (65), 111–120. https://doi.org/10.3916/C65-2020-10

Fisher, A., Exley, K., & Ciobanu, D. (2014). *Using technology to support learning and teaching*. Routledge.

García-Peñalvo, F. J., Corell, A., Abella-García, V., & Grande-de-Prado, M. (2021). Recommendations for mandatory online assessment in higher education during the COVID-19 pandemic. In *Radical solutions for education in a crisis context* (pp. 85–98). Springer.

Gökerik, M., Gürbüz, A., Erkan, I., & Sap, S. (2018). Surprise me with your ads! The impacts of guerrilla marketing in social media on brand image. *Asia Pacific Journal of Marketing and Logistics, 30*(5), 1222–1238. https://doi.org/10.1108/APJML-10-2017-0257

González-Pérez, L., Ramírez-Montoya, M., & García-Peñalvo, F. (2019). Innovación educativa en estudios sobre el desarrollo y uso de la tecnología: Un mapeo sistemático. In M. S. Ramírez-Montoya & J. R. Valenzuela-González (Eds.), *Innovación educativa: Tendencias globales de investigación e implicaciones prácticas* (pp. 171–195).

Gottlieb, M., Egan, D. J., Krzyzaniak, S. M., Wagner, J., Weizberg, M., & Chan, T. (2020). Rethinking the approach to continuing professional development conferences in the era of COVID-19. *Journal of Continuing Education in the Health Professions, 40*(3), 187–191.

Hao, S., Hu, P., Zhao, P., Hoi, S., & Miao, C. (2018). Online active learning with expert advice. *ACM Transactions on Knowledge Discovery from Data, 12*(5), 1–22. https://doi.org/10.1145/3201604

Hassan, M. M., Mirza, T., & Hussain, M. W. (2020). A critical review by teachers on the online teaching-learning during the COVID-19. *International Journal of Education and Management Engineering, 10*(8), 17–27.

Hinson, R., & Mogaji, E. (2020). Co-creation of value by universities and prospective students: Towards an informed decision-making process. In E. Mogaji, F. Maringe, & R. Hinson (Eds.), *Higher education marketing in Africa* (pp. 17–46). Palgrave Macmillan.

Hiremath, P., Kowshik, C. S., Manjunath, M., & Shettar, M. (2020). Covid 19: Impact of lockdown on mental health and tips to overcomes. *Asian Journal of Psychiatry, 51*(102088). https://doi.org/10.1015/j.ajp.2020.102088

Ito, M., Gutiérrez, K., Livingstone, S., Penuel, B., Rhodes, J., Salen, K., & Watkins, S. (2013). *Connected learning: An agenda for research and design*. Digital Media and Learning Research Hub.

Junco, R., Heiberger, G., & Loken, E. (2011). The effect of Twitter on college student engagement and grades. *Journal of Computer Assisted Learning, 27*(2), 119–132.

Kao, C. P., Wu, Y. T., & Tsai, C. C. (2011). Elementary school teachers' motivation toward web-based professional development, and the relationship with Internet self-efficacy and belief about web-based learning. *Teaching and Teacher Education, 27*(2), 406–415. https://doi.org/10.1016/j.tate.2010.09.010

Karim, A., Shahed, F., Rahman, M., & Mohamed, A. (2019). Revisiting innovations in ELT through online classes: An evaluation of the approaches of 10-minute school. *Turkish Online Journal of Online Education, 20*(1), 248–266. https://doi.org/10.17718/tojde.522729

Kieu, T., Mogaji, E., Mwebesa, C., Sarofim, S., Soetan, T., & Vululleh, S. P. (2020). Marketing higher education in Africa: Moving from research to practice. In E. Mogaji, F. Maringe, & R. Hinson (Eds.), *Strategic marketing of higher education in Africa* (pp. 221–237). Routledge.

Kiraka, R., Maringe, F., Kanyutu, W., & Mogaji, E. (2020). University league tables and ranking systems in Africa: Emerging prospects, challenges and opportunities. In E. Mogaji, F. Maringe, & R. Hinson (Eds.), *Understanding the higher education market in Africa* (Routledge studies in marketing). Routledge.

Maina, M. (20 de April de 2020). *E-actividades para un aprendizaje activo*. Obtenido de Universitat Oberta de Catalunya. http://symposium.uoc.edu/50446/detail/e-actividades-para-un-aprendizaje-activo.html

Marinoni, G., Van't Land, H., & Jensen, T. (2020). The impact of Covid-19 on higher education around the world. *IAU Global Survey Report*.

Marshall Crotty, J. (14 de November de 2012). Online learning has been around since 1892, you big MOOC. *Forbes*. https://www.forbes.com/sites/jamesmarshallcrotty/2012/11/14/online-learning-has-been-around-since-1892-you-big-mooc/#9c3357a23187

Mishra, L., Gupta, T., & Shree, A. (2020). Online teaching-learning in higher education during lockdown period of COVID-19 pandemic. *International Journal of Educational Research Open, 1*, 100012.

Mogaji, E., & Jain, V. (2020). Impact of the pandemic on higher education in emerging countries: Emerging opportunities, challenges and research agenda. *SSRN Electronic Journal*. https://doi.org/10.2139/ssrn.3622592

Mogaji, E., & Yoon, H. (2019). Thematic analysis of marketing messages in UK universities' prospectuses. *International Journal of Educational Management, 33*(7), 1561–1581. https://doi.org/10.1108/IJEM-05-2018-0149

Mogaji, E., Maringe, F., & Hinson, R. (2020). Marketisation in higher education in Africa: New directions for a decolonising continent. In E. Mogaji, F. Maringe, & R. Hinson (Eds.), *Understanding the higher education market in Africa* (Routledge studies in marketing). Routledge.

Ndofirepi, E., Farinloye, T., & Mogaji, E. (2020). Marketing mix in a heterogenous higher education market: A case of Africa. In E. Mogaji, F. Maringe, & R. E. Hinson (Eds.), *Understanding the higher education market in Africa*. Routledge.

Nie, J., Li, W., Wang, P., Wang, X., Wang, Y., & Lei, L. (2019). Adolescent type D personality and social networking sites addiction: A moderated mediation model of restorative outcomes and affective relationships. *Psychiatry Research, 271*, 96–104. https://doi.org/10.1016/j.psychres.2018.11.036

Olaleye, S., Ukpabi, D., & Mogaji, E. (2020). Public vs private universities in Nigeria: Market dynamics perspective. In E. Mogaji, F. Maringe, & R. E. Hinson (Eds.), *Understanding the higher education market in Africa*. Routledge.

Prigoff, J., Hunter, M., & Nowygrod, R. (2021). Medical student assessment in the time of COVID-19. *Journal of Surgical Education, 78*(2), 370–374.

Rahiem, M. D. (2020). The emergency remote learning experience of university students in Indonesia amidst the COVID-19 crisis. *International Journal of Learning, Teaching and Educational Research, 19*(6), 1–26.

Rashid, C. A., Salih, H. A., & Budur, T. (2020). The role of online teaching tools on the perception of the students during the lockdown of Covid-19. *International Journal of Social Sciences & Educational Studies, 7*(3), 178–189.

Richardson, J. C., Maeda, Y., Lv, J., & Caskurlu, S. (2017). Social presence in relation to students' satisfaction and learning in the online environment: A meta-analysis. *Computers in Human Behavior, 71*(C), 402–417. https://doi.org/10.1016/j.chb.2017.02.001

Rosell, C. D. (n.d.). Virtual classes: How to teach them on a learning platform. *CAE*. https://www.cae.net/es/como-impartir-clase-en-una-plataforma-virtual/

Salinas, J., & De-Benito, B. (2020). Construction of personalized learning pathways through mixed methods [Construcción de itinerarios personalizados de aprendizaje mediante métodos mixtos]. *Comunicar, 28*(65), 31–42. https://doi.org/10.3916/C65-2020-0

Sharma, H., Jain, V., & Mogaji, E. (2020). Defining developing countries in higher education context. *Research Agenda Working Papers, 2021*(1), 1–9.

Stein, D., Glazer, H., & Wanstreet, C. (2009). The virtual university: Online learning spaces for adult learners. In T. Kidd & J. Keengwe (Eds.), *Adult learning in the digital age: Perspectives on online technologies and outcomes* (pp. 32–39). IGI Global.

van der Spoel, I., Noroozi, O., Schuurink, E., & van Ginkel, S. (2020). Teachers' online teaching expectations and experiences during the Covid19-pandemic in the Netherlands. *European Journal of Teacher Education, 43*(4), 623–638.

Wisniewski, M. A. (2019). Leadership development for academic chairs: Programs for promoting competence in higher education. *Journal of Continuing Higher Education, 67*(1), 48–51. https://doi.org/10.1080/07377363.2019.1642718

Zhang, D., Zhao, J. L., Zhou, L., & Nunamaker, J. F., Jr. (2004). Can e-learning replace classroom learning? *Communications of the ACM, 47*(4), 75–79. https://doi.org/10.1145/986213.986216

12

Emergency Remote Instruction (ERI) in Times of COVID-19 Pandemic: Experiences of Educators at Zimbabwean Higher Education Institutions

Mavis Thokozile Macheka, Josiah Taru, and Fortune Sibanda

Introduction

As part of COVID-19 containment measures, the World Health Organization (WHO) declared the rapidly spreading disease to be a pandemic on 11 March 2020, (WHO, 2020), leading to most countries in Africa declaring a state of emergency. Zimbabwe, in particular, declared a state of emergency on 17 March 2020 and resultantly, higher education and tertiary institutions were to close operation by 24 March 2020. Universities, college campuses, and higher education institutions cancelled classes and closed their doors following government directives that aimed to contain the COVID-19 pandemic (Hodge, 2020). Furthermore, a number of universities worldwide shifted to online virtual learning, cancelled the spring break period, and advised international students to return to their home countries. While everyone has been affected by COVID-19, research and experience have shown that of all the sectors of society, including the education sector, particularly at the tertiary level, appear to have been most greatly affected and, therefore, require a more pragmatic approach to resolution (Anifowoshe et al., 2020).

Against this background, this chapter discusses the challenges that were faced by educators and learners as they adapted, adjusted, and embraced new

M. T. Macheka (✉) • J. Taru • F. Sibanda
Great Zimbabwe University, Masvingo, Zimbabwe

E. Mogaji et al. (eds.), *Re-imagining Educational Futures in Developing Countries*,
https://doi.org/10.1007/978-3-030-88234-1_12

approaches to teaching and learning during lockdown. The chapter examines factors that militated against effective teaching and learning in six higher education institutions in Masvingo and Midlands provinces, Zimbabwe. Furthermore, the chapter explores opportunities and potential strategies for preparing higher education institutions to be resilient and agile in times of uncertainties and shocks. The chapter offers a comparative analysis of each institution's adaptability to the shock caused by COVID-19 and draws lessons from cases of institutions that managed the situation better. The chapter argues that there is a need to build higher education systems that are flexible and creative, and to embrace hybrid teaching and learning. There is a need to strengthen investment in ICT infrastructure development to allow higher education institutions to transit seamlessly during disturbances and also to position them for the fourth industrial revolution (Mogaji & Jain, 2020). Personnel at universities and colleges require capacitate building that positions them to make use of hybrid and creative teaching and learning in times disturbances (Ndofirepi et al., 2020), Further, the chapter suggests that higher education teaching must shift from pedagogical to andragogical approaches that are participatory.

We present our argument through six distinct sections. The introduction is presented in the first section. The subsequent section is literature review that highlighted challenges faced by higher education institutions globally during the pandemic. The methodology guiding the study and the sources of data used are discussed in the third section. The fourth section discusses the experiences and preparedness of educators from Masvingo and Midlands provinces in Zimbabwe in adopting, and adapting to, emergency digital teaching and technology demands in higher education institutions during the COVID-19 pandemic. This section further provides a context to the fifth section, which discusses theoretical and managerial implications and also discusses how to reimagine educational futures in Zimbabwe in ways that would transform the current higher educational systems so that it is resilient, empowering, and enfranchising during times of emergencies. The last section concludes the discussion by highlighting the major arguments, findings of the study and suggestions for further research.

Literature Review

When higher education institutions in Africa closed due to COVID-19, the institutions' management faced challenges in ensuring continuity of learning and developing appropriate responses to the pandemic (Muftahu, 2020).

Furthermore, as the world is upturned by the COVID-19 pandemic, one fundamental aspect of people's rights that has, and remains, so impacted, is their right to affordable education and universal access to a quality higher education as enshrined in the United Nations Sustainable Development Goal 4 (United Nations, 2015) and the Constitution of Zimbabwe (Section 75) of 2013. In addition, most institutions in Africa prefer face-to-face learning to hybrid modes of teaching that combine face-to-face and online platforms. As such, the shift to emergency remote teaching and learning puts pressure on management as they are faced with various challenges such as lack of infrastructure, availing of internet data, online supervision, training of faculty to use e-learning tools, and resistance from students, among others (Nganga et al., 2020). Most institutions in Africa have little or no investment in technological infrastructure that supports online teaching at higher education institutions (Olaleye et al., 2020). Thus, COVID-19 exacerbated the already crippled higher education system that is mainly hinged on face-to-face learning. The COVID-19 pandemic has pushed institutions of higher education beyond their limits, forcing many to search for appropriate methods to ensure that there is continuity of learning.

As argued, COVID-19 has significantly impacted the foundation of the education ecosystem wherein educational institutions worldwide are currently struggling towards identifying options available to them in dealing with the impact of the pandemic (Rieley, 2020). Globally, the education system is in the process of transforming and adapting to new challenges that are putting conventional teaching and learning practices to test (Cuaton, 2020). As higher education institutions transit from conventional learning, most of the institutions were not prepared for the change. Higher education institutions are considering challenges with regard to the quality of online instructions delivered through technology (Smalley, 2020).

In Africa, particularly in Sub-Saharan Africa, the pandemic uncovered both the lack of preparation and little consumption of online platforms by a lot of higher education institutions (Anifowoshe et al., 2020). While some universities managed to offer distance learning or online learning, most of the universities in Africa were unprepared to have immediate responses to mitigating consequences of the total lockdown caused by COVID-19 (Martin & Furiv, 2020). As such, some of the academic staff and students were unprepared for drastic changes in their education system design (Flavell et al., 2019).

With regard to Southern African Development Community (SADC) and Zimbabwe, the response measures against COVID-19 on education were addressed through several guidelines and legal instruments. Recognizing the global threat of the COVID-19 outbreak, the Southern African Development

Community (SADC) and the United Nations Education, Scientific, and Cultural Organisation (UNESCO) have entered into an agreement to ensure that 'Learning-Never-Stops' in the 16 SADC member states (Mukute et al., 2020). Furthermore, under the agreement, SADC countries were to be assisted to mobilize resources and implement context-appropriate and equitable solutions on distance education and learning remotely (SADC & UNESCO, 2020). SADC introduced a phased educational response to COVID-19 which was supposed to be adopted by all member states.[1] Zimbabwe like other SADC member states also developed Education Sector COVID-19 Response plans or strategies. The Zimbabwe Education Cluster COVID-19 Preparedness and Response Strategy (2020) has the following objectives, to (1) ensure continuity of learning through the implementation of key activities aimed at quality of learning and well-being of teachers, learners, and school communities during the COVID-19 emergency, (2) support teachers, learners, and school communities to prevent the transmission and spread of COVID-19, and (3) facilitate the safe return to quality learning for teachers, learners, and school communities after the COVID-19 emergency (Zimbabwe Education Cluster, 2020: 3).

Despite this, the documents do not make reference to the provision of e-learning resources and training to educators. In Zimbabwe, there was and still is a lack of preparedness among educators in adopting, and adapting to, emergency online teaching and technology demands in higher education institutions during the COVID-19 pandemic. This is particularly so because higher education systems lack the leadership ability to provide diverse learning pathways towards supporting sustainable university education (Salihu et al., 2020). Similarly, in a 2008 study of technology acceptance in Malaysia, academics and students faced challenges with regard to technology acceptance and adoption because there were some who found the remote learning environment too difficult (Lim et al., 2008).

Methodology

The data discussed in this chapter was collected through semi-structured interview with participants in Masvingo and Midlands provinces in Zimbabwe. The provinces have a total of nine tertiary institutions, namely, Midlands

[1] The phased approach include: (1) continuing to provide education through distance learning during the pandemic, (2) re-opening the schools and resuming face-to-face teaching when the pandemic is over, and (3) restructuring the organization of teaching and learning to benefit from the lessons (see UNESCO-IESALC, 2020).

State University (MSU), Great Zimbabwe University (GZU), Reformed Church University (RCU), Zimbabwe Open University (ZOU), and Catholic University (CU) satellite; and teacher training colleges, namely, Bondolfi Teachers' College (BTC), Morgenster Teachers' College (RCMTC), Masvingo Teachers' College (MTC), and Mkoba Teachers' College (MKTC). For the purpose of this study, data was gathered from three Teacher Training Colleges and three universities. In selecting the tertiary institutions, we purposively selected state universities and teachers' colleges as well as mission-owned university and teacher training colleges. In stratifying institutions on the basis of control, we aim to understand if there are differences between state-owned and mission-owned institutions in terms of preparedness and support provided to educators in response to the disturbance brought by the COVID-19 pandemic (Farinloye & Adeola, 2020). The study adopted a qualitative research approach which is exploratory in nature (Farinloye et al., 2019). The approach uses any procedures that rely upon primary source materials, where very often the 'data' is not numerical (Yates, 2004). This approach permitted the understanding of lived experiences for different educators employed at different universities during the COVID-19 pandemic. Data for the study was gathered through a combination of in-person interviews, telephone, Skype and Zoom interviews, and online open-ended questionnaire surveys as a COVID-19 containment measure.

The study made use of secondary sources of data on higher education inequalities and pandemics. This information was obtained from blogs, and newspaper and magazine articles that capture the experiences of educators in transitioning to emergency remote instruction during the COVID-19 pandemic. Purposive and convenient samplings were utilized to select six key informants from each participating institution and 30 educators from the six higher education institutions. Six key informants were administrators from these institutions such as registrars, pro-vice chancellors, deans, principals, and human resources managers.

In conducting this study, ethical guidelines for research were strictly adhered to. Data collection followed the WHO and Ministry of Health guidelines of two-metre social distancing, where in-person interviews were conducted. Ethical issues such as informed consent, voluntary participation, privacy, and confidentiality were respected. Data collected was thematically analysed and categorized in accordance with the themes that had emerged.

Demographic Data of Participants

Respondents	Age	Sex	Institution type	Location
Educator B	43	M	State university	Gweru
Educator C	35	F	State university	Masvingo
Educator J	39	F	State University	Masvingo
Educator M	53	F	Mission owned College	Masvingo
Educator P	31	M	Mission-owned university	Masvingo
Educator X	33	F	Government College	Gweru
Educator Z	40	F	Government College	Gweru
Educator X	46	M	State University	Masvingo
Registrar Z	41	M	Mission-owned university	Masvingo
Registrar X	55	M	State university	Gweru

Findings

Experiences of Educators at Zimbabwean Higher Education Institutions

While there are provisions and national statements/documents in adopting online teaching during COVID-19, as we have noted, educators still face challenges in delivering tuition via online platforms. Interviews held with educators and key stakeholders revealed that the most common challenges are that the majority of educators were not ready to adopt ERI in performing their duties. A number of educators and learners are not technologically savvy to cope with the fast-changing trends for online teaching and learning. Furthermore, most institutions in Zimbabwe are structured in a manner that promotes face-to-face learning rather than a hybrid mode of teaching. The following sub-sections discuss the challenges that prevent educators in delivering lectures during the lockdown, namely internet-related challenges, lack of investment on online infrastructure, lack of e-learning training, and low uptake of technology by students.

Internet-Related Challenges

Internet penetration has increased in Zimbabwe, with 27% of the population having access to the internet mainly through pay-as-you-go mobile connections.[2] With slightly over a quarter of the population with internet access and

[2] World Bank data set https://data.worldbank.org/indicator/IT.NET.BBND?locations=ZW

only 204,424 with fixed broadband subscriptions, the majority of the populace lack access to stable and reliable internet connections that can sustain online teaching.[3] Few Zimbabweans enjoy broadband internet since most people opt for the cheaper pay-as-you-go mobile connections that are slow and erratic, especially in rural areas. Lack of reliable internet connection presented challenges for most educators interviewed. Educators from all institutions in the study highlighted that they could not upload videos and audio lectures due to erratic internet connections. Slow connections and erratic internet connection forced educators to opt for alternative ways of delivering lectures. Some educators noted that online teaching was reduced to mere sending of lecturer notes and reading material via emails and WhatsApp. This adversely impacted the interactive learning process that most educators envisage. The frustrations that some educators felt were illustrated in one respondent who noted that:

> The process of uploading videos and audio lectures takes forever… a lot of time is wasted while buffering and processing till it times out. I tried uploading (teaching) material during off-peak hour[s] early in the morning [and] still I could not…. The teaching that I did in 2020 was only sending a pdf copy of lecture notes for students to read and prepare for examination. (Educator B, Gweru)

Slow internet connection adversely affected the quality of teaching and instructional approaches. Educators resorted to pedagogical approaches that limited students' participation and interaction in the learning processes. Effective learning occurs in environments characterized by high student participation and interaction (Townsend et al., 2002). The pandemic is reconfiguring teaching processes in ways that limit student participation. Furthermore, some educators noted that when they teach in face-to-face classrooms, they can assess students' appreciation through body language. Due to erratic internet connections, teaching was reduced to mere forwarding of notes via email. As such, educators were deprived in ways of assessing students and adjusting their teaching accordingly.

Most educators lamented about the high cost of data in Zimbabwe. One gigabyte of data cost on average USD10.00. When understood within the broader context, some institutions did not provide funds for the purchase of data while some institutions provided insufficient funds as little as USD3.00. On average, university educators teach three modules. Without a proper plan

[3] Ibid.

of how educators would access data, online teaching was affected. Educators noted that most universities chose Google Classroom as the official online platform. Google Classroom requires and expends more data, especially when assessing assignments online. More research is required on the amount of data expended per module on various online platforms. This will give university administrators estimates on the amount of data required for each module to be taught. Online teaching was crippled by lack of resources for the purchase of data. During the first half of 2020, Zimbabwe declared a total lockdown during which movements were outlawed (Taru, 2020). Educators had no access to institutional internet network, making it difficult to smoothly transition to internet-based teaching. Several weeks into the lockdown, some educators had not accessed learners or posted activities for learners. Educators in Zimbabwe are struggling, caught between duty and the economic situation that does not allow them to provide their services to learners.

Educators interviewed expressed concern over issues of privacy and academic freedom when they teach through online platforms. Educators' privacy is limited due to digital imprints that can be traced to their homes through Internet Protocol addresses and Local Area Networks. Furthermore, some educators were worried that online teaching exposes them to hackers, trolls and cyber bullies whose conduct affect the smooth flow of lectures. One educator narrated her experience when a non-student managed to obtain log-in details from students. The non-student disrespected the educator and interjected during the lecture. Through online platforms, educators fall victim to outsiders who may gain unauthorized access to the private teaching sessions.

Universities under study prefer Google Classroom as the official Learning Management System because this platform gives administrators full control to oversee and monitor learning processes. At one institution, educators were not administrators of the class they taught. In order for them to add students, correct module code or narration, they had to engage a third-party administrator. In a way, online platforms disempowered educators and directly placed them under the control of administrators and middle-level managers who otherwise would not directly monitor them in face-to-face learning. One educator noted that the pandemic has opened opportunities for administrators to exercise control over educators and also, to some extent, limit academic freedom. More and more content is coming under the scrutiny of administrators who have the power to remove and repackage the content that educators choose. Administrators now discuss module content, style of teaching, approaches, and conduct during online session because they oversee what happens during online teaching. These shifts in power and authority may remain even after society returns to normalcy and face-to-face learning resumes.

COVID-19 exposed the assumption that educators are middle class and elite and therefore should have abodes fit for working from home. This attitude was reflected in institution administrator's failure to inquire and assist educators in creating a proper at-home work environment. All educators highlighted that there are challenges that come with teaching from home. Some highlighted that their homes did not have conducive working space from where they can conduct online teaching. The living arrangement and space in certain homes do not accommodate teaching at home. Female educators noted that the pandemic has opened a portal which allowed them to assess the possibility of working from home in the future. For female educators, home chores and child minding are processes that take all day. Earmarking and reserving time for teaching from home was difficult for female educators (Taru, 2020). These challenges were not foreseen or anticipated by university and college management and administrators.

Lack of Investment on Online Infrastructure

Zimbabwe has experienced economic challenges since the late 1990s (Bond, 1998). The economic crisis was characterized by high inflation rates, collapse of domestic currency, and closure of businesses (Bond & Manyanya, 2003). The crisis adversely impacted operations on most institutions, educational institutions included. Concomitantly, universities and colleges in Zimbabwe failed to fully embrace the use of technology in teaching and learning. Most education institutions in Zimbabwe prefer face-to-face learning to online teaching. Little investment has been made to prepare educators and students for online teaching. Universities have neither provided educators with computers nor developed software for online teaching. The pandemic found Zimbabwean education institutions ill-prepared for online teaching due to lack of necessary infrastructure required for online teaching. For instance, pertaining to some Catholic-run educational institutions such as Bondolfi Teachers' College, it was acknowledged that COVID-19 pandemic caught them unawares but they were prepared to learn and redefine the way learners continued with studies under the current emergency situation (Karombo, 2020). Therein, the pandemic was an opportunity for rediscovery in the educational sector.

Most institutions resorted to emergency remote instruction that was neither organized nor coordinated in a structured manner. Furthermore, necessary software for video recording, plagiarism checks, and document processing are not in place in majority of state-run and church-run institutions. Lack of necessary hardware and software adversely affected the lecture delivery. Going forward, investment in online teaching infrastructure is essential for effective teaching as society embraces the new normal.

Despite the fact that most universities and colleges were ill-prepared infrastructurally, one church-run university in Masvingo bought laptops for the teaching staff as a way of promoting online teaching. In terms of ICT infrastructure, one church-run teacher training college had a head-start. Since 2018, the institution took a phased approach in providing its staff with laptops, starting with lecturers in Information Technology department and followed by Commerce department. As such when abrupt closure was forced by COVID-19, lecturers already had gadgets to use during online teaching. In state-run institutions, the process of transitioning to online teaching was marred by a number of challenges, namely most lecturers had old laptops that had no webcam and faster processors. State-run universities do not provide lecturers with laptops; most lecturers depend on desktop computers in computer laboratories and offices. When movement was restricted due to lockdown, lecturers could not access offices and laboratories, disrupting continuation of teaching during lockdown.

Transition to online teaching was also affected by one-size-fit-all approach that was taken by some institutions in providing data packages for lecturers and instructors. In some cases institution opted for data packages from services provider whose services are cheaper than other services providers but also slower and with limited coverage. In such cases, online teaching was a challenge, as noted by interviewees from one state-run institution of higher education. The interviewees noted that poor coverage and connectivity made real-time teaching impossible with machines buffering for long. Learning was postponed until wee hours when connectivity improved in some locations in Masvingo.

Lack of e-Learning Training for Educators

COVID-19 has become a threat to higher education sectors in Zimbabwe as there was demand for emergency transition to online teaching and learning. In addition to providing online resources to students and educators, there was a need for training educators on online teaching, especially on Zoom and Google Classroom. Interviews with educators from universities and colleges indicate that most of the educators did not have experience in online teaching, but were expected to start teaching their courses online during the pandemic. A majority of these institutions can only go to the extent of providing internet data to educators without any efforts to train educators on how to use online platforms. The following interview excerpts shed more light on the matter:

> Our university management expected us to learn overnight to move from face-to-face learning to virtual classroom. Imagine the Chairpersons were asking us to ensure that teaching continues via Google classroom, yet I do not know what Google classroom is and how it works. We had a very difficult experience. (Educator J, Gweru)

These same sentiments are expressed by another educator based in Masvingo who noted that:

> The bursary department provided us with data for online teaching. No one cares about training the college lecturers about skills on how to use the internet for zoom classrooms and Google classroom. How do they expect us to deliver lectures successfully to our students? Our academic leaders are always encouraging us to teach and post material online, but no measures were taken to ensure that we know how to do it. (Educator M Masvingo)

As many educators were not technologically savvy to cope with the fast-changing trends for online teaching and learning, and as training was not offered by their institutions, it was unlikely for the educators to effectively deliver lectures during the pandemic. In view of this, it can be argued that the COVID-19 pandemic exposed higher education unpreparedness in capacity building of its staff and this has left many educators unable to respond effectively. In relation to this, universities should have started to require academic staff to attend technical workshops and training in order to prepare them for handling online courses or using online materials and tools (Muftahu, 2020). The main drawback for e-learning at higher education institutions in Zimbabwe was the digital divide. The challenge was exacerbated by the idea that many academics are slow to embrace new technologies due to a range of issues (Watty et al., 2016) such as risks associated with their potential failure (Howard, 2013), their perceived value/relevance (Debuse et al., 2008), workload and time constraints (Wingo et al., 2017), a lack of confidence as well as a lack of resources/support, and constant new technologies to master (Adams et al., 2017).

It is also worth noting that at some higher education institutions where efforts were made to train educators to use online teaching platforms, efforts were still foiled by infrastructure limitations. The following excerpts detail some training experiences that still presented barriers to online teaching:

> We received communication from the Information and Communication Technology (ICT) Directorate that we were supposed to be trained on how to use Google Classroom and Zoom platform in lecture delivery. To our surprise, the training did not take off because of challenges of internet connectivity. We then wonder[ed] how they expect us to teach online, yet their internet was poor. (Educator X, Masvingo)

Another respondent, Educator Z, Gweru, has this to say:

> I was shocked when the 50 of us gathered in a computer room with 15 machines. Honestly our management expected us to use inadequate resources. To make matters worse, the economic environment in the country has affected us to the extent that we do not have personal gadgets for the e-learning training and teaching of students. It was not an easy task to adopt remote teaching. (Educator Z, Gweru)

This situation was prevalent, with Educator C from Masvingo noting that,

> The email we received was just inviting us to be ready for online training on Google classroom, but there was no provision of data, no access to University facilities to access wifi, [and] no gadgets such as computers, laptops or smart phones. It was an ill-planned decision. University management just wanted students to continue receiving tuition at all costs, but they did not have resources to realise that goal. (Educator C Masvingo)

On the other hand, institutional management had their explanations on training of educators. Key informant interviews revealed that most institutions were facing financial challenges during the pandemic that could not be easily overcome. As one University Registrar notes,

> The pandemic affected us badly, we were caught unprepared financially. As a result there was no funding to provide resources to train academics such as the provision of laptops and related gadgets. The situation was made worse by the current economic challenge in the country that did not spare tertiary institutions. We had no choice but to work with existing resources such as few desktops that we used to have in the laboratories. (Registrar Z, Masvingo)

At other institutions, management members felt that educators were supposed to understand that the times were difficult. The economic environment coupled with the COVID-19 pandemic has made it very difficult for higher and tertiary education institutions to continue. This is illustrated by the vignette below:

> We understand that we were supposed to train our lecturers but the situation was very difficult for the college. To gather lecturers at one place to train them was very difficult since the COVID-19 lockdown was not allowing a gathering of more than 50 participants and requires a physical distance of one meter. This means that we needed more days to train them. This was an additional financial burden to an already crippled college. As a result we failed to train all our educators. Some educators were to learn on their own via several online platforms. (Registrar X, Gweru)

With their limited or no online training in delivering lectures to students during the COVID-19 pandemic, many educators failed to effectively deliver lectures through online platforms such as Google Classroom or Zoom. As argued, some academics and students are not comfortable with the adoption of technology towards facilitating remote learning due to unfamiliarity thereby influencing technology acceptance behaviours (Muftahu, 2020). The experiences and challenges faced by educators have affected continuation of tuition by higher and tertiary education.

Training of educators for online teaching goes beyond training them to navigate teaching platforms. Educators require training on lecture delivery when teaching on online platforms. Studies have shown that voice and management skills are crucial when delivering lectures. Voice and management, the ability to develop online exercises and activities, and monitoring students while teaching online are important (Bao, 2020). Educators must be trained on vocal functions such as speaking gently and pronouncing words in way that students can comprehend and capture for notes. Some educators noted that they faced difficulties in adjusting some practical subjects such as woodwork, metal work, and observations to online platforms. Educators who were interviewed noted that administrators neglected this component in training, yet it influences how students comprehend what they are taught. We see gaps in the training processes as university and college administrators are mainly concerned with equipping educators with skills on navigating online teaching platforms without equipping them with necessary skills for effective and successful teaching.

Low Uptake by Students

In addition to the aforementioned challenges faced by educators at higher education institutions, they also face low uptake by students. Similar challenges of lack of online resources were also experienced by higher and tertiary education students. With closure of colleges and universities, higher and tertiary education students were expected to work virtually from home. This means that disadvantaged pupils and students from poor and marginalized communities were less likely to have access to technological resources such as internet, computers, or tablets. The introduction of Google classes, online lectures, and Zoom lectures, among others, further impoverished the poor. Interviews revealed that the educational attainment gap escalated between the poor students and the more affluent ones. Educators from different institutions revealed the following,

> My class has 156 registered students but only 67 registered successfully on Google classroom. Most of the students could not afford data to access the classes. I realised that I was wasting my time if more than 50% of the students are not receiving tuition yet they have paid the fees. (Educator X, Gweru)

Educator P, Masvingo raised the same concerns of accessibility. This is illustrated in the following verbatim:

> I failed to create a Google classroom because of lack of data. I then resorted to Whatsapp platform where I thought it will be easy to discuss and deliver lectures to my students. I was surprised that 30% of students were not on Whatsapp. Some students do not have proper phones for Whatsapp. Some of the students do not have phones. So practically, not all students managed to access tuition during the COVID-19 lockdown. (Educator P, Masvingo)

The other challenge noted is that though some students have internet data for the available platform such as Google Classroom and Zoom, they were not technologically savvy. As argued, school closures and the other impacts of disease outbreaks have a disproportionately negative impact on the learning, safety, and wellbeing of the most vulnerable children in the poorest families (Hallgarten, 2020). Further, those from poor families were more likely to die or have a family member die; they are likely to learn less, eat less, and may be subject to other safeguarding issues and risky behaviour (World Bank, 2020). With reference to COVID-19 pandemic lockdown, these digital divides have prompted student bodies such as the South African Students Congress

(SASCO), the University of Malawi Students Union (UMSU), and the Zimbabwe National Students Union (ZINASU) to reject e-learning as the educational solution in Africa (Mukeredzi et al., 2020).

Discussion

Reimagining Educational Futures in Zimbabwe: Critical Reflections

In this section, the chapter proffers suggestions towards reimagining educational futures that would transform the current higher educational systems so that they are resilient, empowering, and enfranchising during times of emergencies in Zimbabwe. As Zimbabwean higher education institutions readjust and adapt in light of COVID-19, there is need for creative and pragmatic approaches of delivering. Hybrid approaches must be customized to suit institution-specific challenges and strengths. The implementation of Education 5.0 that emphasizes innovation must cascade to ways in which content is delivered within higher education institutions. Universities and colleges need to develop learning systems that combine face-to-face teaching as well as online teaching. Such approaches reduce disruption that come with unforeseen events. COVID-19 has opened a portal through which we can envision higher education under Fourth Industrial Revolution (4IR).

Furthermore, ICT skill sets in learners and teachers must be upped. ICT skills must be a requirement for teachers and instructors. These skills are useful even in post-COVID-19 era. Teaching must continue remotely even when teachers are away attending conferences and workshops. This is an area that institution of higher learning must invest in. On another point, higher education institutions must develop customized platforms for remote teaching and learning that expend less data, are easy to navigate, and are highly accessible. The pandemic has opened up opportunities for higher education institutions to realize their potential to link virtually with established scholars across the globe for combine lectures and seminars (Hinson & Mogaji, 2020; Kieu et al., 2020). Higher education institutions must promptly avail infrastructure that support online teaching and learning. As discussed earlier, non-state institutions fared better than state-run institution in provision of infrastructure that support online teaching and learning. There is need for heavy investment in state higher education institutions in this regard.

In terms of teaching approaches there is a need for further development of participatory approaches to teaching and learning (Mogaji et al., 2020). Higher education teaching must shift from pedagogical to andragogical approaches that are participatory to allow learners to contribute to the learning processes. Participatory approaches are best suited for online teaching. There is need for intensive training and refresher courses for educators. Educators must be trained in new approaches to teaching, especially hybrid teaching and methods that encourage collective learning and teaching. COVID-19 demands paradigm shifts in management and administration of higher education institutions. Higher education institutions should build virtual learning environments that guarantee access to internet and availability of computers, laptops, or tablets to educators and learners. Much effort must be channelled towards refocusing research departments and teaching and learning centres towards envision hybrid learning. These departments must develop homegrown approaches, software, and teaching material that require less internet bandwidth. Furthermore, these departments must actively consult educators and identify missing skill set that are required in situation where face-to-face learning is impossible (Agbo et al., 2020).

Conclusion

This chapter demonstrated that there was and still is lack of preparedness among educators in adopting, and adapting to, emergency online teaching and technology demands in higher education institutions during the COVID-19 pandemic in Zimbabwe. In addition, the chapter exposed the challenging experiences of educators in adopting, and adapting to, emergency remote instruction on one hand, and the availability of infrastructure that facilitates ERI, on the other hand. The main challenges identified include: lack of reliable internet connection, lack of adequate investment in online infrastructure, lack of e-learning training for educators, and low uptake by students. The data from key informants at tertiary institutions shows the lack of preparation and little consumption of online platforms by higher education management. While the educators expect to be provided with internet-related material and training from the institution, the management assumed that all educators have abodes fit for working from home and learning should continue as normal. Such attitudes, moreover, are part of the institution's failure to create a proper at-home work environment for educators. Unless addressed through deliberate institutional intervention and legislation, these shortcomings are likely to continue to compromise educators' lecture delivery during pandemics.

The data we discussed in this chapter was collected from a few institutions located in central and south-eastern parts of Zimbabwe, and our findings cannot be generalized to all institutions in Zimbabwe. There is need for extensive study that covers wider geographical area and institutions by including polytechnics and vocational centres. The Zimbabwean education system is opening and learners at all levels are returning to schools; there is a need to further research to understand interactions in the classroom set-up, assess if educators and learners continue to rely on online teaching and comparative assessments of learners' performance when learning via online platforms.

References

Adams, B. S., Cummins, M., Davis, A., Freeman, A., Hall, G. C., & Ananthanarayanan, V. (2017). NMC horizon report: 2017 Higher Education Edition. https://www.nmc.org/publication/nmc-horizon-report-2017-higher-education-edition/

Agbo, F. J., Olawumi, O., Oyelere, S. S., Kolog, E. A., Olaleye, S. A., Agjei, R., & Olawuni, A. (2020). Social media usage for computing education: The effect of tie strength and group communication on perceived learning outcome. *International Journal of Education and Development using Information and Communication Technology, 16*(1), 5–26.

Anifowoshe, O., Aborode, A. T., Ayodele, T. I., Iretiayo, A. R., & David, O. O. (2020). Impact of COVID-19 on education in Sub-Saharan Africa. *Preprints*, (www.preprints.org). https://doi.org/10.20944/preprints202007.0027.v1

Bao, W. (2020). COVID -19 and online teaching in higher education: A case study of Peking University. *Human Behaviour and Emerging Technologies, 2*(2), 113–115.

Bond, P. (1998). *Uneven Zimbabwe, a study of finance, development, and underdevelopment*. Africa World Press Inc.

Bond, P., & Manyanya, M. (2003). *Zimbabwe's plunge. Exhausted nationalism, neoliberalism and the search for social justice*. Weaver Press.

Cuaton, G. P. (2020). Philippine higher education institutions in the time of COVID-19 Pandemic. Working Paper No. 001. https://doi.org/10.13140/RG.2.2.12511.61603

Debuse, J. C. W., Lawley, M., & Shibl, R. (2008). Educators' perceptions of automated feedback systems. *Australasian Journal of Educational Technology, 24*(4), 374–386. https://doi.org/10.14742/ajet.1198

Farinloye, T., & Adeola, O. (2020). Typology of Nigeria universities: A strategic marketing and branding implication. In E. Mogaji, F. Maringe, & R. E. Hinson (Eds.), *Understanding the higher education market in Africa*. Routledge.

Farinloye, T., Aririguzoh, S., & Kieu, T. A. (2019). Qualitatively exploring the effect of change in the residential environment on travel behaviour. *Travel Behaviour and Society, 17*(1), 26–35.

Flavell, H., Harris, C., Price, C., Logan, E., & Peterson, S. (2019). Empowering academics to be adaptive with eLearning technologies: An exploratory case study. *Australasian Journal of Educational Technology, 35*(1), 1–15.

Hallgarten, J. (2020). Evidence on efforts to mitigate the negative educational impact of past disease outbreaks. In *K4D Helpdesk report 793*. Education Development Trust.

Hinson, R., & Mogaji, E. (2020). Co-creation of value by universities and prospective students: Towards an informed decision-making process. In E. Mogaji, F. Maringe, & R. Hinson (Eds.), *Higher education marketing in Africa* (pp. 17–46). Palgrave Macmillan.

Hodge, E. (2020). The impact of coronavirus on higher education. Retrieved April 21, 2020, from https://www.keystoneacademic.com/news/the-impact-of-coronavirus-on-higher-education

Howard, S. K. (2013). Risk-aversion: Understanding teacher's resistance to technology integration. *Technology, Pedagogy and Education, 22*(3), 357–372. https://doi.org/10.1080/1475939X.2013.802995

Karombo, T. (2020). Zimbabwe's Bishops say Coronavirus disruptions an opportunity for rediscovery. Retrieved September 12, 2020, from https://www.ncronline.org/news/coronavirus/zimbabwes-bishops-say-coronavirus-disruptions-opportunity-rediscovery

Kieu, T., Mwebesa, C., Sarofim, S., Soetan, T., & Vululleh, S. P. (2020). Marketing higher education in Africa: Moving from research to practice. In E. Mogaji, F. Maringe, & R. Hinson (Eds.), *Strategic marketing of higher education in Africa* (pp. 221–237). Routledge.

Lim, B-C. Y., Sam, H. K., & Wah, T. K. (2008). Acceptance of e-learning among distance learners: A Malaysian perspective. *Proceedings ascilite Melbourne*, pp. 541–551.

Martin, M., & Furiv, U. (2020). COVID-19 shows the need to make learning more flexible. Retrieved August 21, 2020, from https://www.universityworldnews.com/post.php?story=20200324115802272

Mogaji, E., & Jain, V. (2020). Impact of the pandemic on higher education in emerging countries: Emerging opportunities, challenges and research agenda. *SSRN Electronic Journal.* https://doi.org/10.2139/ssrn.3622592

Mogaji, E., Maringe, F., & Hinson, R. (2020). Marketisation in higher education in Africa: New directions for a decolonising continent. In E. Mogaji, F. Maringe, & R. Hinson (Eds.), *Understanding the higher education market in Africa.* Routledge Studies in Marketing. Routledge. ISBN 978-0367344382.

Muftahu, M. (2020). Higher Education and Covid-19 Pandemic: Matters arising and the challenges of sustaining academic programs in developing African universities. *International Journal of Educational Research Review, 5*(4), 417–423.

Mukeredzi, T., Kokutse, F., & Dell, S. (2020). Student bodies say e-learning is unaffordable and elitist. Retrieved April 24, 2021, from https://www.universityworldnews.com/post.php?story

Mukute, M., Francis, B., Burt, J., & de Souza, B. (2020). Education in times of COVID-19: Looking for silver linings in Southern Africa's educational responses. *Southern African Journal of Environmental Education, 36*, 62–79.

Ndofirepi, E., Farinloye, T., & Mogaji, E. (2020). Marketing mix in a heterogenous higher education market: A case of Africa. In E. Mogaji, F. Maringe, & R. E. Hinson (Eds.), *Understanding the higher education market in Africa*. Routledge.

Nganga, G., Waruru, M., & Nakweya, G. (2020). Universities face multiple challenges in wake of COVID-19 closures. Retrieved November 21, 2020, from https://www.universityworldnews.com/post.php?story=20200407162549396

Olaleye, S., Ukpabi, D., & Mogaji, E. (2020). Public vs private universities in Nigeria: Market dynamics perspective. In E. Mogaji, F. Maringe, & R. E. Hinson (Eds.), *Understanding the higher education market in Africa*. Routledge.

Rieley, J. B. (2020). Coronavirus and its impact on higher education. Retrieved January 15, 2021, from https://www.rieley.com

SADC & UNESCO. (2020). *SADC &UNESCO sign agreement to ensure learning never stops*. Press Release. SADC & UNESCO.

Salihu, M. J., Nayel, M. R., & Rabiatul-Adawiah, A. R. (2020). Sustainable higher education leadership: A conceptual approach from the functionalist paradigm for higher institutions of learning. *Humanities and Social Sciences Reviews – (HSSR), 8*(2), 8–12.

Smalley, A. (2020). *Higher education responses to Coronavirus (COVID-19)*. Retrieved April 21, 2020, from https://www.ncsl.org/research/education/higher-education-responses-to-coronavirus-covid-19.aspx

Taru, J. (2020). You can work from home if the situation at home allows: Teaching in times of the pandemic. *Education International*. Retrieved January 19, 2021, from https://www.worldsofeducation.org/en/woe_homepage/woe_detail/16818/'you-can-work-from-home-if-the-situation-at-home-allows'-teaching-in-times-of-the-pandemic-by-josiah-taru#gsc.tab=0

Townsend, E., Campbell, C., Curran-Smith, J., McGinn, F., Persaud, D., & Peters, P. (2002). Accessibility and interactivity in distance education programs for health professions. *Journal of Distance Education, 17*(2), 1–24.

UNESCO-IESALC (United Nations Educational, Scientific and Cultural Organisation – International Institute for Higher Education in Latin America and the Caribbean). (2020). COVID-19 and higher education: Today and tomorrow. Impact analysis, policy responses and recommendations. Retrieved April 9, 2021, from http://www.iesalc.unesco.org/en/wp-content/uploads/2020/04/COVID-19

United Nations (2015, 25 September). Transforming our world: The 2030 Agenda for Sustainable Development' Resolution adopted by the General Assembly, United Nations.

Watty, K., McKay, J., & Ngo, L. (2016). Innovators or inhibitors? Accounting faculty resistance to new educational technologies in higher education. *Journal of Accounting Education, 36*, 1–15. https://doi.org/10.1016/j.jaccedu.2016.03.003

Wingo, N. P., Ivankova, N. V., & Moss, J. A. (2017). Faculty perceptions about online teaching exploring the literature using the technology acceptance model as an organizing framework. *Online Learning, 21*(1), 15–35. https://doi.org/10.24059/olj.v21i1.761

World Bank. (2020). Managing the impact of COVID-19 on education systems around the world: How countries are preparing, coping, and planning for recovery. Retrieved December 10, 2020, from https://blogs.worldbank.org/education/managing-impact-covid-19-education-systems-around-world-how-countries-are-preparing

World Health Organization (WHO). (2020). *Coronavirus disease (COVID-19) outbreak situation.* Retrieved July 25, 2020, from https://www.who.int/emergencies/diseases/novel-coronavirus-2019

Yates, J. S. (2004). *Doing social science research.* Sage Publications in association with the Open University Press.

Zimbabwe Education Cluster. (2020). Humanitarian response and COVID-19 situation report. Retrieved April 23, 2021, from https://www.humanitarianresponse.info/en/operations/zimbabwe/education

Theme IV

Reimagining the Future

13

Role of Culture in Developing Transformative Leadership for Higher Education in Emerging Economies

Pooja Sharma and Varsha Jain

Introduction

Organizations are bound together with a glue which is known as culture. Higher education institutions such as colleges and universities, just like any other organizations, have to effectively communicate their culture in terms of their mission, vision, and purpose in an ever-changing world (Vasudeva & Mogaji, 2020). During the COVID-19 pandemic, higher education institutions have been confronted with keeping their culture intact and remaining relevant to the students and the workforce (leadership, instructors, researchers, administrators, and the support staff) while they work from home. The pandemic has affected higher education institutions severely as attracting and enrolling new students has become more difficult in this financially unstable time, as has engaging existing students who do not have the resources to connect virtually (McCarthy, 2020; Moody's, 2020). Such challenges faced by higher education institutes are heightened in developing economies as they have been under the stress of poor infrastructure, governmental support (Olaleye et al., 2020), and lower literacy rates. Learners are socially disadvantaged with minimal access to technology, thereby impacting their ability to engage with the online learning environment (Zhong, 2020).

P. Sharma • V. Jain (✉)
Marketing, MICA, Ahmedabad, India
e-mail: poojasharma.fpm20@micamail.in; varsha.jain@micamail.in

E. Mogaji et al. (eds.), *Re-imagining Educational Futures in Developing Countries*,
https://doi.org/10.1007/978-3-030-88234-1_13

Recognizing the socio-economic, educational, and health challenges arising from the COVID-19 pandemic, this chapter presents the urgency to formulate transformational leadership within higher education institutes in emerging and developing economies. The administration has to keep intact the institution's vision and mission while taking care of the learners and their needs, which is one of the critical challenges faced by institutes. The shift from the traditional classroom model of teaching to online platforms (Govindarajan & Srivastava, 2020) such as Zoom and WebEx as a medium of instruction brings a set of challenges and opportunities, which has become the center of attention for leaders across educational institutions (Lake & Buelow, 2021; Seltzer, 2020). Since 2020, almost all institutes have adopted remote learning through various digital platforms or a blended approach which constitutes the combination of on-campus and remote education (Selingo & Silagadze, 2021). Educational institutions are the foundation that promotes community building where young people engage with each other, indulging in dialogues regarding ideas, innovations, and social and scientific breakthroughs resulting in the development of human potential across different areas. Hence, the role of leaders across institutions becomes more crucial while navigating through challenges presented by the COVID-19 pandemic. Transformational leadership works effectively by providing support, encouraging team spirit, enabling decision-making autonomy among stakeholders, and generating creative and innovative ideas through continuous brainstorming, resulting in all the stakeholders working as a team (Li et al., 2019). Naqshbandi et al. (2019) explain that transformational leadership in an organization helps the employees develop new ideas and concepts through constant motivation and encouragement.

The cultural fabric of the institutions plays a significant role in interweaving these ideas and breakthroughs. Navigating cultural fabric (Athavale, 2020) includes the shared values and beliefs by leaders, which are consequently communicated and reinforced through various methods that influence employee behaviors and understanding, which becomes tricky in the present pandemic scenario. Still, the institutions have to take the risk of separating the history, traditions, beliefs, and norms that are beginning to contradict the modern-day values and practices. However, it is equally essential for organizations to communicate their cultural fabric in a manner that honors their vision and mission and at the same time capture the future aspirations of stakeholders focusing on the changing world order. This focus can be achieved through transformational leadership. All stakeholders and their viewpoints are valued, agile structures are established, and processes are followed under the stewardship of a dynamic leader. Hence, transformational leadership leads to attaining the institutional purpose that focuses on integrated learning, collective goals, community-oriented objectives, and collective wellbeing. This learning helps in the maintenance of quality standards in higher education through the interactive and socializing process.

The present chapter aims to provide a framework for understanding the role of the cultural fabric within higher educational institutions, bringing about quality education to the forefront in developing countries post-pandemic through transformational leadership. The chapter focuses on higher education and is divided into four sections. The first section explains the role that an organization plays in developing higher education institutions with the introduction of the framework. The second section mentions the concept of leadership, where agile structures and processes, stakeholder inclusiveness, and distributed leadership play in bringing about transformational leadership and its impact on higher education. The third section illustrates the implications that culture and transformational leadership have on the institutions of higher education. Finally, in the fourth section, implications and conclusion are made based on the proposed framework.

The Need for a Framework for Transformational Leadership

During the COVID-19 pandemic, higher educational institutes have witnessed cultural dilemmas. McCarthy (2020) explains the management of COVID-19, higher education institutions have been shut down for physical classroom-based learning, an act that has devastatingly impacted the global educational systems. Another impact of the pandemic on learners has been the financial implications of the world due to lower recruitments of prospective students (Moody's, 2020). This transition has been tough on higher education in developing economies. They already had to contend with poor infrastructure, low governmental support (Olaleye et al., 2020), and lower literacy rates. The pandemic has also demonstrated the limitations of higher education institutions in developing countries due to inadequate resources. Learners are socially disadvantaged with minimal access to technology, thereby impacting their ability to engage in the online learning environment (Zhong, 2020). Recognizing the socio-economic, educational, and health challenges arising from the COVID-19 pandemic, this chapter presents the urgency for the formulation of transformational leadership in developing economies focusing on higher educational institutions. Leaders can use the following

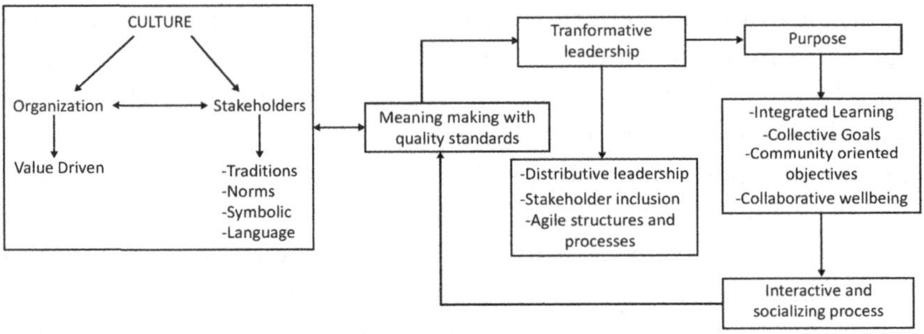

Source: Author

Fig. 13.1 Role of culture in developing transformative leadership leading to improved quality standards of higher education in developing nations. (Source: Author)

framework (Fig. 13.1) in higher educational institutions to understand the importance of organizational culture, the role of transformative leadership, and steps in adapting to the changing educational environment that is witnessing a drastic shift towards remote (online) learning.

Culture and Higher Education

With the changing societal and technological developments, innovation and flexibility are the key factors that determine the expanding knowledge base and the success of an organization. Additionally, organizations and their leaders constantly work towards formulating frameworks that help motivate and guide individuals' behaviors that are acceptable to the organization based on cultural norms. Organizational culture, therefore, influences how individuals regard identity and openness to change. This culture is essential for higher education institutions in various aspects. These aspects include environment (defined by the stakeholders of the organization and their attitude towards it), vision, and mission (the symbolic functions that hold the members together under a unified common belief and identity and the usage as the basis for the decision-making process). It also includes structures, processes, goals, and strategies (to attain those goals) through leadership development influenced by political, economic, and demographic conditions (Tierney, 1988). How an institution of higher education works and is involved in its functioning is reflected in its culture. Tierney (1988) explains that these aspects are not the operationalizations of cultural concepts. Instead, they form the critical dimensions of the culture within organizations emanating from their history, deriving motivation from their values, processes, and goals (Hinson & Mogaji,

2020). Highlighting the importance of symbolic meanings attached to the organization's culture, Dill (1982) points out that academics and leadership should be inclined towards the higher education institutions as a whole rather than identifying themselves with their domain-based individualistic careers. Masland (1985) discusses the central role of culture in the organization and focuses on the symbols, rituals, saga, and heroes' aspects of the cultural fabric for the higher education institutions to understand the influences of both past and present. This understanding provides the institution with stability and continuity within emerging economies through transformative leadership focusing on collaborations and inclusiveness of stakeholders in decision-making processes.

Finally, Maassen (1996) explains the academic culture as an amalgamation of values, beliefs, practices, and attitudes leading to the integration of a specific group of academics. Kalkan et al. (2020) emphasize that leadership, strategy and information norms, values, beliefs, and socialization are also the aspects that are determined based on an organization's culture. The economic and political factors influence the world and transform educational institutions, resulting in the educational services being weighed in sale and purchase. They compete for funding from the governments instead of selling their services. In the Indian Institute of Management, Ahmedabad (IIMA), considerable importance in explaining the role of culture is given at this higher education institution. The institution is from an emerging and developing economy—India. Taking forward the cultural fabric of the institution, the institution is working towards creating an all-inclusive higher educational environment. IIMA, in its vision and mission of the institute of higher education, focuses on a work environment that yields high performance through the support of its culture of autonomy, collaboration, and creativity amongst different stakeholders, namely the students, staff, and faculty instructors. To achieve its objective in becoming an institute on par with those in developed countries, IIMA ensures that its research and teaching activities address diverse areas that concern society.

In the present pandemic times and the time to come, higher education institutes across developing countries need to embrace transformative leadership, which can help in the institution's success. To compete with institutions in the developed world, they need to cultivate strategies, attitudes, shared values, behavior, and tools that may foster a culture that is open to creativity and innovation. Here, the concept of network university, proposed by Lewis et al. (2005), is crucial. In a network university, the changing education patterns are based on collaborations, a decentralized approach of the institution, and leadership development. The practices include the stakeholders' concerns resulting in a contemporary higher education institution where borderless learning, open community, and different social values and norms determine the institution's culture. Such phenomena are being observed in educational institutions worldwide due to the novel coronavirus, which has pushed the institutions to shut down the classrooms and move towards remote learning. However, it has played an essential role in contributing to the global knowledge infrastructure and expanding higher education institutions' shared values and beliefs.

The migration of students to different countries has been an important phenomenon that needs to be addressed by the developing countries in higher education. It has created a melting pot (Castiello-Gutiérrez, 2019) of different cultures in the same classroom environment. Collectivism instead of individualism (Manikutty et al., 2007) will play an essential role in bringing about all-inclusive learning among migrant students. The collectivist and collaborative learning environment among students would create an integration of different cultures, shared values, and beliefs resulting in the formation of agile higher education institutions. For instance, Some universities in Nigeria have adopted mobile learning that embraces the importance of various stakeholders such as academics, information technology personnel, and administrative leadership in shifting from the traditional teacher-driven classroom learning to flexible learning enabled by technology. Mobile phones are readily available in Nigeria and can easily access online platforms at reasonable tariff charges. During this pandemic, mobile technology has enabled virtual learning, thus, bridging the digital divide among the developing and developed countries. The mission, vision, and consequently the culture of the higher educational institutions can be maintained and enhanced through integration with essential values and belief systems that the learners from across the world bring about while participating in Nigeria's higher education institutions' mobile platforms. This appropriate use of technology for educational advancement made the Nigerian universities use transformative leadership with all relevant stakeholders (internal and external). These stakeholders are consulted for a thorough integration of technology and pedagogy, which is more student-centered, focusing on student-student, student-content, student-instructor, and student-outside-resource interactions (Ozdamli, 2012).

In the present times, higher education institutes are adopting a cross-cultural approach to open educational resources to learners and instructors across the globe. This approach can explain two long-established cross-cultural frameworks, namely Hall's (1976) high-context and low-context cultural theory and Hofstede's (2001) cultural values framework. Hall's high-context cultures depend on unspoken tacit communication such as body language, voice tones, facial expressions, and high value on interpersonal relationships. These parameters are the contextual cues that are central to understanding those belonging to the same culture the importance of a close-knit community. On the other hand, low-context cultures depend on clear verbal communication, emphasizing interpersonal dynamics and community-based interactions. Therefore, contextual cues based on common cultures do not play any part in interactions among the people. Hofstede (2001) defines the cultural dimensions as masculinity/femininity (denotes the extent to which culture values the motivations, achievements, and effectiveness of higher education), uncertainty avoidance (indicates culture's tolerance towards uncertainty and ambiguity), and individualism/collectivism (which denotes the individual's relationships within and across different groups) with precise meanings.

Leadership and Higher Education

The social and economic transformations through the growth and development of human capital can be attributed to higher education in a country (Kuzminov et al., 2019). There has been a rise in the number of students enrolled in institutes of higher education. However, this positive development has been undercut by low employability, lack of good-quality instructors, and weak governance in developing countries (Kieu et al., 2020; Ndofirepi et al., 2020). Howells et al. (2014) explain that factors such as globalization, disruption in technology (the gap between developing and developed countries), increased student migration, and diverse demographics, funds, and regulatory frameworks have impacted higher education institutions' credibility. Kezar (2017) explains how the governance within higher education institutes have undergone three significant changes in the context of leadership—in the form of increased scrutiny due to active participation of the stakeholders resulting in an inclusive decision-making environment and additional accountability; diverse faculty; and the need for immediate response to the changing societal needs and structures. For example, the University of Cape Town (UCT), belonging to an emerging and developing economy, emphasizes an inclusive and engaging research-intensive environment. Creativity is all about the achievements in education that enhance the lives of the students, staff, and faculty, leading to a more equitable and sustainable social order ascending towards a global higher education landscape. The university aims to advance the distinctiveness of academic scholarship by engaging in strategic partnerships across Africa, the Global South, and the world. It highlights the importance of transformative leadership in its advancement towards nurturing an inclusive institutional culture embracing diversity.

Agile Structures and Processes

Agility is the ability of an organization to respond to the needs and wants at a particular time without compromising the quality of the product or service in a cost-effective manner (Ganguly et al., 2009). An organization's agility can be achieved through continuous observations of market conditions and adapting strategies and functions in line with the internal and external environments of the organization. According to Wendler (2016), organizational agility can be classified under three broad categories. The first is agility related to organization which includes norms, beliefs, values, and principles shared among the stakeholders of an organization. The second is people agility consisting of the workforce's capabilities and strategies to manage the changes. The third is structure-enhancing agility, where the organization can adapt to the changing market conditions by making necessary changes quickly and efficiently (Crocitto & Youssef, 2003).

Stakeholder Inclusiveness

Organizational leadership plays an essential role in bringing all the stakeholders (internal and external) together to form an all-inclusive structure. Higher educational institutes are known to maintain the relationship with different stakeholders inside and outside the institute (Vasyakin et al., 2016) based on their involvement (active or passive), location (internal or external), cooperation potential, and exercise of influence over the working of the institution (Avci et al., 2015). Mukerjee (2014) explains that educational institutions showcase partner agility through collaboration with industry stakeholders through engaging in research, internships, and placement programs. They demonstrate customer agility by banking on the feedback generated by multigenerational consumers on the changing requirements in terms of ideas, competencies, and skillsets that the employers will seek in the students (Kiraka et al., 2020). Thus, stakeholder inclusion is essential in bringing about agile structures and processes in higher educational institutions similar to any business organization.

Distributed Leadership

McCully and McDaniel (2007) explain that leadership in agile organizations should be distributed across different levels and not be centralized to understand and respond to the changes essential for effective functioning. Higher education institutions, similar to business organizations, flourish when they foster a shared vision, mission, and collaborations, aligning the structures and process according to changing global dynamics under the stewardship of a flexible and dynamic leader in terms of decision-making. According to Mukerjee (2014), the decision-making process in higher education institutions is primarily under the control of leadership presiding over different committees or departments. This multilevel governance under dynamic leadership is critical towards achieving the environment of shared learning through collaboration and cooperation. Thus, distributed leadership, stakeholder inclusion, and agile structures and processes formulate the foundation for a transformative leadership working towards realizing the larger good for the educational system in developing countries. These are achieved by attaining collective goals grounded under community-based objectives for integrated learning and collaborative wellbeing.

Transformative Leadership

The concept of transformational leadership was introduced by James V. Downton in 1973 and further developed by Burns (2004), who explains that transformational leadership can be witnessed when "leaders and followers make each other advance to a higher level of morality and motivation." Transformational leaders inspire their colleagues, followers, and stakeholders to work towards the common goals and objectives, going beyond their areas of interest by motivating them and changing how they perceive and expect things to happen in the organization. They bring about change in the organization by practicing and articulating energizing vision and objectives for the organization instead of just preaching about the need to transition. They work towards the overall benefit and advancement of the organization. Transformational leaders enhance the morale, performance, and motivation of their colleagues and stakeholders in an organization through their mission, vision, skills, and attitude and garner the trust, admiration, and respect of their counterparts (Bass, 1985). It is the indispensable need of the stakeholders in an organization that, along with inspirational leadership that helps them guide through the uncertain environment, requires leadership that challenges them, inspires them, empowers them, and, consequently, nurtures them into becoming loyal, hardworking, aspirational individuals. This leadership emerges from charismatic, inspirational leaders who constantly work towards strengthening the organization's culture by motivating and encouraging the stakeholders.

The four components of transformational leadership known as the four I's are explained below:

- **Idealized Influence (II)**—the leader is admired for being an ideal role model for colleagues and stakeholders by following the principle of walking the talk. He/she challenges and motivates them to perform well and take ownership of their actions. The followers trust the leader and are motivated by the qualities of the transformational leader.
- **Inspirational Motivation (IM)**—through their vision and mission, transformational leaders inspire and encourage the different stakeholders in an organization. Through the idealized influence and emotional motivation, a transformational leader can convince his/her followers who aspire to attain their leader's charisma.
- **Individualized Consideration (IC)**—the transformational leader is always ready for understanding and helping the followers with their needs and feelings and has genuine concern towards them. He/she helps them self-actualize their aspirations by motivating them to work hard and achieve the goals and objectives by giving them personalized attention. This personalization helps the leader in garnering the trust of the stakeholders in the organization. An example of transformational leadership through individualized consideration can be a situation where a leader points out the issues and problems of a particular member in a group and, consequently, helps the member work towards rectifying the problem through training and inspiration. Here, the team members help each other through working together, generating positive outcomes leading to progress in the work through the constant support of the leader.
- **Intellectual Stimulation (IS)**—by constantly challenging the organization's members, the leader generates higher performance levels by being creative and innovative. A transformational leader is never a soft leader. Instead, he/she inspires the members to be open to challenges for achieving their true potential.

Transformational Leadership in Higher Education

Educational leaders and instructors should use transformational leadership as a model to lead by example. Transformational leadership places a high emphasis on forming strong community ties that motivate both students and instructors to achieve higher levels of success. Therefore, it is used by educational leaders and teachers as a model to lead by example. Two leading figures in transformational leadership theory, Bass and Avolio (1994) describe these leaders as individuals who mentor, encourage, and inspire all the stakeholders associated with educational institutions (students, colleagues, and staff). Bass and Avolio (1994) view transformational leadership as a crucial building block for the relationship development among different stakeholders in an organization. It helps form a nurturing environment leading to the growth and expansion of the learning community as it builds on the stakeholders' combined efforts. A transformational leader inspires all stakeholders to become a better version of themselves. They direct their energy and attention towards the increased efficiency and working of the educational community. In this process of motivating and inspiring the members and stakeholders, the transformational leader forgoes his/her self-interest and self-promotion, allocating utmost attention to the development and advancement of the educational institution keeping in mind the vision and mission. Instilling a passion for change and challenging the status quo following the changing world educational environments, a transformational leader motivates all the stakeholders to achieve the larger goal of developing a sense of community in education and capacity building for the younger generations to come.

Characteristics of Transformational Leadership

Thomas J. Sergiovanni (1984) focuses on five aspects of transformational leadership: cultural, symbolic, educational, human, and technical. These aspects collectively emphasize the need for passion for overall development instead of just the educational aspect. The technical element focuses on good strategic management practices where planning and organization play an essential part. Change in learning and education patterns becomes challenging and trying for an educational institution when the leadership and stakeholders are less effective and less evidence-based. The social and interpersonal resources available in the educational institution's setting constitute the human aspect. These resources help improve the morale and motivation among different stakeholdersS, where the participatory decision-making process helps bring in transformational leadership. Under the educational element, transformational leadership brings professional competence and effective implementation of teaching strategies. By finding and evaluating the problems within the educational design of the institution and providing practical solutions to them through collaboration with different stakeholders, leaders bring about change that is in line with the changing quality standards of education across the globe. The transformational leadership theory recognizes instructors and stakeholders as playing an essential role of being the bearers and conveyors of rituals, traditions, norms, and beliefs of the educational institutions. Therefore, they act as the symbolic leaders of the institutional community. This symbolic meaning attached to the leadership helps bring about the best possible ecosystem for the institution where learning and personal growth are supported. Shared values, beliefs, and practices in higher education institutions form the cultural aspect of transformational leadership (Agbo et al., 2020). It helps in articulating the vision and mission of the institution and the mythos of the educational milieu.

According to Avolio et al. (1991), transformational leadership risks elevating leaders to the level where they are indispensable. To avoid a situation when the withdrawal or going away of one member leads to the crumbling of the institution's structures, transformational leaders help build and strengthen the institution through participatory dialogue among stakeholders and not accruing any power to themselves. Thus, a genuinely transformative leadership would develop educational institutions where there is a participatory, collaborative culture at all levels.

Implications

Culture plays a significant role in developing leadership in an organization, especially in emerging and developing market economies. The present chapter deals with the cultural influence in the development of transformational leadership in the institutes of higher education in these developing countries, where a considerable gap in terms of quality of education. An instructor who works towards bringing about change in educational quality while adhering to the symbolic meaning, values, vision, and mission of the educational institution nurtures the youth by assisting them with generating a framework that can help them find their passions.

The implications about the role of culture in higher education for emerging economies are at three levels: policymaking, societal, and scholarly development. Policymakers would use collectivistic culture promoting an inclusive environment for all in the higher education institutions in emerging and developing market countries' collaborations. Continuous interaction between different stakeholders (internal and external) will create avenues for socialization and formulate a comprehensive community value-driven policy where symbolic meanings are derived from across cultures. This amalgamation of values derived from different cultures in higher educational institutions could only be possible through transformational leadership, which collaborates with all stakeholders.

At a societal level, the continuous interactions among internal and external stakeholders navigated through leaders transforming the relationship between different cultures and subcultures of the emerging and developing countries would result in the overall capacity building and upliftment of communities' standards to global level. At the academic development level, this chapter has contributed to bridging the gap between quality education in developed and developing countries by identifying mobile phones as a valuable criterion for education attainment in emerging economies to allow for greater access to a more interactive learning ecosystem. This ecosystem results from low-context cultural amalgamation based on collaborations where agile leadership plays an important role. This leadership engages with different stakeholders, understands changing market conditions, and adapts strategies and functions that align with the collective institutional education development (fostering new and innovative instructional techniques) in emerging and developing countries.

Conclusion

The COVID-19 pandemic has affected the overall development and advancement of world economies. However, the emerging and developing economies have been the worst hit worldwide. These economies, unlike the developed economies, do not have the adequate resources and infrastructure to deal with a pandemic (Mogaji & Jain, 2020). This chapter focuses on the role of culture in bringing about transformational leadership and argues that culture plays a significant role in advancing higher education in emerging and developing countries. The collectivist and collaborative learning environment among students would help bridge the gap between developed and developing countries, bringing the amalgamation of different cultures, shared values, and beliefs resulting in the formation of agile higher education institutions with agile structures and processes under transformational leadership. The chapter calls for transformational leadership in emerging and developing economies and provides theoretical and practical insights from live examples. Countries such as Nigeria and India focus on the need for technological advancements in higher educational institutions, primarily in a mobile learning environment providing education to every young aspiring individual. This transformational leadership will help attain the institutional purpose that focuses on integrated learning, collective goals, community-oriented objectives, and collective wellbeing. This goal will support maintaining quality standards in higher education through the interactive and socializing process.

References

Agbo, F. J., Olawumi, O., Oyelere, S. S., Kolog, E. A., Olaleye, S. A., Agjei, R. O., & Olawuni, A. (2020). Social media usage for computing education: The effect of tie strength and group communication on perceived learning outcome. *International Journal of Education and Development using Information and Communication Technology, 16*(1), 5–26.

Athavale, E. (2020, April 15). Six predictions for higher education in a post COVID-19 world. McKim Communications Group. Retrieved April 26, 2021, from https://mckimcg.ca/ideas/six-predictions-for-higher-education-in-a-post-covid-19-world/

Avci, Ö., Ring, E., & Mitchell, L. (2015). Stakeholder in U.S higher education: An analysis through two theories of stakeholders. *Bilgi Ekonomisi ve Yönetimi Dergisi, 10*(2).

Avolio, B. J., Waldman, D. A., & Yammarino, F. J. (1991). Leading in the 1990s: The Four I's of transformational leadership. *Journal of European Industrial Training, 15*(4). https://doi.org/10.1108/03090599110143366

Bass, B. M. (1985). Leadership: Good, better, best. *Organizational Dynamics, 13*(3), 26–40. https://doi.org/10.1016/0090-2616(85)90028-2

Bass, B. M., & Avolio, B. J. (1994). *Improving organizational effectiveness through transformational leadership*. SAGE.

Burns, J. M. (2004). *Transforming leadership: A new pursuit of happiness*. Grove Press.

Castiello-Gutiérrez, S. (2019). Beyond the melting pot: International students on campus. Inside Higher Ed. Retrieved April 26, 2021, from https://www.insidehighered.com/blogs/world-view/beyond-melting-pot-international-students-campus

Crocitto, M., & Youssef, M. (2003). The human side of organizational agility. *Industrial Management & Data Systems, 103*(6), 388–397. https://doi.org/10.1108/02635570310479963

Dill, D. D. (1982). The management of academic culture: Notes on the management of meaning and social integration. *Higher Education, 11*(3), 303–320.

Ganguly, A., Nilchiani, R., & Farr, J. V. (2009). Evaluating agility in corporate enterprises. *International Journal of Production Economics, 118*(2), 410–423. https://doi.org/10.1016/j.ijpe.2008.12.009

Govindarajan, V., & Srivastava, A. (2020, March 31). What the shift to virtual learning could mean for the future of higher ed. *Harvard Business Review*. Retrieved April 26, 2021, from https://hbr.org/2020/03/what-the-shift-to-virtual-learning-could-mean-for-the-future-of-higher-ed

Hall, E. T. (1976). How cultures collide. *Psychology Today, 10*(2), 66.

Hinson, R., & Mogaji, E. (2020). Co-creation of value by universities and prospective students: Towards an informed decision-making process. In E. Mogaji, F. Maringe, & R. Hinson (Eds.), *Higher education marketing in Africa* (pp. 17–46). Palgrave Macmillan.

Hofstede, G. (2001). *Culture's consequences: Comparing values, behaviors, institutions and organizations across nations*. SAGE Publications.

Howells, J. R., Karataş-Özkan, M., Yavuz, Ç., & Atiq, M. (2014). University management and organisational change: A dynamic institutional perspective. *Cambridge Journal of Regions, Economy and Society, 7*(2), 251&270.

Kalkan, Ü., Altınay Aksal, F., Altınay Gazi, Z., Atasoy, R., & Dağlı, G. (2020). The relationship between school administrators' leadership styles, school culture, and organizational image. *Sage Open, 10*(1), 2158244020902081.

Kezar, A. (2017). Leadership in higher education, concepts and theories. In J. C. Shin & P. Teixeira (Eds.), *Encyclopedia of international higher education systems and institutions* (pp. 1–8). Springer Netherlands. https://doi.org/10.1007/978-94-017-9553-1_537-1

Kieu, T., Mogaji, E., Mwebesa, C., Sarofim, S., Soetan, T., & Vululleh, S. P. (2020). Marketing higher education in Africa: Moving from research to practice. In E. Mogaji, F. Maringe, & R. Hinson (Eds.), *Strategic marketing of higher education in Africa* (pp. 221–237). Routledge.

Kiraka, R., Maringe, F., Kanyutu, W., & Mogaji, E. (2020). University league tables and ranking systems in Africa: Emerging prospects, challenges and opportunities. In E. Mogaji, F. Maringe, & R. Hinson (Eds.), *Understanding the higher education market in Africa*. Routledge Studies in Marketing. Routledge. ISBN 978-0367344382.

Kuzminov, Y., Sorokin, P., & Froumin, I., 2019. Generic and specific skills as components of human capital: New challenges for education theory and practice. *Форсайт, 13*(2 (eng)).

Lake, F., & Buelow, R. (2021). From surviving to thriving. *Insider Higher Ed*. Retrieved April 26, 2021, from https://www.insidehighered.com/views/2021/01/06/pandemic-has-forced-institutions-reckon-value-higher-education-student-perspective

Lewis, T., Marginson, S., & Snyder, I. (2005). The network university? Technology, culture and organisational complexity in contemporary higher education. *Higher Education Quarterly, 59*(1), 56–75. https://doi.org/10.1111/j.1468-2273.2005.00281.x

Li, H., Sajjad, N., Wang, Q., Muhammad Ali, A., Khaqan, Z., & Amina, S. (2019). Influence of transformational leadership on employees' innovative work behavior in sustainable organizations: Test of mediation and moderation processes. *Sustainability, 11*(6), 1594.

Maassen, P. A. M. (1996). The concept of culture and higher education. *Tertiary Education and Management, 2*(2), 153–159. https://doi.org/10.1007/BF02354009

Manikutty, S., Anuradha, N. S., & Hansen, K. (2007). Does culture influence learning styles in higher education? *International Journal of Learning and Change, 2*(1), 70–87.

Masland, A. T. (1985). Organizational culture in the study of higher education. *The Review of Higher Education, 8*(2), 157–168. https://doi.org/10.1353/rhe.1985.0026

McCarthy, N., (2020). COVID-19's staggering impact on global education. *World Economic Forum*. https://www.weforum.org/agenda/2020/03/infographic-covid19-coronavirus-impact-global-education-health-schools/

McCully, M. S., & McDaniel, E. A. (2007). College transformation through enabling agility. *Issues in Informing Science & Information Technology, 4*, 703–712.

Mogaji, E., & Jain, V. (2020). Impact of the pandemic on higher education in emerging economies: Emerging opportunities, challenges and research agenda. *SSRN*. http://apers.ssrn.com/sol3/papers.cfm?abstract_id=3622592

Moody's. (2020). Moody's – Covid-19 puts pressure on higher education finances. *Moody's*. https://www.moodys.com/research/Moodys-Covid-19-puts-pressure-on-higher-education-finances%2D%2DPBC_122296.3

Mukerjee, S. (2014). Agility: A crucial capability for universities in times of disruptive change and innovation. Australian Universities' Review, National Tertiary Education Union (NTEU). Retrieved April 25, 2021, from https://search.informit.org/doi/abs/10.3316/ielapa.870516339761060

Naqshbandi, M. M., Tabche, I., & Choudhary, N. (2019). Managing open innovation: The roles of empowering leadership and employee involvement climate. *Management Decision, 57*(3), 703–723.

Ndofirepi, E., Farinloye, T., & Mogaji, E. (2020). Marketing mix in a heterogenous higher education market: A case of Africa. In E. Mogaji, F. Maringe, & R. E. Hinson (Eds.), *Understanding the higher education market in Africa*. Routledge.

Olaleye, S., Ukpabi, D., & Mogaji, E. (2020). Public vs private universities in Nigeria: Market dynamics perspective. In E. Mogaji, F. Maringe, & R. E. Hinson (Eds.), *Understanding the higher education market in Africa*. Routledge.

Ozdamli, F. (2012). Pedagogical framework of m-learning. *Procedia – Social and Behavioral Sciences, 31*, 927–931. https://doi.org/10.1016/j.sbspro.2011.12.171

Selingo, J., & Silagadze, M. (2021, January 28). The pandemic hit colleges hard, but surfaced the potential of blended learning. *Harvard Business Publishing*. Retrieved April 26, 2021, from https://hbsp.harvard.edu/inspiring-minds/the-pandemic-hit-colleges-hard-but-surfaced-the-potential-of-blended-learning

Seltzer, R. (2020, September 9). Who leads colleges after COVID-19? *Inside Higher Ed.* Retrieved April 26, 2021, from https://www.insidehighered.com/news/2020/09/09/what-college-presidents-say-about-leading-covid-19-era

Sergiovanni, T. J. (1984). Leadership and excellence in schooling. Report No Pub Date Note Available from, 41, 45.

Tierney, W. G. (1988). Organizational culture in higher education. *The Journal of Higher Education, 59*(1), 2–21. https://doi.org/10.1080/00221546.1988.11778301

Vasudeva, S., & Mogaji, E. (2020). Paving the way for world domination: Analysis of African universities' mission statement. In *Understanding the higher education market in Africa* (pp. 145–167). Routledge.

Vasyakin, B. S., Ivleva, M. I., Pozharskaya, Y. L., & Shcherbakova, O. I. (2016). A Study of the Organizational Culture at a Higher Education Institution [Case Study: Plekhanov Russian University of Economics (PRUE)]'. *International Journal of Environmental and Science Education, 11*(10), 11515–11528.

Wendler, R. (2016). Dimensions of organizational agility in the software and IT service industry: Insights from an empirical investigation. *Communications of the Association for Information Systems, 39*(1). https://doi.org/10.17705/1CAIS.03921

Zhong, K. (2020). A research on the effect of learner attribution on performance under the mediation of online learning environment. *Journal of Educational Technology Development and Exchange, 13*(1), 21&38 https://doi.org/10.18785/jetde.1301.02

14

Universities' Endowments in Developing Countries: The Perspectives, Stakeholders and Practical Implications

Nguyen Phong Nguyen and Emmanuel Mogaji

Introduction

An endowment is a collection of assets invested to generate revenue for a non-profit organisation or to support specified activities (Stepanova et al., 2020). It has become common for higher education institutions, such as colleges and universities, to rely on permanently invested funds to yield income for current expenses.

Endowments originated in England in the fifteenth and sixteenth centuries, and they have supported colleges and universities for over three centuries (Kimball & Johnson, 2012). The development of endowments can be traced back to the United States (US), and the longest record of investment belongs to Harvard College (Histphil, 2017). Harvard College is the undergraduate college of Harvard University. Despite recent studies highlighting the

N. P. Nguyen
School of Accounting, University of Economics Ho Chi Minh City, Ho Chi Minh City, Vietnam
e-mail: nguyenphongnguyen@ueh.edu.vn

E. Mogaji (✉)
Department of Marketing, Events and Tourism, University of Greenwich, London, UK
e-mail: e.o.mogaji@greenwich.ac.uk

E. Mogaji et al. (eds.), *Re-imagining Educational Futures in Developing Countries*,
https://doi.org/10.1007/978-3-030-88234-1_14

significance of endowments in higher education, the fundamental significance of, competition of and emphasis on its increments were not recognised until the 1890s and then again in the 1930s (Histphil, 2017). During this period, certain institutions, including the Harvard and Yale universities, increased their financial capital to establish an upper tier of endowed universities (Kimball & Johnson, 2012). Their elite statuses have lasted for over a century.

Many universities—especially in the Western world—were established as a result of the concept of endowments. Learning institutions have different motivations for taking endowments, and available data indicates that over 43 per cent of non-profit organisations have received endowments (Calabrese & Ely, 2017). Higher education institutions receive the most endowment assets—about 64 per cent—with other education non-profits, such as private secondary and elementary schools, following. About 33 per cent of endowment funds held by learning institutions are unrestricted, while permanently restricted funds account for 41 per cent (Calabrese & Ely, 2017). Among these institutions, the average annual pay-out rates exceed 5 per cent. These rates cover, on average, 4.1 per cent of the institutions' net organisational expenses, signifying how much higher education institutions depend on endowment revenue (Calabrese & Ely, 2017).

The power of generous provisions for higher education in the form of endowments has led some governments to the conclusion that endowments offer the only means to finance higher education (Mahamood & Ab Rahman, 2015). This form of funding causes the higher education sector to be less dependent on a single source of funding (Olaleye et al., 2020). Some countries, such as Israel, generate a large quantity of resources through endowments. These endowments mainly come from the global diaspora community, which operates under the umbrella of overseas registered non-profit organisations. In 2000, the American Friends of the Hebrew University raised over $600 million (Teferra, 2015). Chinese universities have also opted for similar ventures despite less organised and robust initiatives. A suitable example of this is the Peking University Education Foundation, and part of this foundation (regarding North America) focuses on strengthening the ties between the university in question and all the areas of North America to raise funds and promote technological, cultural and educational cooperation (Teferra, 2015).

This chapter recognises the benefits of endowment for universities, especially during the pandemic, which has caused global health challenges. Universities' source of income has been affected. In particular, for many universities in developing countries, it is becoming vital that they seek additional sources of income to remain viable. Therefore, the aim of this research is to contextualise endowments in developing countries during the Covid-19 pandemic and to provide practical recommendations for key stakeholders. This chapter presents a theoretical framework for stakeholders who are involved in managing the endowment process. We identify four stakeholders: the endowment provider, the endowed university, the endowment team and the endowment enablers. We highlight the managerial implications for university managers who are exploring endowments as an additional source of income.

The subsequent section provides an overview of endowments in higher education. This is followed by a specific focus on the endowments in the higher education institutions of developing countries. The need for endowments is identified in the subsequent chapters, and the four stakeholders in the endowment process are presented. The concluding section provides an overview of the discussion.

Endowments in Higher Education

An endowment involves assets that are invested to generate a steady income stream for universities (Baum & Lee, 2019). Notable examples of endowments include the $3.5 million property grant that was given to Johns Hopkins University in 1873 and the $34.7 million that was given to the University of Chicago by Rockefeller in 1910 (Kimball & Johnson, 2012). According to Lerner et al. (2008), the top 20 endowment values have grown each year, and by 2007, the largest endowments were $35 billion for Harvard University and $22 billion for Yale University.

Initially, an endowment income was regarded as a dividend income or as interest, but legal and regulatory practices have been updated to include a loss of assets and unrealised gains. Endowment accumulation is of key interest for higher education institutions; it can act as a great source of tax revenue, especially during a period of budget constraints. Endowment funds are mostly established by donor-restricted gifts and bequests to provide permanent sources of income or as a short-term source of income for an institution (Calabrese & Ely, 2017). Endowments are utilised as rainy-day funds that help an institution to sustain certain programmes during tough economic periods. They comprise both restricted and unrestricted funds, whereby an institution can only spend earnings that have been accumulated from the assets of the former type of fund (Bowman, 2002). Under temporary restrictions, an institution can only spend its donations after a certain period or after the occurrence of a particular event. Unrestricted endowments can be designated as quasi-endowments—they lack binding restrictions, yet the board still proceeds with caution when spending the funds (Sloan et al., 2016). During financial difficulties, institutions may require a court's approval to use restricted endowments as collateral for borrowing, which is based on the fact that it may be permissible to collateralise endowment funds and loan proceeds when they are used in strict adherence to the donor's intent (Mason & Caufield, 2010). An example of an institution requiring court approval is the Seattle Arts Museum—case no. 10-2-30952-7—in 2010 (Calabrese & Ely, 2017).

According to Gentry (2002), the tax arbitrage incentives associated with endowments generate an increased use of tax-exempt borrowing by non-profit organisations due to their being defined as net assets. This motivation arises from the influence of special tax rules that enable the state's authorities to issue tax-exempt bonds, which affect financing and investment decisions. These tax exemptions are common in non-profit organisations that offer various social services. This enables higher education institutions to increase their investment portfolio through physical assets and, when the need arises, engage in tax arbitrage opportunities by capitalising on tax-exempt debts while retaining their endowment assets (Gentry, 2002).

Endowments are also regarded as investments that increase leverage on decisions related to borrowing. The management of endowments can be complex; some institutions may decide to manage the funds through separate entities (Baum & Lee, 2019). This restricts a board from inappropriately collecting endowment funds during emergencies. Since non-profit organisations can hold endowments in several separate legal entities, using a separate entity provides leeway to aggregate the investments for efficient management.

The general description of endowments can refer to a single fund despite comprising a collection of discrete funds. These discrete funds have individual stipulations concerning the purposes for which they can be used. The public's attention is usually focused on the small number of higher education institutionsS that have large endowments, but most institutions have either modest endowments or none at all (ACE, 2021). Most public universities have minimal endowments despite ranking among the largest beneficiaries. Endowments include funds provided by donors with the main condition that the principal fund should not be spent—this is under the expectation that its value will increase over time. An increase in their value arises from a responsible balance between the expenditure and reinvestment of the fund. Endowments can be invested in different ways, including stocks, real estate and bonds as well as other illiquid assets, such as hedge funds (ACE, 2021). Trustees oversee the allocation and management of these assets, and they are under a legal obligation to prudently manage the investment.

The increased sophistication in investments in recent years, fuelled by market changes, has led to the inclusion of non-traditional investments, such as venture capital and other natural resources, in endowment funds' investment portfolios. Most endowments in higher education institutions yield earnings that are exempt from taxation. This tax exemption is based on the recognition of the public functions served by these institutions. It also increases the confidence of donors; they are confident that the institution in question will use their endowment to support its designated purposes. The tax exemption is also as the result of the institution's societal contribution toward supporting higher education in the specified country.

The management of these endowments is mostly at the discretion of the institution. In most cases, the institution devises rules and strategies to maximise the endowment's potential, which will help to support current and future spending needs (ACE, 2021). Some institutions manage these funds with their own staff, while others depend on contracted professional managers or trustees. Formal spending rules are common in most institutions, which ensure a flowing stream of revenue from the endowments and sufficient reinvestments to support the endowments' value over time (Hinson & Mogaji, 2020).

Endowments in Higher Education in Developing Countries

Among developing countries, South Africa has been one of the main countries that has capitalised on endowments (Teferra, 2015). These endowments account for the recent drive in the development of scholarly institutions and programmes. Overseas partners, such as the UCT Trust of the United Kingdom (UK) and of the US, respectively, are major contributors toward achieving development by means of endowments. Through a significant raising of funds, universities have been able to initiate or continue building endowments for other chairs of universities. The collaboration between philanthropic institutions accounts for the major endowment initiatives that have been channelled toward African higher education institutions (Teferra, 2015). These philanthropic institutions have committed endowment grants for higher education institutions in Egypt, South Africa and Kenya. An analysis of this activity in selected universities of these three countries indicates that endowments in developing countries can be managed appropriately, can contribute to the institution's viability and can increase collaborations between the faculty, its students and its administrators.

In Peru, rationalisation from the credit markets has meant that institutions are dependent on endowments to finance the direct and opportunity costs of education (Castro et al., 2016). The Peru State College is among the higher education institutions that are benefiting from endowments in Latin America. It had an endowment that valued in the region of $13.8 million at the end of the 2019 fiscal year, and the return on this endowment was $276,000, accounting for 1.9 per cent, which was below the 4.44 per cent average (Data USA, 2021). The Brazil Foundation is conducting a similar initiative by transforming engineering education in Brazil. This foundation was inspired by the endowments in renowned American universities and has supported over 60 projects and impacted 3500 students through $20 million in donations, which was raised in the nine years following its establishment (Brazil Foundation, 2018).

The National University of Singapore (NUS) has received the largest university endowment to date, which was valued at $1.05 billion in 2008 (Ong, 2009). The NUS is considered the most successful fundraiser, having accumulated $227 million in donations in 2018 alone. According to Singapore Minister Ong Ye Kung, Singaporean universities have been building endowments over the last 20 years, and their endowments are not excessively large when compared to other international universities (Tan, 2019). In contrast, endowments are not common in India, yet the increasing costs of education have compelled some Indian institutions to scale up efforts to increase endowments (Parmar, 2011).

Endowments are essential to higher education institutions. Most of the institutions in this Southeast Asian region have followed European educational policies, but the growing costs of education have compelled them to recover some of these costs from their students. According to a 2011 report by the World Bank, the escalating costs of education in North Africa have been the result of an increasing demand for higher education, the higher education sector's inability to compete with other economic sectors and increments in the overall educational cost per student (Khemani, 2020). The report further highlights that education is a labour-intensive sector, owing to the immense labour required to combat resistance to advancements in productivity.

It has also been established that countries in North Africa lack adequate administrative capacities to increase revenue through taxation or to effectively collect imposed taxes. Such a challenge results in a reduction in how much funding is available to support higher education, for most institutions rely on governments for additional funding. The policies involved in mass higher education, adopted since the 1960s, are a major cause of the crises implicated in financing higher education (Khemani, 2020). These challenges make it necessary for higher education institutions to consider endowments as another suitable source of funding (Ndofirepi et al., 2020).

The Need for Endowments in Higher Education

Endowment funds serve as a financial buffer to cushion an institution against periodic hardships that arise from business cycles (Hansmann, 1990). They also serve to maintain its long-term organisational reputation as well as allowing the passage of particular standards between generations of decision-makers. Endowments, especially in a higher education setting, reflect the donors' desire to contribute to the institution's long-term viability. In developing countries, higher education institutions do not have as many sources of income or endowments; endowments therefore serve as contributors toward long-term viability (Robinson & Maitra, 2020). This situation leads to the deduction that endowments can serve as reserves for smoothing out fluctuations in revenue and other forms of support. Income arising from endowments establishes a spending limit so as to prevent the ceasing of basic services despite not being able to offset spending cutbacks or to replace additional operating revenues.

Permanent endowments impact the perpetual success and perceived quality of education in higher education institutions (Kimball & Johnson, 2012). This impact is associated with the benefits of endowments in enhancing the autonomy and competitive advantage of the university in the long term. In most universities, major sources of revenue, such as grants, tuition fees or gifts for current expenditure, deplete immediately, which means that the institutions have to depend directly on external support. Endowments allow an institution to expand its self-determination capability by availing revenue that is directly controlled by the university (Kimball & Johnson, 2012). The revenue generated from these ventures enhances stability in the institution due to its associated reliability and facilitates long-term and short-term planning. Additionally, larger endowments enhance the capacity to pursue discretionary goals and other opportunities, which increase an institution's comparative advantage against its competition. This support for competition between higher education institutions is especially important to enhance the quality of service delivery. The comparative advantage arising from larger endowments is mainly associated with increases in accomplishments and elevated prestige.

The increasing costs of education for succeeding generations account for another crucial factor that contributes to endowments (Mogaji & Varsha, 2020). This increase in costsS is associated with a lack of increments in productivity in the educational sector compared to other goods (Hansmann, 1990). These escalating costs imply that if other funding sources remain constant, they would only cover a smaller fraction of the cost of education. These changes suggest that the real value of endowments must be increased over time. The cumulative amount of real income spent from the endowment annually will also rise at a rate that is just sufficient to cover a significant portion of the cost of education (Hansmann, 1990). Since the demand for education is inelastic, stronger endowments are the only suitable option to compensate for the increase in costs associated with enrolment rates. Increasing endowments will also help to retain the endowment's income as a constant fraction of the cumulative cost of education.

Endowments can serve as a suitable tool for educational fundraising in entrepreneurial universities. The rise in entrepreneurial universities in recent decades has been associated with social transformations (Krasulia, 2014). These transformations have escalated the priorities accorded to higher education institutions regarding public policy developments in both developing and developed countries. Therefore, countries are now paying greater attention to this situation in the higher education system to devise the most effective ways to help these institutions survive the crisis, develop and implement their knowledge-imparting mission and strengthen the scientific and regional potential of the country and region. Historically, endowments have been regarded as the most suitable form of educational fundraising (Krasulia, 2014). The current situation, in terms of market relations, has led to a decrease in funding for higher education institutions. This change comes alongside an increase in competition in the educational service market, which has resulted in an urgent need for universities in developing countries to diversify their sources of income (Mogaji & Varsha, 2020; Sharma et al., 2021).

Fundraising through endowments involves soliciting funds from different donors, including charity funds, alumni, friends and corporations. Endowments are a key mechanism of educational fundraising and represent the number of financial assets donated to higher education institutions and those invested to yield profits on the principal, which are used to finance various operations (Krasulia, 2014). This is based on the donors' individual philanthropic motives. For instance, alumni may donate based on the desire to aid their alma mater or as a token of appreciation for the education that they received. Foundations are mainly motivated by the need to support the research activities that are carried out in the universities; they provide crucial financial support to the research and educational processes that are intended to achieve certain defined goals (Krasulia, 2014). Corporations also channel their support toward higher education institutions due to their interest in qualified young professionals. These different motives among donors demonstrate the different aspects of educational fundraising. The effective utilisation of endowments as a form of educational fundraising accounts for a significant source of income for higher education institutions to fund their daily operations.

According to Stepanova et al. (2020), endowments are a suitable tool for fundraising in research universities as they play a crucial role in the country's innovative development. Innovative development is of major significance to developing countries due to its contributions to the economy. Research universities promote education, incorporate scientific systems and shift technology into production. As a fundraising tool for higher education institutions, endowments fulfil the main principles of fundraising activities. These principles include transparency, honesty, integrity, empathy and respect (Stepanova et al., 2020). Fundraising in higher education institutions helps to accomplish the major functions of public charities, including solving social issues and supporting crucial social development programmes. This is in line with the principles of voluntariness, irretrievability and gratuitousness. Endowments also account for the most effective modern educational fundraising tools, which world practice has confirmed. They enable research universities to transition to new quantitative levels and establish a business–science–society relationship. Thus, educational endowments have a direct impact on the innovative economic development of a country.

The pandemic has exposed the need for new sources of funding in higher education. This assertion is based on the observation that the challenges brought about by this healthcare emergency have had far-reaching impacts on the sources of funding for universities. In many developing countries, governments have had to redirect funding toward mitigating the pandemic's socio-economic impact as well as fulfilling the health sector's requirements (Friga, 2020). The re-appropriation of funds implies that there will be fewer financial resources available for the governments to support higher education institutions. This scarcity of funds may be a key reason for higher education institutions to capitalise on endowments as a more viable source of funding after the pandemic. According to former World Bank tertiary education coordinator Jamil Salmi, there is an urgent need for African universities to design and implement a sustainable financing strategy to support their higher education systems. This observation is based on the postulation that African universities will be hit hard by the economic recession resulting from the pandemic, as will be the case in other parts of the world.

According to Krishnamurthy (2020), the economic and social challenges arising from the Covid-19 pandemic have led to many rapid changes in the higher education sector. Some of these changes are associated with the unpredictability of key factors in higher education, such as enrolment rates. This uncertainty implies that many institutions will face financial pressures as a result of the inability to ascertain the exact financial contributions from students in the form of tuition fees and other levies. Blankenberger and Williams (2020) also established that the Covid-19 crisis came when funding in higher education was already in decline. Many countries have reduced higher education funding in the midst of growing budget challenges.

Further cuts to budgets fuelled by the pandemic will have serious implications on degree completion and other educational attainment factors in higher education. Major universities, such as Harvard University, anticipate an increase in demand for financial aid based on the economic fallout caused by the pandemic (Blankenberger & Williams, 2020). This situation is faced by both developed and developing countries, but the developing countries may be worse off compared to developed countries. In the context of these uncertainties, universities will have to evaluate additional funding sources, such as endowments, to enhance sustainability.

According to Robinson and M(2020), many universities will experience challenges in preserving core academic functions due to funding challenges. An increasing body of evidence indicates that higher education is in a crisis, and all sources of revenue will decrease in both public and private universities. Recent surveys indicate that four-year colleges may experience a decrease of between 10–20 per cent in enrolment rates in 2021 (Robinson & Maitra, 2020). Tax collections in many countries are also expected to not meet projections, which will result in budgets experiencing shortfalls.

Although financial challenges have escalated much faster during the pandemic, many universities had already begun to experience declines in enrolment rates due to changes in demographics. Therefore, it is sufficient to say that the Covid-19 pandemic has led to the development of a worst-case scenario in terms of funding in higher education. It is predicted that the pandemic will raise numerous existential questions for small and mid-tier institutions, which is a common characteristic in developing countries. Postulations from industry experts indicate that universities with large endowments and highly competitive admission rates are the only institutions expected to survive the funding challenges associated with the pandemic. Based on this hypothesis, it is valid to conclude that higher education institutions in developing countries must take advantage of endowments to survive the financial challenges associated with the pandemic.

Stakeholders in Higher Education Endowment Post Covid-19

Developing countries need to recognise the need for endowments and higher education and explore the prospects of endowment. With endowments for universities expected to outlive their benefactors and continue to educate students for centuries, it is important for universities to explore how they can cause them to become optimal, long-term investment entities (Achtypi et al., 2021). This section presents a theoretical framework of the stakeholders involved in managing these processes and presents practical implications, which are relevant for universities. As illustrated in Fig. 14.1, we identify four stakeholders: the endowment provider, the endowed university, endowment team and the endowment enablers.

Endowment Provider

An endowment provider is an individual, philanthropist, corporation or charity organisation who is willing to give an endowment to a university. It is important to recognise that endowment providers may come in different shapes and sizes. It will not always be a rich philanthropist in the country; it could simply be an alumnus who feels the urge to give back to their university or organisation. These endowments could be in form of cash donations or resources for teaching and research. In 1114, Markgraf (Count) Leopold III endowed Stift Klosterneuburg, a monastery near Vienna, with valuable assets that included real estate and vineyards, which still support the monastery today (Cejnek et al., 2015). These endowment providers must understand why the university deserves the endowment. This suggests that the provider may wish to be associated with the university for a specific reason, which the university must provide.

Integrating these endowments may also be utilised as a display of corporate social responsibility; the endowment provider uses an opportunity to endow a university to demonstrate their commitment to their society. Thus, these endowments are used as a way to give back to society. This can also enhance the positioning and perception of the provider; often a building that is donated as part of an endowment could be named after its provider. However,

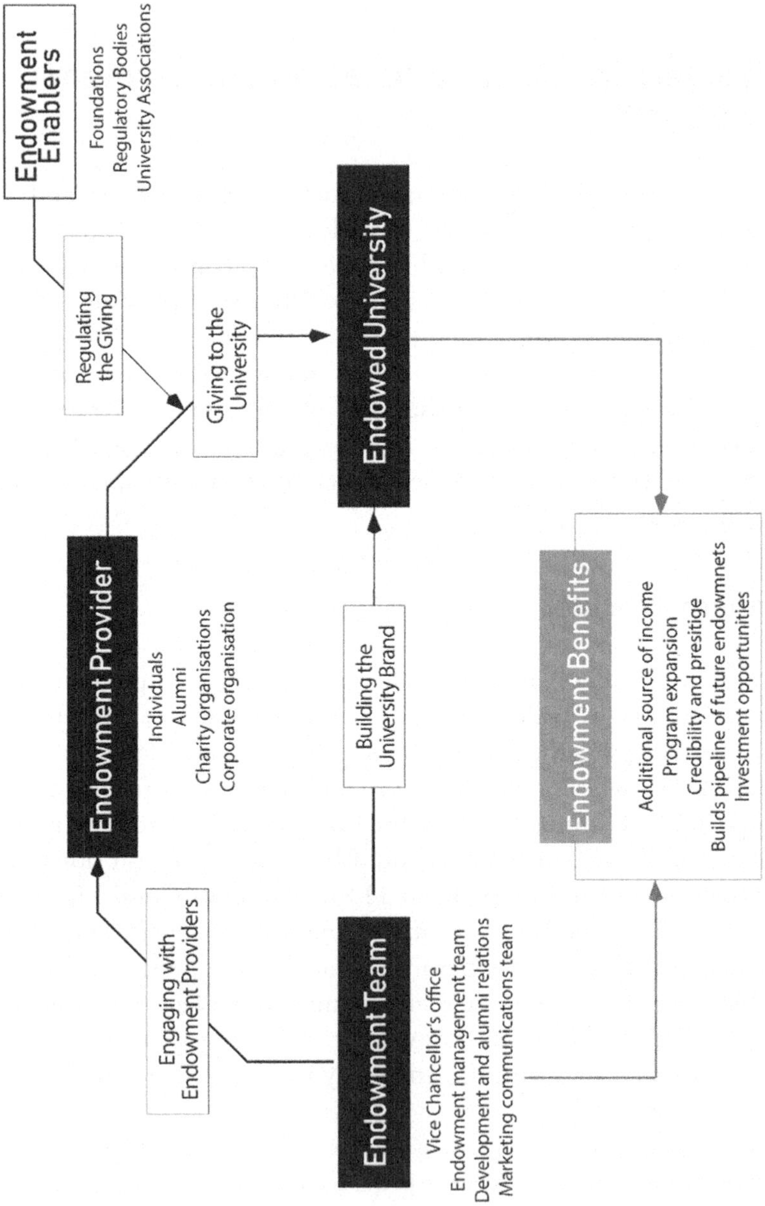

Fig. 14.1 Theoretical framework of stakeholders involved in university endowment

this also presents challenges. After Black Lives Matter protests spread across the US, many universities faced ongoing floods of petitions to change campus building names that were named to honour many endowment providers who had ties to slave ownership or racist policies (Weissman, 2020).

There are also legal implications for an endowment provider so as to ensure that they are not using the endowment as a form of money laundering and that there are no other forms of controversy attached to the individual or group. The School of Oriental and African Studies (SOAS) University of London came under much criticism when it was found that the Sultan of Brunei was introducing laws in his country that would make gay sex punishable by stoning to death. The university had to make an official statement, declaring that 'The Sultan of Brunei made a donation to SOAS in 1995 to build the gallery[,] and the gift was received before any introduction of Sharia Law in that country. The donor has no role, influence or involvement in the policy or operation of the gallery or the wider School'. In 2018, the Tate group of British art galleries also announced that they would no longer accept any gifts offered by members of the Sackler family, who own the US production of OxyContin, as this prescription painkiller was under fire amid an opioids public health crisis (Walters et al., 2019).

In certain cases, some philanthropic institutions and foundations may be restricted by fundamental policy guidelines regarding committing their resources to endowments (Eaton, 2020; Mogaji et al., 2020). Such a hindrance necessitates suitable policy interventions to eliminate these limitations and make it easier to channel endowment funds to designated institutions. The limitations can also be addressed by creating partnerships between philanthropic organisations and foundations to establish new ventures with disparate guidelines and missions in order to deflect the inherent restrictive policies that affect individual foundations.

Endowed University

There are many universities around the world, and in certain countries, that are competing for endowment funds from endowment providers. It is therefore important for a university to recognise this competition, making the effort to stand out and put themselves in a strong position to receive funds (Adeyanju et al., 2020; Kieu et al., 2020). As earlier indicated, though many of the top American universities have been endowed by different endowment providers, there are many reasons for universities in developing countries to consider endowments as a way to support their delivery of education.

No doubt, some of the more established universities in a developing country may be considered more suitable for endowment, for it will enhance how the endowment provider is perceived. Other universities must make the effort to build a reputation, becoming more recognised and presenting a compelling offer to the endowment provider (Farinloye et al., 2020). However, this will require a long-term strategy; reputations are not built in a day. A good reputation requires investments in research and development to improve the institution's ranking and worldwide recognition. A university must improve their students' experiences, producing graduates with high employability prospects and, thus, alumni who are willing to give back to their university.

Endowed universities must also consider socially responsible investing (SRI) and environmental, social and governance (ESG) investing for their endowment funds. The Hechinger Report (2020) suggests that universities can capitalise on increasing their endowment income to compensate for diminishing sources of income (Eaton, 2020). It outlines that universities can increase their endowment income by capitalising on private equity and hedge funds to manage their investments. Though it is acknowledged that endowment management is relatively rare in the UK compared to the US (OUEM, 2021), it is even rarer in developing countries, but there are still options for universities in these countries to consider. The University of Oxford is one of a handful of institutions in the UK that is fortunate to have a large enough endowment to require an investment team (OUEM, 2021). OUem Ltd is a subsidiary company of the University of Oxford. It is regulated and authorised by the UK Financial Conduct Authority and manages charitable endowments in excess of £4 billion (€4.5 billion) for over 40 investors in the Oxford Endowment Fund.

Endowment Team

Endowment teams include individuals and teams who work with endowed universities and are responsible for engaging with the endowment provider and other stakeholders. They are responsible for improving the prospects of the endowed universities. Vice chancellors (VCs) are considered the chief fundraisers for the universities. They should be able to use their office to build connections and networks with prospective endowment providers. The role of the VC as the chief fundraiser also involves leading the university in a way that will attract prospective endowment providers and making the work of other endowment teams easier.

Universities can also employ an endowment manager to lead endowment management teams. In most cases, this should be separate from the alumni's office. Endowment management teams will solely focus on securing more endowments for the university. According to the Uniform Prudent Management of Institutional Funds Act (UPMIFA) in the US, which provides fundamental rules for the investment of funds held by charitable institutions and the expenditure of funds donated, an endowment management team is expected to prudently invest endowments through diversified investments that seek growth as well as income for the university.

The alumni team also has a huge role in building connections with alumni and keeping them updated on the university. This team works on developing a database of alumni and developing effective communication. Social media will surely play a crucial role here. The alumni team, as part of the endowment team, may also work with alumni teams in different countries, allowing them the opportunity to contribute through charity organisations created in their home countries. The University of Cape Town in South Africa has registered charities and trusts in Australia, Canada, the UK and the US. These charities support and connect alumni and collect endowments and donations for the university. This intervention increases the universities' access to donors and, consequently, increases their endowment reserves.

The marketing team of a university also forms an integral part of the endowment team. It has the responsibility of placing the university in a good position for endowment, sharing positive stories about the university and creating the needed awareness. The efforts of this marketing team in shaping the reputation of the university will enhance the work of the endowment management team when reaching out to prospective endowment providers. The provider should then have seen the university and heard about what they are doing; thus, they will be more willing to work with a known organisation.

Endowment Enablers

One possible solution to increasing endowments for higher education institutions in developing countries is to mobilise the major players. Major players are described as endowment enablers. They include major foundations, who can devise initiatives to revitalise higher education in developing countries, and regulators—both financial and higher education quality regulators. An example of an endowment enabler is the initiative devised in 2000 by the Ford, Rockefeller and McArthur foundations and the Carnegie Corporation of New York. They implemented their initiative under the banner 'Partnership for Higher Education in Africa' to support selected African universities by strengthening their teaching and research capacities, infrastructure development and strategic planning activities and by holding major conferences (PHEA, 2021).

The main drive for mobilising major players to improve the higher education of developing countries is the fact that the achievements associated with higher education are crucial for a country's development. Such interventions should be continuously expanded to include more institutions and to increase the resources at its disposal. Continuous increments in endowments will also serve to ensure that the supported programmes remain stable.

These endowment enablers (particularly higher education regulatory bodies in developing countries like the University Grants Commission [UGC] in India, the National Universities Commission [NUC] in Nigeria and the Council on Higher Education [CHE] in South Africa) should create an environment that can support endowment providers in giving to and supporting the universities. These enablers should also devise mechanisms to mobilise resources of other entities combined with their committed funds regarding the endowment drive (Whitford, 2020). While a government may still fund some forms of higher education, these bodies should develop initiatives and opportunities to support the endowment drive of the universities. This will help to generate more resources from other sources, such as matching funds.

Other interventions include organising major international conferences to popularise and create awareness of the need for endowments in higher education in developing countries. These conferences will bring together major development partners, including foundations, agencies, major multinational corporations, non-governmental organisations (NGOs), private business entities and representatives of diaspora communities. The new ventures devised from such initiatives will help to attract national, regional and international attention.

Endowment Benefits

There are certain benefits to effectively exploring endowment opportunities. Newman (2005) identified significant benefits for stakeholders—especially the endowed university. The endowed university receives access to additional revenue for teaching, research and public service. With the additional funds, programmes and courses can be expanded thanks to funding for scholarships, faculty chairs, staff positions, research, facility maintenance and equipment.

This creates more opportunities for students and enhances the positioning of the university (Hagood, 2019; Newman, 2005).

Endowments create an ongoing source of income for the endowed university. In addition, the endowment status of the university enhances the reputation of the institution, attracting merits and other forms of endorsements. Endowment does not act as deterrent to other funding sources; rather, it increases the endowment provider's confidence in the university. Newman (2005) noted that a well-managed endowment suggests planned long-term stability, fiscal responsibility and financial viability, enhancing the university's prestige and credibility. This growing confidence and credibility enhance the prospect of acquiring more income (Kiraka et al., 2020; Mogaji et al., 2021).

This additional funding can also be invested to guaranteed income for many years ahead. The 2020 study of endowments by the National Association of College and University Business Officers (NACUBO) and the Teachers Insurance and Annuity Association of America (TIAA), which gathered data from 705 US colleges, universities and affiliated foundations, found that endowments' average one-year returns were 1.8 per cent and that the 10-year average reached 7.5 per cent. There are also expendable endowments that can be invested. The UK Charity Commission also recognised this: 'Expendable endowment, when invested, can provide a relatively secure stream of income[,] but the trustees also have the option of spending all, or part, of the endowment'. The return from these investments provides vital and permanent operating support to universities (Conley, 2017). A summary of these stakeholders and implications are presented in Table 14.1.

Conclusion

Universities in developing countries can implement various reforms and long-term restructuring initiatives to help mitigate the revenue shortfalls caused by the Covid-19 pandemic. These reforms will help to reduce pressure on existing endowment funds to account for a decrease in enrolment rates and a reduction in revenue from state appropriations (Robinson & Maitra, 2020). Implementing these reforms will help to preserve the core academic functions through reductions in administration costs and services and in auxiliary services.

This chapter has provided a theoretical contribution to study endowment in higher education (Calabrese & Ely, 2017; Kimball & Johnson, 2012), especially in developing countries, which is an under-researched area. Specifically, we developed a framework that highlights four stakeholders

Table 14.1 Summary of stakeholders and implications

Stakeholders	Subgroup	Implications
Endowment provider	• Individuals • Alumni • Charity organisations • Corporate organisations	• Nature of endowment—cash or gift • Legal implications • Corporate social responsibility • Brand position
Endowed university		• The university's reputation • Positioning the university to receive endowments • Creating graduates with high employability prospects and advertently alumni • SRI and ESG investing of their endowment funds
Endowment team	VC's office Endowment management team Development and alumni relations Marketing communications team	• The VC as the chief fundraiser • Endowment team focusing on getting more endowments for the university and managing existing funds • Development and alumni relations working with alumni across the world, opening and operating charity foundations. • Marketing team advertising and shaping the brand of the university
Endowment enablers	Foundations Regulatory bodies University associations	• Foundations driving funds to universities in developing countries. • Regulatory bodies to ensure funds are collected and managed ethically. • University regulatory bodies should create an environment that can support endowment providers to give to and support the universities.

involved in managing the processes of endowment. This framework shows the relationship between the endowment provider, the endowed university, the endowment team and the endowment enablers. Using this framework, university managers involved in managing the endowment process will find relevant practical implications that can enhance the process.

This study has not been contextualised in any country. This may be considered a limitation, but it opens an opportunity for future research. Empirical research into the prevalence of endowments in these developing countries is encouraged. In addition, future research should explore stakeholders' levels of perception toward and understanding of endowment. The challenges for universities in developing countries regarding seeking endowment can also be empirically explored. This understanding will further verify the theoretical framework presented in this chapter and advance knowledge regarding endowment in universities in developing countries.

References

ACE. (2021). Understanding College and University Endowments. American Council on Education. https://www.acenet.edu/Documents/Understanding-College-and-University-Endowments.pdf

Achtypi, E., Ashby, N. J. S., Brown, G. D. A., Walasek, L., & Yechiam, E. (2021). The endowment effect and beliefs about the market. *Decision, 8*(1), 16–35.

Adeyanju, S., Mogaji, E., Olusola, J., & Oyinlola, M. (2020). Factors influencing students' choice of a federal university: a case study of a Nigerian federal university. In *Higher education marketing in Africa* (pp. 135–163). Palgrave Macmillan.

Baum, S., & Lee, V. (2019). *The role of College and University endowments.* Urban Institute.

Blankenberger, B., & Williams, A. (2020). COVID and the impact on higher education: The essential role of integrity and accountability. *Administrative Theory & Praxis, 42*(3), 404–423. https://doi.org/10.1080/10841806.2020.1771907

Bowman, W. (2002). The uniqueness of nonprofit finance and the decision to borrow. *Nonprofit Management and Leadership, 12*(3), 293–311.

Brazil Foundation. (2018). The Endowment Fund is transforming engineering education in Brazil. BrazilFoundation. Retrieved May 13, 2021, from https://www.brazilfoundation.org/the-endowment-fund-is-transforming-engineering-education-in-brazil/

Calabrese, T., & Ely, T. (2017). Understanding and measuring endowment in public charities. *Nonprofit and Voluntary Sector Quarterly, 46*(4), 859–873. https://doi.org/10.1177/0899764017703712

Castro, J., Yamada, G., & Arias, O. (2016). Higher education decisions in Peru: On the role of financial constraints, skills, and family background. *Higher Education, 72*(4), 457–486. https://doi.org/10.1007/s10734-016-0040-x

Cejnek, G., Franz, R., & Stoughton, N. (2015). *An integrated model of university endowments.* Working Paper. https://doi.org/10.2139/ssrn.2348048

Conley, A. T. (2017). Securing donor support for unrestricted endowments: A case study in higher education. *Philanthropy & Education, 1*(1), 48–63.

Data USA. (2021). Peru State College | Data USA. Datausa.io. Retrieved May 13, 2021, from https://datausa.io/profile/university/peru-state-college

Eaton, C. (2020). Opinion: How to use university endowments for coronavirus recovery. The Hechinger Report. Retrieved May 8, 2021, from https://hechingerreport.org/opinion-how-to-use-university-endowments-for-coronavirus-recovery/

Farinloye, T., Adeola, O., & Mogaji, E. (2020). Typology of Nigeria universities: A strategic marketing and branding implication. In E. Mogaji, F. Maringe, & R. E. Hinson (Eds.), *Understanding the higher education market in Africa*. Routledge.

Friga, P. (2020). Under Covid-19, university budgets like we've never seen before. Retrieved May 8 , 2021, from F.hubspotusercontent00.net

Gentry, W. (2002). Debt, investment and endowment accumulation: The case of not-for-profit hospitals. *Journal of Health Economics, 21*(5), 845–872. https://doi.org/10.1016/s0167-6296(02)00056-5

Hagood, L. P. (2019). The financial benefits and burdens of performance funding in higher education. *Educational Evaluation and Policy Analysis, 41*(2), 189–213.

Hansmann, H. (1990). Why do universities have endowments? *The Journal of Legal Studies, 19*(1), 3–42. Retrieved May 8, 2021, from http://www.jstor.org/stable/724411

Hinson, R., & Mogaji, E. (2020). Co-creation of value by universities and prospective students: Towards an informed decision-making process. In E. Mogaji, F. Maringe, & R. Hinson (Eds.), *Higher education marketing in Africa* (pp. 17–46). Palgrave Macmillan.

Histphil. 2017. A "Thoroughly Satisfactory and Permanent Remedy": The Twentieth Century Invention of the American University Endowment. [Online]. https://histphil.org/2017/11/06/a-thoroughly-satisfactory-and-permanent-remedy-the-twentieth-century-invention-of-the-american-university-endowment/

Khemani, S. (2020). *An opportunity to build legitimacy and trust in public institutions in the time of COVID-19*. World Bank Group. https://ssrn.com/abstract=3602352

Kieu, T., Mogaji, E., Mwebesa, C., Sarofim, S., Soetan, T., & Vululleh, S. P. (2020). Marketing higher education in Africa: Moving from research to practice. In *Strategic marketing of higher education in Africa* (pp. 221–237). Routledge.

Kimball, B., & Johnson, B. (2012). The inception of the meaning and significance of endowment in American higher education, 1890–1930. Teachers College Record, 114(100302). Retrieved May 8, 2021, from https://www.tcrecord.org/books/Content.asp?ContentID=16669

Kiraka, R., Maringe, F., Kanyutu, W., & Mogaji, E. (2020). University league tables and ranking systems in Africa: Emerging prospects, challenges and opportunities. In E. Mogaji, F. Maringe, & R. Hinson (Eds.), *Understanding the higher education market in Africa*. Routledge Studies in Marketing. Routledge. ISBN 978-0367344382.

Krasulia, A. (2014). Endowment as an educational fundraising tool for entrepreneurial university: The US experience versus Ukrainian reality and perspectives. *Kultura-Społeczeństwo-Edukacja, 6*(2), 57–73.

Krishnamurthy, S. (2020). The future of business education: A commentary in the shadow of the Covid-19 pandemic. *Journal of Business Research, 117*, 1–5.

Lerner, J., Schoar, A., & Wang, J. (2008). Secrets of the academy: The drivers of University endowment success. *Journal of Economic Perspectives, 22*(3), 207–222. https://doi.org/10.1257/jep.22.3.207

Mahamood, S., & Ab Rahman, A. (2015). Financing universities through waqf, pious endowment: Is it possible? *Humanomics, 31*(4), 430–453. https://doi.org/10.1108/h-02-2015-0010

Mason, C. M., & Caufield, C. R. (2010, March). Charities in distress: Governance and standards in troubled times. On Philanthropy. http://onphilanthropy.com/2010/charities-in-distress-governance-and-standards-of-care-in-troubled-times/#respond

Mogaji, E., Adamu, N., & Nguyen, N. P. (2021). Stakeholders shaping experiences of self-funded international PhD students in UK business schools. *The International Journal of Management Education, 19*(3), 10054.

Mogaji, E., Maringe, F., & Hinson, R. (2020). Marketisation in higher education in Africa: New directions for a decolonising continent. In E. Mogaji, F. Maringe, & R. Hinson (Eds.), *Understanding the higher education market in Africa*. Routledge Studies in Marketing. Routledge. ISBN 978-0367344382.

Mogaji, E., & Varsha, J. (2020). *Impact of the pandemic on higher education in emerging countries: Emerging opportunities*. Challenges and Research Agenda. https://doi.org/10.2139/ssrn.3622592

Ndofirepi, E., Farinloye, T., & Mogaji, E. (2020). Marketing mix in a heterogenous Higher Education Market: A case of Africa. In E. Mogaji, F. Maringe, & R. E. Hinson (Eds.), *Understanding the higher education market in Africa*. Routledge.

Newman, D. S. (2005). *Nonprofit essentials: Endowment building*. John Wiley & Sons.

Olaleye, S., Ukpabi, D., & Mogaji, E. (2020). Public vs private universities in Nigeria: Market dynamics perspective. In E. Mogaji, F. Maringe, & R. E. Hinson (Eds.), *Understanding the higher education market in Africa*. Routledge.

Ong, B. (2009). Key insights for managing an Asian Endowment Fund (from one who knows). IPE. Retrieved May 13, 2021, from https://www.ipe.com/key-insights-for-managing-an-asian-endowment-fund-from-one-who-knows/10003912.article

OUEM. (2021). Oxford University Endowment Management. About OUem, Available at https://www.ouem.co.uk/about-ouem/

Parmar, B. (2011). Endowment funds – Current scenario in India. Eduvisors. https://eduvisors.com/dwnld_assets/PDF/Eduvisors_Monograph_-_Endowment_Funds_-_August_20112.pdf

PHEA. (2021). The partnership for higher education in Africa. [Online]. http://www.foundation-partnership.org/linchpin/introduction.php

Robinson, J., & Maitra, S. (2020). Higher education after COVID-19 – Policy brief. *SSRN Electronic Journal*. https://doi.org/10.2139/ssrn.3604670

Sharma, H., Jain, V., & Mogaji, E. (2021). Defining developing countries in higher education context. *Research Agenda Working Papers, 2020*(1), 1–9.

Sloan, M. F., Charles, C., & Kim, M. (2016). Nonprofit leader perceptions of operating reserves and their substitutes. *Nonprofit Management & Leadership, 26*, 417–433.

Stepanova, A., Horbas', I., Derkach, O., & Ovcharenko, T. (2020). Endowment as a fundraising tool of the research university. *European Journal of Sustainable Development, 9*(2), 366–374. https://doi.org/10.14207/ejsd.2020.v9n2p366

Tan, T. (2019). Local universities' endowment funds not excessively large: Ong Ye Kung. The Straits Times. Retrieved May 13, 2021, from https://www.straitstimes.com/singapore/local-universities-endowment-funds-not-excessively-large-ong

Teferra, D. (2015). African endowments: Implementation policies. *International Higher Education, 38*. https://doi.org/10.6017/ihe.2005.38.7451

Walters, M., Gee, D., & Mohammed, S. (2019). A Literature Review-Digital Citizenship and Elementary Education. *International Journal of Technology in Education, 2*(1), 1–21.

Weissman, A. K. (2020). Striving to Include the Excluded: A Case Study of a Special Education Initiative in Rural Honduras. *FIRE: Forum for International Research in Education, 6*(1), 64–84.

Whitford, E. (2020). Colleges faced with whether to increase endowment spending as finances grow more dire. Insidehighered.com. Retrieved May 8, 2021, from https://www.insidehighered.com/news/2020/05/22/colleges-faced-whether-increase-endowment-spending-finances-grow-more-dire

15

Reimagining the Place of Physical Buildings in Higher Education in Developing Countries in a Post-COVID-19 Era

Yemi Oginni, Emmanuel Mogaji, and Nguyen Phong Nguyen

Introduction

Before the outbreak of COVID-19, most of the learning activities in higher education institutions relied on physical infrastructure, including classrooms and lecture theatres (Azubuike et al., 2021). Higher education institutions were run traditionally, with a lecturer and students in the same physical space. In addition, universities were investing in their physical teaching spaces to

Y. Oginni
Department of Architecture, University of Lagos, Lagos, Nigeria
e-mail: Yemi.oginni@uniilag.edu

E. Mogaji (✉)
Department of Marketing, Events and Tourism, University of Greenwich, London, UK
e-mail: e.o.mogaji@greenwich.ac.uk

N. P. Nguyen
School of Accounting, University of Economics Ho Chi Minh City, Ho Chi Minh City, Vietnam
e-mail: nguyenphongnguyen@ueh.edu.vn

E. Mogaji et al. (eds.), *Re-imagining Educational Futures in Developing Countries*,
https://doi.org/10.1007/978-3-030-88234-1_15

enhance teaching experiences (Mogaji & Yoon, 2019). However, teaching landscapes have changed because of safety precautions taken during the pandemic and the growing online teaching and learning trends.

COVID-19 led to the closure of learning institutions and a sudden shift towards online learning. Initially, online learning was considered an option to complement traditional face-to-face learning (Coman et al., 2020). However, it has been transformed during the coronavirus pandemic to become an essential mode for sustaining learning activities in higher education institutions. The Association of University Directors of Estates' (AUDE, 2020) management report found that 65% of member universities responding to their survey had paused or cancelled capital development projects, while 54% had stopped maintenance work that was not connected to statutory compliance. There are huge concerns about the need to invest in teaching spaces while considering the changing learning landscape. Universities are busy working and re-working investment plans (AUDE, 2020).

This significant change is expected to alter the students' perceptions of traditional face-to-face learning (Vasudeva & Mogaji, 2020), adoption of technology for teaching and learning and the relevance of physical teaching spaces in higher education (Adekola et al., 2017). Changes in the students' views of their physical learning spaces are associated with the perceived benefits of online learning, which will, in turn, inform the perceptions towards the classrooms and lecture theatres after COVID-19 (Closs et al., 2021). Li et al. (2020) found that university students are demanding more flexible learning that goes beyond the on-campus/online dichotomy. They also noted that blended learning offers learning opportunities and supports university students' flexible learning.

The increased use of online learning during the pandemic has also exposed its strengths and weaknesses. While the strengths of online learning include opportunities for content support, content creation, student management, engagement and learning analytics (Liu et al., 2020; Verawardina et al., 2020), there are still concerns about the digital divide. This is often further enhanced by the poor socio-economic situation of individuals in some countries (Abdulquadri et al., 2021). Lembani et al. (2020) found that students in marginalised and peripheral communities struggle with inadequate ICT access. This disparity is also evidenced in the quality of teaching and learning when comparing developing and developed countries. Poor access to technology often affects the attitudes of students in many developing countries when it comes to online classes (Azubuike et al., 2021). Further, it supports the debate on the need for physical teaching spaces (Reinius et al., 2021).

The major focus of online learning seems to be on practical courses, like health sciences and creative courses (Nortvig et al., 2020). However, these courses require a practical approach to teaching and learning, which cannot be easily achieved through online learning modalities (Kauppi et al., 2020). Soares et al. (2020) presented the daily-life reality faced by professionals engaged in chemistry education in Brazil, recognising the significant absence of adequate technological equipment. The pedagogical limitations of instructors without sufficient training to use online technologies and the inherent limitations of video classes as factors that negatively affected teaching were acknowledged. Torda (2020) reflected on how COVID-19 has pushed a revolution in medical education. Saputra et al. (2021) also noted their online innovations for learning music in Indonesia and, while they recognised the need for physical spaces for practical work, they highlighted how they used recorded video to deliver teaching materials.

The perceived effectiveness of online learning necessitates the need to explore the prospects of classrooms and lecture theatres post COVID-19 and the possibility of decreased frequency of their use (Mogaji & Jain, 2020; Nortvig et al., 2020). How will the scope of the university architecture adapt to the new scheme of things? Will universities need to build more classrooms and lecture theatres as the education system is now mainly becoming virtual or hybrid? These are questions that university leadership and estates teams need to explore and consider across developing countries.

This chapter recognises the benefits of physical teaching spaces in higher education—the need to engage in social interaction, interacting with peers and the lecturers' physical presence in the classroom to enhance learning. However, with the increasing prospects of technology and redefining higher education post-COVID-19, this chapter questions the possibilities of physically building additional facilities in developing countries. In this theoretical, crucial evaluation, the report recognises the universities, students and staff as key stakeholders in evaluating the prospects of physical building projects.

Specifically, this study has three aims. First, it will critically evaluate the relevance of physical buildings in higher education in developing countries in a post-COVID-19 setting. Second, the critical evaluation will be expanded into a conceptual framework that highlights the key stakeholders and the specific context in which these universities in emerging countries are operating. Third, it will provide relevant managerial implications for university leaders and managers to adapt their building programmes for post-pandemic higher education.

The subsequent section summarises the key stakeholders while examining the value of university buildings in post-COVID-19 higher education, recognising the students engaging with the facilities, staff facilitating teaching and learning in the facilities and the universities providing these facilities. The country context (developing countries with inherent economic and financial challenges) and the course context (practical and non-practical courses) are further discussed. A conceptual framework integrating all these stakeholders is presented in the penultimate section. Finally, the concluding section provides an overview of the discussion, highlighting the theoretical and managerial implication.

The Stakeholders

The Student

The use of online learning has eroded the long-held perceptions of the classrooms and lecture theatres in developing countries. Online learning, whose use increased exponentially during the pandemic, has been received positively by both the students and faculties (Mukhtar et al., 2020). Most cite its manageability, and students have indicated the levels of convenience in accessing the instructors and teaching materials (Kauppi et al., 2020). It also reduced additional expenses, such as travel costs (Azubuike et al., 2021). Lecturers found online learning to ease various administrative tasks, such as marking attendance and recording lectures (Saputra et al., 2021; Soares et al., 2020). Other advantages of online learning modalities include encouraging student-centredness in the learning process as the students are transformed into self-directed learners (Mukhtar et al., 2020). These specific advantages associated with online learning were often absent in the face-to-face learning that dominated before COVID-19. The perceived benefits of online education have led to a shift in preferences that might not favour regular face-to-face learning again. Consequently, the students might have less favourable perceptions of the classrooms and lecture theatres after the pandemic.

Student learning preferences about online courses determine their perceptions of the classroom. According to Simonds and Brock (2014), younger students prefer face-to-face classes, while older ones prefer online courses. Older students often prefer watching pre-recorded video lectures. Some of them have indicated that they find them interesting, and most learn from both face-to-face lectures and by watching pre-recorded videos (Simonds & Brock, 2014). The instructor's comments during video lectures help them remain engaged in the online learning sessions. Others find they gain more knowledge when watching and listening to the professor in uninterrupted lecture formats through recordings (Thakkar & Nair, 2021). Younger students are of the opposite opinion and are more inclined towards face-to-face classes, indicating that the comments and interactions during face-to-face classes are valuable. Some also find the pre-recorded lecture videos slow and multitask with other activities (Simonds & Brock, 2014). Thus, the students' perceptions of the classrooms and lecture theatres depend on their age, as older students generally prefer online learning while younger students often prefer face-to-face classes.

The Subject

The standard model of delivering practical-based education has been the traditional content-centred, design-oriented and hands-on approach that majorly focuses on the development of critical thinking skills (Bourne et al., 2005). Some effective pedagogical methodologies in teaching and learning practical courses include project-based learning, active learning and flipped classrooms (Mills & Treagust, 2003). However, these methodologies can only be adequately used in the traditional face-to-face classroom learning environment. The sudden transition to online learning has affected the effectiveness of delivering education in these fields. According to Vielma and Brey (2021), there is a need for evidence-based planning interventions to mitigate the effects of COVID-19 on health sciences, engineering and creative education. Faculties also face challenges in developing rigorous learning assessments, which have never been a challenge during conventional face-to-face learning (Asgari et al., 2021). The prospect of online teaching for engineering after the pandemic is limited because hands-on training is among the integral components of engineering education. Other limitations include the high cost of home lab kits necessary for practical activities and the challenges associated with recording lab experiments (García-Alberti et al., 2021). This limitation is exacerbated by the time-consuming nature of the practical exercises, making them less convenient when conducted in an online setting.

A study by Khan and Abid (2021) investigated the challenges and opportunities associated with online learning in engineering education in Pakistan. This study indicates that online learning in developing economies is less feasible because of the limited resources and limited availability of internet services. Part of this observation can be accounted for, as engineering education is among the most challenging domains and requires proper integration of classroom tutoring and synchronised laboratory instructions (Rubin &

Fernandes, 2013). Studies on the efficacy of remote laboratories in engineering education indicate a series of challenges that limit the implementation and subsequent use of this system. For instance, laboratory engineers and faculty members conducting the remote sessions require extra training by the institution to undertake this learning activity (Tucker et al., 2013). Online evaluation for engineering students also poses many difficulties. According to Ardid et al. (2015), institutions need to devise new evaluation techniques alongside redefining examinations in this setting, which is a considerable challenge. The instructors also face challenges in designing questions to test the students' application of knowledge, critical thinking and interpretation of ideas in the online assessments (Howarth et al., 2004).

Teaching and learning these practical courses can be intensive and fast-paced, requiring hand-on teaching (Ndofirepi et al., 2020), and might not be adequately fulfilled through online learning. According to Mukhtar et al. (2020), faculty members and students have expressed concerns about the inability to teach and learn clinical and practical work. Faculties indicate the challenges in teaching and assessing knowledge components through the online learning modalities (Mukhtar et al., 2020). This is a significant disadvantage for the students because the learning outcomes extend beyond mere acquisition and reproduction. Additional limitations include a lack of immediate feedback and the inability of the instructors to assess the students' comprehension during online lecturing (Mukhtar et al., 2020).

There will be significant changes in the instructional methods with the emergence of a hybrid educational model for higher education institutions. The emergence of the hybrid model is associated with the belief that online learning will persist post-COVID-19 (El Said, 2021). These online learning modalities will only favour business and other faculties that do not require intensive practical learning activities. However, music, medicine and engineering courses will benefit from the hybrid model. It will allow the instructors to fuse some online learning modalities with the traditional face-to-face system to maximise learning outcomes.

Olum et al. (2020) investigated the preferences, awareness, attitudes and barriers among undergraduate medicine and nursing students at Makerere University in Uganda. According to this study, online teaching for medicine will not be feasible post-COVID-19 as the removal of restrictions on physical learning will allow for the use of more convenient face-to-face learning programmes. The primary factor limiting the feasibility of online learning for medicine arises from the findings that teaching medicine has practical physiology, anatomy and biochemistry sessions (Okhovati, 2015). These practical sessions can only be effectively achieved in laboratories, making face-to-face learning the only viable option for this course. Additionally, students must undergo clinical bedside training as part of the learning process, which requires constant contact with the faculty and peers (Lakbala, 2016). Medical students acknowledge that online learning reduces the quality of knowledge and is inefficient (Olum et al., 2020). A significant proportion of the students prefer the hybrid learning model that incorporates online learning with the traditional classroom lectures (Azubuike et al., 2021). The findings coincide with another study among medical and dental students in Pakistan who indicated less favourable perceptions towards online learning (Abbasi et al., 2020). A hybrid learning model will maximise teaching efficiency by ensuring that the students can engage with faculty and peers in practical sessions while utilising online learning for theoretical sessions that do not require intensive, physical interactions.

The Classroom

The traditional college classroom design has not shown any significant changes since medieval times, except in size (Park & Choi, 2014). This aspect has been crucial to the learners' educational environment and attitudes towards the classroom educational philosophy. Yelkpieri et al. (2011) found that the students' perceptions of the classrooms matter because it entails the primary physical services provided by the university to support physical learning. Findings indicate that a 'golden zone' and a 'shadow zone' exist in traditional classrooms and are vital to the level of satisfaction with the area (Park & Choi, 2014). The golden zone is considered the front area of the classroom that provides optimal learning conditions. In contrast, the shadow zone is regarded as the back of the class, offering limited engagement with the whiteboard and the lecturer. Based on findings in active learning classrooms evaluating student learning, there are preferred seating positions such as the golden zone, which positively impacts learning. However, it also implies that the students occupying the shadow zone seats may experience challenges during the delivery of a lecture (Park & Choi, 2014). The competition for preferred seats affects the students' learning processes as it limits the levels of relationships between the students, motivation for learning and their sense of belonging to the class (Chiu & Cheng, 2017). Such limitations will affect the students' perceptions of classrooms and lecture theatres post-COVID-19 because of the availability of online learning as another suitable platform.

Larger class sizes in higher education institutions in developing countries result from increased population and the subsequent demand for higher education. This phenomenon eventually affects the quality of teaching and assessment of the students and the quality of graduates entering the job market (Effah et al., 2014). Another study by Anderson (2000) also indicates that class size and student achievements are directly related to the quality of teaching. This impact mainly manifests through the disparities in the student-teacher ratio. Higher student-teacher ratios arise from staffing challenges in public universities, which compel the management to have large class sizes for general courses to compensate for the limited staff available (Hinson & Mogaji, 2020). Furthermore, with the advent of COVID-19, most students have realised the convenience of online learning, which might be vital to their perceptions of the classrooms and lecture theatres after the pandemic.

The lecturers' perceptions of classrooms and lecture theatres after the pandemic might not be favourable, based on the perceived difficulty of handling larger classes. Most lecturers indicate that the major challenges in managing large classrooms include audibility challenges, difficulty marking the students' scripts, low contributions from the students and limited interactions with the students (Webb et al., 2007). These challenges eventually translate into the overall quality of teaching and assessment in higher education institutions. The difficulties in handling large classes, common in developing countries, may take precedence in determining the perceptions towards classrooms and lecture theatres after COVID-19. The availability of online learning as a more favourable alternative could be chosen. Considering an alternative mode of learning will also minimise pressure on the institutions to employ more staff. The pressure mainly arises from the increase in expenses against dwindling finances (Yelkpieri et al., 2011). Thus, the perceptions of classrooms and lecture theatres in higher education institutions in developing countries will depend on the challenges associated with the large class sizes and the facilities.

The Country

This chapter focuses on universities in developing countries to understand their inherent characteristics that may challenge redefining teaching spaces and supporting hybrid learning. What defines a developing country? Using income classifications to group countries, the World Bank represents 'developing countries' as the ones associated with low- and middle-threshold levels of gross national income (GNI) per capita (World Bank, 2021). The International Monetary Fund (IMF) classifies 37 counties as advanced economies against the remaining countries globally, categorised as emerging or developing economies (IMF, 2021). Statistically organised data support this classification. However, while the United Nations (UN) has no formal definition for developing countries it still addresses 159 countries across the world as developing. These countries are categorised based on GNI, human capital and economic positioning (Sharma et al., 2020). The Economic Analysis and Policy Division of the United Nations (2020) divides the world into three categories: developed economies, economies in transition and developing economies.

In all these classifications, developing countries are measured by their economic capabilities, development prospects and social integration (Abdulquadri et al., 2021; Mogaji & Jain, 2020). However, developing nations still face dilemmas in expanding higher education, quality trade-offs, equity and life-long learning culture (Ndofirepi et al., 2020). This is often due to limited funding by the government, which may influence investment in teaching spaces (Olaleye et al., 2020). Therefore, it is not surprising that there are insufficient teaching areas, many of which may not be adequate for hybrid learning (Mogaji & Jain, 2020). A study by Yelkpieri et al. (2011) on the impact of large class sizes on effective teaching in Ghana established that the large sizes of classes constitute one of the significant challenges crippling the education sector in developing countries. Crawford et al. (2020) provided higher education responses to COVID-19 across 20 developing countries. They acknowledged the challenges based on the limited availability of resources to cater to the students' needs.

The digital divide and inadequate access to technology in many developing countries do not encourage students to engage in hybrid learning (Azubuike et al., 2021). The International Association of Universities (IAU) (2020) report on the impact of COVID-19 on higher education worldwide highlights the disparities of access to technology among students in developing countries. Online learning faces many challenges because students do not have access to a laptop or smart device, and there is limited access to the internet and an inadequate electricity supply (El Said, 2021; Mogaji & Jain, 2020). According to a study investigating barriers to online learning in Nigeria and the Philippines, the erratic electricity supply is among the major hindrances to the adoption of online learning (Oluyinka & Endozo, 2019). In addition, many students in developing countries desire the ability to engage effectively in online learning without disruption due to high traffic and connectivity (Azubuike et al., 2021). Crawford et al. (2020) cited the case of Jordan, where a faculty had to adopt several low-technology solutions to support online teaching. This disparity presents a challenge to how universities can adopt hybrid learning extensively without total reliance on face-to-face teaching on campus.

There are concerns about the disparities in the perceived usefulness of technology and its ease of use (Azubuike et al., 2021). The willingness for a faculty to integrate hybrid learning into their course delivery depends on several factors, including their class size (Gratz & Looney, 2020). Some might not be comfortable because of a lack of training (Kumar et al., 2020) or might have concerns that their students may not have the resources to engage fully (Motala & Menon, 2020). Institutionally, there are concerns about the ability to support and enhance hybrid learning in developing countries, demonstrating the impact of poorly resourced institutions and socially disadvantaged students with limited access to technology (Crawford et al., 2020; Agbo et al., 2020). McCormack et al. (2021) question a university's agility and adaptability in responding to the COVID-19 pandemic, suggesting universities could do more to provide an enabling environment for students to continue learning irrespective of the pandemic. Tang et al. (2021) described this as organisational agility and an ability to effectively transfer and remodel teaching and learning in response to the global pandemic. Houlden and Veletsianos (2020) queried if higher education was prepared for the forthcoming digital era of learning. It can be said that universities in developing countries are aware of the trend and are taking action (Crawford et al., 2020). However, the inherent challenges may make higher education institutions reluctant to adopt online learning (Mogaji & Jain, 2020).

Conceptual Framework

The prospects of developing more classrooms and lecture theatres in higher education institutions post-COVID-19 will depend on the perceived effectiveness of conventional lectures. According to Schmidt et al. (2015), the efficacy of traditional lectures is limited to the attainment of certain curriculum objectives. It does not account for the promotion of critical thinking or cognitive engagement or for the fact that lectures cannot adequately cover the essential subject matter. While lecture theatres and classrooms cannot be removed entirely from the delivery of learning in higher education, a better understanding of their value is worth exploring (Hinson & Mogaji, 2020).

This section of the chapter presents a conceptual framework for reimagining the place of physical buildings in higher education in developing countries in a post-COVID-19 era. As illustrated in Fig. 15.1, the conceptual framework integrates the universities' staff and students as the key stakeholders in shaping the need for physical teaching space. In addition, the course and country context are illustrated within the framework. These two contexts

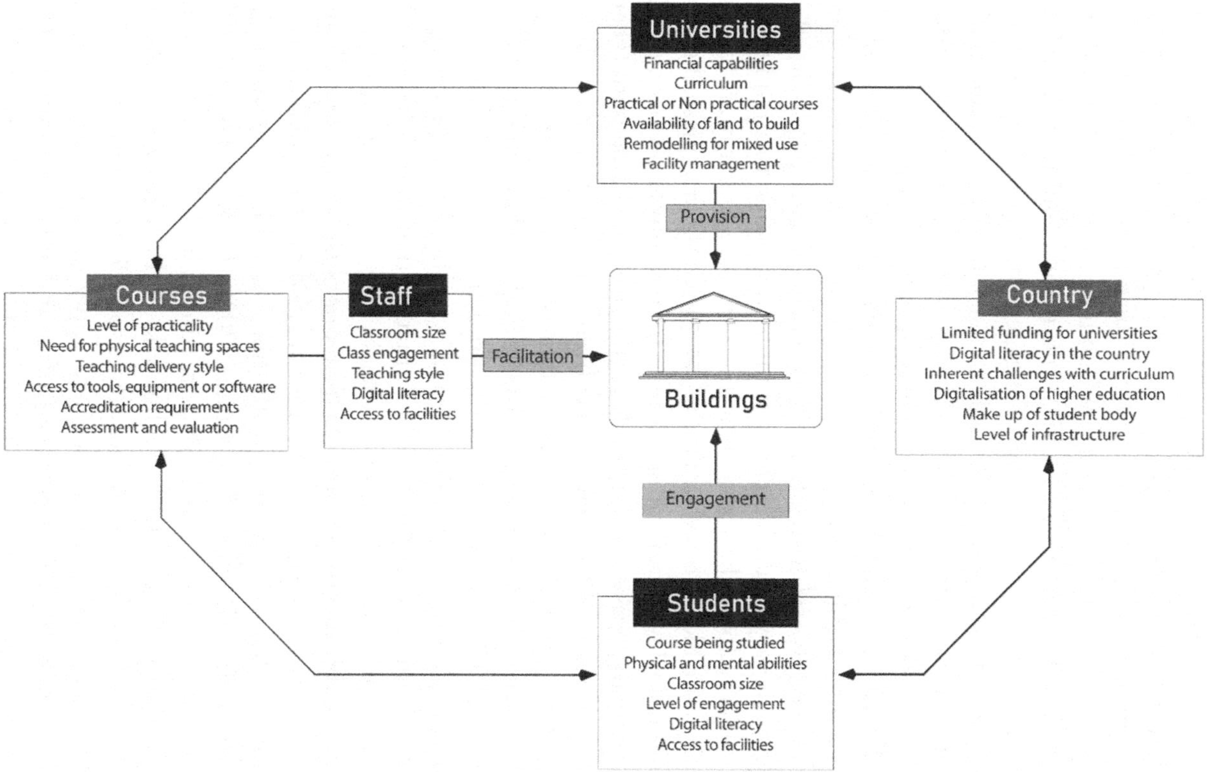

Fig. 15.1 Conceptual framework for reimagining the place of physical buildings in higher education in developing countries in a post-COVID-19 period

specifically explored the relevance of the teaching spaces and balance between the purpose of the university, to deliver knowledge, and the inherent challenges of the universities in developing countries. These challenges pose a considerable obstacle to achieving the purpose of a university post-COVID-19.

With the physical building at the centre of the framework, students engage and interact with the building and the building spaces aligned with their courses (Zhou & Li, 2019). The physical and mental abilities of the student can also pose a challenge in their level of engagement, especially for physically disabled students who may often struggle to make their way around the university buildings. They may prefer an online teaching mode where they do not have to interact with any physical teaching spaces. Classroom size can also pose a challenge, especially when students struggle to get a seat in an overcrowded teaching facility. Using online classes to relieve the stress of overcrowding in the physical structure is also a post-pandemic possibility. A low level of digital literacy could present even more motivation to attend physical classes. If students do not have sufficient internet access or hardware for learning, they are more likely to favour face-to-face teaching in a physical space.

With staff tasked with facilitating learning in these physical spaces, the class sizes and ability to engage with the student effectively are paramount (Feraria, 2019). Lack of student engagement has been cited by numerous scholars, including Bligh (1998), who suggested that lectures are a generally poor method for teachers who wish to promote critical thinking among their students. Kelly et al. (2007) also observed that student engagement is usually the lowest in lecture theatres. The major factor accounting for the perceived ineffectiveness of lectures arises from the 'information transmission fallacy' characteristic of conventional lecturing, whereby the instructors believe that information can be directly transmitted from one person to another (Schmidt et al., 2015). Many scholars have recommended developing hybrid learning environments in higher education institutions to achieve transformational learning outcomes (Mumford & Dikilitaş, 2020; Gratz & Looney, 2020). Providing the course allows it, hybrid instruction is presented as the future of higher education (Selingo, 2013; Skulmowski & Rey, 2020). According to Henry (2008), hybrid instruction encourages social interactions and independent learning and enables the students to apply the content in real-world problems. It entails the use of both face-to-face and online platform for teaching and learning (Gratz & Looney, 2020). Hybrid learning or blended learning has immense potential to improve the students' satisfaction with the course by using a dynamic learning model that enables the students to be actively involved in their educational experience (Osorio-Gómez, 2010;

Mogaji et al., 2021). Thus, the lower perceived effectiveness of conventional lecture implies that the prospects of investing in classrooms and lecture theatres after COVID-19 may be limited.

The challenges in many of these developing countries are considered by exploring the value of buildings in a post-COVID-19 period. Although, recently, with online platforms such as Zoom and Google Meet, a recent surge has been experienced in virtual learning use globally (Adeyanju et al., 2022). Many of these developing countries are still grappling with these realities and falling short of these expectations. Some government institutions and public schools have been unable to actualise this sufficiently. Therefore, the physical teaching method cannot be replaced immediately, so a hybrid or blended learning system is currently being introduced. This requires an assessment of the capabilities of the teaching staff, the building facilities and the need for infrastructure to support physical teaching (Cahapay & Anoba, 2020).

With the hybrid system, what will the architecture of classrooms look like in the near future? Classrooms are equipped with interactive whiteboards, projectors or audio-visual display equipment, digital boards and green screens for video production and online teaching. Classrooms will probably transition to more technical spaces to support the hybrid system. There will be less segmented space and more open and flexible, mixed-use areas rather than fixed classrooms. The buildings will require more digital viewing spaces, interactive boards for Zoom lectures, etc., and will become more high-tech to meet online learning requirements. In effect, the design of buildings will transform to have less enclosed spaces and walls and have more open-plan areas for mixed or flexible use. The buildings will look more like theatres for viewing large touch screen computers with less bulky furniture and storage spaces.

This conceptual framework provides an insight into the key stakeholders and allows for a critical evaluation of the need for physical teaching spaces. Unfortunately, there is no blanket approach to reimagining higher education spaces in a post-COVID-19 period as this depends on different factors that must be interwoven and integrated. For example, the university may be offering a non-practical course like business administration, and it may be more effective to invest in technology for teaching rather than physical spaces. Likewise, a university with predominantly adult students interested in and focusing on open learning and Massive Open Online Courses (MOOC) may have a different approach. Ultimately, university managers need to examine the unique features of their universities, the capabilities of their staff and students and the courses being offered, all within the context of the country in which they are operating.

Theoretical Contribution

This chapter has provided a theoretical contribution to reimagining education in a post-COVID-19 period in developing countries. First, the study critically evaluated the relevance of physical buildings in higher education in developing countries (Closs et al., 2021). Second, while the focus of research has often been on the teaching experiences and the role of technology (Limniou, 2021; Thomas & Bryson, 2021), this study has explored classroom and physical teaching spaces for the future. Third, we recognise that while technology is important, the basic teaching concepts within a physical space need to be re-evaluated. Finally, the study contributes to pedagogical insight by exploring the role of teaching spaces and by understanding the students' characteristics and the challenges faced by universities' in developing countries when it comes to supporting their students.

The study contributes to the literature on facility management in higher education institutions (Edirisinghe et al., 2017; Mwando et al., 2021). With the enormous implications for developing infrastructure for universities, this study further evaluates the role of buildings and the design of the buildings to accommodate the growing possibility of hybrid teaching and learning. It recognises that in the time of austerity in a post-COVID-19 period and the increase in technology adoption, universities need to ensure optimal use of space, lower operating costs and improved work productivity (Mwando et al., 2021).

The study expands the critical evaluation into a conceptual framework highlighting the key stakeholders and the specific context in which these universities in emerging countries are operating. Our conceptual framework presents ideas for consideration by the universities providing the learning spaces, the faculties facilitating teaching in the rooms and the students engaging with the physical spaces to learn. This framework further shows the relationship between these stakeholders (universities, staff and students) and the course and the country context in which they are operating. Using this framework, university managers involved with the buildings and other physical facilities will find relevant practical implications to enhance planning.

Managerial Implications

This study presents practical implications for university managers, particularly those in a leadership role responsible for building and infrastructure development decisions. These suggestions also apply to the facility managers responsible for monitoring the inventories and assets of the university and to timetabling staff who need to know the capacity of the physical facilities and how they fit into the course teaching styles. Architects and environment developers interested in higher education will also find this relevant in providing their clients with updated, learning-enhancing teaching spaces.

In summary, we recognise the importance of the financial limitations of universities in emerging countries, the pedagogical approach to hybrid learning and striking the right balance between investing in the physical and/or the digital estate. Identifying this balance will continue to influence how universities invest to achieve an excellent student experience (AUDE, 2020). Physical teaching spaces will still be relevant, but higher education institutions in developing countries need to invest in information technology infrastructures to support online learning and complement existing physical teaching areas. Developments during the pandemic have rendered online learning a necessity rather than an option (Watat et al., 2021).

While we acknowledge inadequate online learning information technology infrastructures in most developing countries due to socio-economic and technological challenges (Palvia et al., 2018), the financial difficulties associated with developing more physical teaching spaces and the growing trends for hybrid learning may compel the institutions to opt for technological advancement. Operating costs of existing areas will be a significant challenge for universities in maintaining their physical estate in a post-COVID-19 era (AUDE, 2020). It is therefore essential for universities to reconsider their priorities to meet the learning needs of their students. Seeking financial support and endowments (Nguyen & Mogaji et al., 2021), private partnership initiatives and shared resources (AUDE, 2020) are options to achieve their objectives.

Despite the call for more investment, universities have financial limitations in developing countries (Mogaji & Jain, 2020). Therefore, universities need to explore options to manage their meagre resources in meeting the learning needs of their students. The universities should be exploring the opportunity to work collaboratively as a sector, perhaps sharing their physical spaces, teaching technology and other resources. Farinloye et al. (2020) proposed that universities within close geographical proximity can share creative teaching spaces and libraries and create multi-institutional online digital resources that can be accessed from technology in any physical space in any of the universities instead of all the universities spending money to build their spaces. AUDE (2020) also noted that the pandemic had shown an unprecedented, impressive, collaborative response within the UK higher education sector. Many other universities could consider this combined approach in developing countries.

From a pedagogical point of view, prospects of future investments in classrooms and lecture theatres may be influenced by the findings indicating numerous challenges associated with large class sizes (Whisenhunt et al., 2019). Large classrooms have been associated with many limitations that eventually affect the students' learning outcomes. Some challenges include difficulties in handling large classes, such as audibility challenges, the low level of student contributions and challenges in administering assessments (Webb et al., 2007). These challenges imply the institutions might not find further reasons to invest in larger lecture theatres but to create smaller teaching spaces that can be used for tutorials (Foley & Masingila, 2014). For example, instead of having large lecture classes, the teaching could be recorded and shared with the students, who would then come to small tutorial classes to better engage with the lecture content.

Universities need to recognise the individual needs of their students, particularly when considering physical ability. Blended learning will mean a greater need for physically flexible spaces (AUDE, 2020). Dianito et al. (2021) shared insights about the lived experiences and challenges faced by disabled students. They found that they had experienced social exclusion since the rise of online learning during the pandemic. Ryan (2021) also noted the need to adapt physical spaces to meet the needs of students with disabilities. Students in practical courses also need to be considered in decisions about investment in physical teaching spaces. Most pedagogical methodologies for delivering education in these subjects include active learning, project-based learning and flipped classrooms, which can be effectively implemented in the face-to-face learning environment (Asgari et al., 2021; Mills & Treagust, 2003).

Conclusion

Future developments in higher education in developing economies should doubtless focus on establishing a suitable infrastructure to support online learning. Based on the diversity of preferences for online learning among different age groups and course-specific variables, the institutions should devise mechanisms that will enable adopting a hybrid learning system. This system will accommodate the needs of all students, including the older ones who prefer online learning, while providing face-to-face education for the younger students. The same approach will also accommodate students taking practical courses, which are limited to face-to-face classes. In addition, higher education institutions with adequate physical classrooms may offer premium classes because lecturer-student interaction is a crucial component in teaching courses such as languages, and it is essential for enhancing content comprehension and language development. Thus, students in the fields that require mandatory physical classes may have to pay more for such courses because of these advantages.

This is a theoretical study about reimagining the usefulness of physical buildings in higher education in developing countries during the post-COVID-19 era. Though relevant academic sources have been used to buttress the positions made in this chapter, further empirical research is proposed to establish these positions. This study has not been contextualised for any country, and this may be considered a limitation, but it opens opportunities for future research. Empirical research into the need for physical areas, student engagement with physical spaces and the cost implications of remodelling learning spaces are advised. The challenges for universities in developing countries regarding space management to provide quality teaching can also be empirically explored. This understanding will further verify the conceptual framework presented in this chapter and advance our knowledge regarding the relevance of physical buildings in higher education in developing countries.

References

Abbasi, S., Ayoob, T., Malik, A., & Memon, S. (2020). Perceptions of students regarding E-learning during Covid-19 at a private medical college. *Pakistan Journal of Medical Sciences, 36.* (COVID19-S4). https://doi.org/10.12669/pjms.36.covid19-s4.2766

Abdulquadri, A., Mogaji, E., Kieu, T. A., & Nguyen, N. P. (2021). Digital transformation in financial services provision: A Nigerian perspective to the adoption of chatbot. *Journal of Enterprising Communities: People and Places in the Global Economy., 15*(2), 258–281.

Adekola, J., Dale, V. H., & Gardiner, K. (2017). Development of an institutional framework to guide transitions into enhanced blended learning in higher education. *Research in Learning Technology, 25*, 1973–1989.

Adeyanju, S., Ajilore, O., Ogunlalu, O., Onatunji, A., & Mogaji, E. (2022). Innovating in the face of the COVID-19 pandemic: Case studies from Nigerian universities. *STAR Scholar Book Series*, 104–120.

Agbo, F. J., Olawumi, O., Oyelere, S. S., Kolog, E. A., Olaleye, S. A., Agjei, R. O., … Olawuni, A. (2020). Social media usage for computing education: The effect of tie strength and group communication on perceived learning outcome. *International Journal of Education and Development using Information and Communication Technology, 16*(1), 5–26.

Anderson, L. W. (2000). Why should reduced class size lead to increased student achievement? In M. C. Wang & J. D. Finn (Eds.), *How small classes help teachers do their best* (pp. 3–24). Temple University Center for Research in Human Development.

Ardid, M., et al. (2015). Online exams for blended assessment. Study of different application methodologies. *Computers & Education, 81*, 296–303.

Asgari, S., Trajkovic, J., Rahmani, M., Zhang, W., Lo, R., & Sciortino, A. (2021). An observational study of engineering online education during the COVID-19 pandemic. *PLOS ONE, 16*(4), e0250041. https://doi.org/10.1371/journal.pone.0250041

AUDE. (2020). *AUDE higher education estates management report 2020*. Association of University Directors of Estates.

Azubuike, O. B., Adegboye, O., & Quadri, H. (2021). Who gets to learn in a pandemic? Exploring the digital divide in remote learning during the COVID-19 pandemic in Nigeria. *International Journal of Educational Research Open, 2*, 100022.

Bligh, D. A. (1998). *What's the use of lectures?* Intellect Books.

Bourne, J., Harris, D., & Mayadas, F. (2005). Online engineering education: Learning anywhere, anytime. *Journal of Engineering Education, 94*(1), 131–146.

Cahapay, M. B., & Anoba, J. L. D. (2020). The readiness of teachers on blended learning transition for post COVID-19 period: An assessment using parallel mixed method. *PUPIL: International Journal of Teaching, Education and Learning, 4*(2), 295–316.

Chiu, P. H. P., & Cheng, S. H. (2017). Effects of active learning classrooms on student learning: A two-year empirical investigation on student perceptions and academic performance. *Higher Education Research & Development, 36*(2), 269–279.

Closs, L., Mahat, M., & Imms, W. (2021). Learning environments' influence on students' learning experience in an Australian Faculty of Business and Economics. *Learning Environments Research*, 1–15.

Coman, C., Mesesan-Schmitz, L., Stanciu, C., & Bularca, M. (2020). Online teaching and learning in higher education during the coronavirus pandemic: Students' perspective. *Sustainability, 12*(24), 10367. https://doi.org/10.3390/su122410367

Crawford, J., Butler-Henderson, K., Rudolph, J., Malkawi, B., Glowatz, M., Burton, R., … Lam, S. (2020). COVID-19: 20 countries' higher education intra-period digital pedagogy responses. *Journal of Applied Learning & Teaching, 3*(1), 1–20.

Dianito, A. J., Espinosa, J., Duran, J., & Tus, J. (2021). A glimpse into the lived experiences and challenges faced of PWD students towards online learning in the Philippines amidst COVID-19 pandemic. *International Journal of Advance Research and Innovative Ideas in Education, 7*(1), 1206–1230.

Edirisinghe, R., London, K. A., Kalutara, P., & Aranda-Mena, G. (2017). Building information modelling for facility management: Are we there yet? *Engineering, Construction and Architectural Management, 24*(6), 1119–1154. https://doi.org/10.1108/ECAM-06-2016-0139

Effah, B., Boampong, E., Adu, G., Anokye, R., Asamoah, J. N., & Ashanti, G. W. A. (2014). Issues of the industrial training programme of polytechnics in Ghana: The case of Kumasi Polytechnic. *Journal of Education and Practice, 5*(5), 39–46.

El Said, G. (2021). How did the COVID-19 pandemic affect higher education learning experience? An empirical investigation of learners' academic performance at a university in a developing country. *Advances in Human-Computer Interaction, 2021*, 1–10. https://doi.org/10.1155/2021/6649524

Farinloye, T., Adeola, O., & Mogaji, E. (2020). Typology of Nigerian universities: A strategic marketing and branding implication. In *Understanding the higher education market in Africa* (pp. 168–198). Routledge.

Feraria, P. J. (2019). Flip and retrofit university lecture theatre into Caribbean classrooms: Turning teacher education and training inside-out. In *Innovative trends in flipped teaching and adaptive learning* (pp. 38–54). IGI Global.

Foley, A. R., & Masingila, J. O. (2014). Building capacity: Challenges and opportunities in large class pedagogy (LCP) in Sub-Saharan Africa. *Higher Education, 67*(6), 797–808.

García-Alberti, M., Suárez, F., Chiyón, I., & Mosquera Feijoo, J. C. (2021). Challenges and experiences of online evaluation in courses of civil engineering during the lockdown learning due to the COVID-19 pandemic. *Education Sciences, 11*(2), 59.

Gratz, E., & Looney, L. (2020). Faculty resistance to change: An examination of motivators and barriers to teaching online in higher education. *International Journal of Online Pedagogy and Course Design (IJOPCD), 10*(1), 1–14.

Henry, R. (2008). *Hybrid learning environments in higher education can transformational learning outcomes be achieved?* Trevecca Nazarene University

Hinson, R. E., & Mogaji, E. (2020). Co-creation of value by universities and prospective students: Towards an informed decision-making process. In *Higher education marketing in Africa* (pp. 17–46). Palgrave Macmillan.

Houlden, S., & Veletsianos, G. (2020). Coronavirus pushes universities to switch to online classes—but are they ready. *The Conservation.* https://theconversation.com/coronavirus-pushesuniversities-to-switch-to-online-classes-but-are-they-ready-132728

Howarth, J., Messing, J., & Altas, I. (2004). Delivering online examinations: A case study. *Turkish Online Journal of Distance Education, 5*(3), 23–45.

IMF. (2021). *World economic outlook.* [Online]. Retrieved May 5, 2021, from https://www.imf.org/external/pubs/ft/weo/faq.htm

Kauppi, S., Muukkonen, H., Suorsa, T., & Takala, M. (2020). I still miss human contact, but this is more flexible—Paradoxes in virtual learning interaction and multidisciplinary collaboration. *British Journal of Educational Technology, 51*(4), 1101–1116.

Kelly, S. (2007). Classroom discourse and the distribution of student engagement. *Social Psychology of Education, 10*(3), 331–352.

Khan, Z., & Abid, M. (2021). Distance learning in engineering education: Challenges and opportunities during COVID-19 pandemic crisis in Pakistan. *The International Journal of Electrical Engineering & Education*. https://doi.org/10.1177/0020720920988493

Kumar, J. A., Bervell, B., & Osman, S. (2020). Google classroom: Insights from Malaysian higher education students' and instructors' experiences. *Education and Information Technologies, 25*(5), 4175–4195.

Lakbala, P. (2016). Barriers in implementing E-learning in Hormozgan University of Medical Sciences. *Global Journal of Health Science, 8*(7), 83.

Lembani, R., Gunter, A., Breines, M., & Dalu, M. T. B. (2020). The same course, different access: The digital divide between urban and rural distance education students in South Africa. *Journal of Geography in Higher Education, 44*(1), 70–84.

Li, X., Yang, Y., Chu, S. K. W., Zainuddin, Z., & Zhang, Y. (2020). Applying blended synchronous teaching and learning for flexible learning in higher education: An action research study at a university in Hong Kong. *Asia Pacific Journal of Education*, 1–17.

Limniou, M. (2021). The effect of digital device usage on student academic performance: A case study. *Education Sciences, 11*(3), 121.

Marinoni, G., Van't Land, H., & Jensen, T. (2020). *The impact of Covid-19 on higher education around the world.* IAU Global Survey Report. https://www.iauaiu.net/IMG/pdf/iau_covid19_and_he_survey_report_final_may_2020.pdf

McCormack, T. J., Lemoine, P. A., Waller, R. E., & Richardson, M. D. (2021). Global Higher Education: Examining Response to the COVID-19 Pandemic Using Agility and Adaptability. *Journal of Education and Development, 5*(1), 10.

Mills, J. E., & Treagust, D. F. (2003). Engineering education—Is problem-based or project-based learning the answer. *Australasian Journal of Engineering Education, 3*(2), 2–16.

Mogaji, E., & Jain, V. (2020). Impact of the pandemic on higher education in emerging countries: Emerging opportunities, challenges and research agenda. *Research Agenda Working Papers*. https://doi.org/10.2139/ssrn.3622592

Mogaji, E., & Yoon, H. (2019). Thematic analysis of marketing messages in UK universities' prospectuses. *International Journal of Educational Management, 33*(7), 1561–1581. https://doi.org/10.1108/IJEM-05-2018-0149

Mogaji, E., Adamu, N., & Nguyen, N. P. (2021). Stakeholders shaping experiences of self-funded international PhD students in UK business schools. *The International Journal of Management Education, 19*(3), 100543–100553.

Motala, S., & Menon, K. (2020). In search of the 'new normal': Reflections on teaching and learning during Covid-19 in a South African university. *Southern African Review of Education with Education with Production, 26*(1), 80–99.

Mukhtar, K., Javed, K., Arooj, M., & Sethi, A. (2020). Advantages, limitations and recommendations for online learning during COVID-19 pandemic era. *Pakistan Journal of Medical Sciences, 36*. (COVID19-S4). https://doi.org/10.12669/pjms.36.covid19-s4.2785

Mumford, S., & Dikilitaş, K. (2020). Pre-service language teachers reflection development through online interaction in a hybrid learning course. *Computers & Education, 144*, 103706.

Mwando, S. M., Issa, A., & Kangotue, V. (2021). Staff and students' perception of implementing flexible working arrangements in institution of higher education. *Journal of Facilities Management*. https://doi.org/10.1108/JFM-07-2020-0040

Ndofirepi, E., Farinloye, T., & Mogaji, E. (2020). Marketing mix in a heterogenous higher education market: A case of Africa. In *Understanding the higher education market in Africa* (pp. 241–262). Routledge.

Nguyen, P., & Mogaji, E. (2021). Universities' endowments in developing countries: The perspectives, stakeholders and practical implications. In E. Mogaji, J. Varsha, F. Maringe, & R. E. Hinson (Eds.), *Re-imagining educational futures in developing countries: Lessons from global health crises*. Palgrave.

Nortvig, A. M., Petersen, A. K., Helsinghof, H., & Brænder, B. (2020). Digital expansions of physical learning spaces in practice-based subjects-blended learning in Art and Craft & Design in teacher education. *Computers & Education, 159*, 104020.

Okhovati, M. (2015). Attitude, knowledge and skill of medical students toward e-learning Kerman University of Medical Sciences. *Education Strategies in Medical Sciences, 8*(1), 51–58.

Olaleye, S., Ukpabi, D., & Mogaji, E. (2020). Public vs private universities in Nigeria: Market dynamics perspective. *Understanding the Higher Education Market in Africa*, 19–36.

Olum, R., Atulinda, L., Kigozi, E., Nassozi, D., Mulekwa, A., Bongomin, F., & Kiguli, S. (2020). Medical education and e-learning during COVID-19 pandemic: Awareness, attitudes, preferences, and barriers among undergraduate medicine and nursing students at Makerere University, Uganda. *Journal of Medical Education and Curricular Development, 7*, 2382120520973212. https://doi.org/10.1177/2382120520973212

Oluyinka, S., & Endozo, A. N. (2019). Barriers to e-learning in developing countries: A comparative study. *Journal of Theoretical and Applied Information Technology, 97*(9).

Osorio-Gómez, L. (2010). Characteristics of blended learning environments: Case study of a postgraduate programme in Los Andes University. *RUSC. Universities and Knowledge Society Journal, 7*(1). https://doi.org/10.7238/rusc.v7i1.655

Palvia, S., Aeron, P., Gupta, P., Mahapatra, D., Parida, R., Rosner, R., & Sindhi, S. (2018). Online education: Worldwide status, challenges, trends, and implications. *Journal of Global Information Technology Management, 21*(4), 233–241.

Park, E., & Choi, B. (2014). Transformation of classroom spaces: Traditional versus active learning classroom in colleges. *Higher Education, 68*(5), 749–771. https://doi.org/10.1007/s10734-014-9742-0

Reinius, H., Korhonen, T., & Hakkarainen, K. (2021). The design of learning spaces matters: Perceived impact of the deskless school on learning and teaching. *Learning Environments Research*, 1–16.

Rubin, B., & Fernandes, R. (2013). Measuring the community in online classes. *Journal of Asynchronous Learning Networks, 17*(3), 115–136.

Ryan, F. (2021). *Remote working has been life-changing for disabled people, don't take it away now.* [Online]. Retrieved June 3, 2021, from https://www.theguardian.com/commentisfree/2021/jun/02/remote-working-disabled-people-back-to-normal-disability-inclusion?fbclid=IwAR3mu7fTSyJtJpsvRcYWgIlRVsFeEmy2kkRWv7BQSc7n_Ix-NOBl2yXbNmU

Saputra, M. A., Mohruni, A. S., & Yani, I. (2021). Work scheduling program design for lecture attendance control and lecturer workload calculation with fingerprint and RFID identification device. *Indonesian Journal of Engineering and Science, 2*(3), 1–10.

Schmidt, H., Wagener, S., Smeets, G., Keemink, L., & van der Molen, H. (2015). On the use and misuse of lectures in higher education. *Health Professions Education, 1*(1), 12–18. https://doi.org/10.1016/j.hpe.2015.11.010

Selingo, J. J. (2013). *College (un) bound: The future of higher education and what it means for students.* Houghton Mifflin Harcourt.

Sharma, H., Jain, V., & Mogaji, E. (2020). Defining developing countries in higher education context. *Research Agenda Working Papers, 2021*(1), 1–9.

Simonds, T., & Brock, B. (2014). Relationship between age, experience, and student preference for types of learning activities in online courses. *The Journal of Educators Online, 11*(1). https://doi.org/10.9743/jeo.2014.1.3

Skulmowski, A., & Rey, G. D. (2020). COVID-19 as an accelerator for digitalization at a German university: Establishing hybrid campuses in times of crisis. *Human Behavior and Emerging Technologies, 2*(3), 212–216.

Soares, R., De Mello, M. C. S., Da Silva, C. M., Machado, W., & Arbilla, G. (2020). Online Chemistry education challenges for Rio de Janeiro students during the covid-19 pandemic. *Journal of Chemical Education, 97*(9), 3396–3399.

Tang, Y. M., Chen, P. C., Law, K. M., Wu, C. H., Lau, Y. Y., Guan, J., ... Ho, G. T. (2021). Comparative analysis of Student's live online learning readiness during the coronavirus (COVID-19) pandemic in the higher education sector. *Computers & Education, 168*, 104211.

Thakkar, K., & Nair, P. (2021). An Empirical Analysis Of Online Learning Over The Face-To-Face Learning. *Psychology and Education Journal, 58*(5), 754–764.

Thomas, M., & Bryson, J. R. (2021). Combining proximate with online learning in real-time: Ambidextrous teaching and pathways towards inclusion during COVID-19 restrictions and beyond. *Journal of Geography in Higher Education*, 1–19.

Torda, A. (2020). How COVID-19 has pushed us into a medical education revolution. *Internal medicine journal, 50*(9), 1150–1153.

Tucker, B., Kazmer, D., Pierrakos, O., Swan, C., Bielefeldt, A., Paterson, K., & Soisson, A. (2013). *Faculty perspectives on service-learning in engineering education:*

Challenges and opportunities. 2013 ASEE Annual Conference & Exposition Proceedings. https://doi.org/10.18260/1-2%2D%2D19610

Vasudeva, S., & Mogaji, E. (2020). Paving the way for world domination: analysis of African universities' mission statement. In *Understanding the higher education market in Africa* (pp. 145–167). Routledge.

Verawardina, U., Asnur, L., Lubis, A. L., Hendriyani, Y., Ramadhani, D., Dewi, I. P., & Sriwahyuni, T. (2020). Reviewing online learning facing the Covid-19 outbreak. *Journal of Talent Development and Excellence, 12*(3s), 385–392.

Vielma, K., & Brey, E. M. (2021). Using evaluative data to assess virtual learning experiences for students during COVID-19. *Biomedical Engineering Education, 1*(1), 139–144.

Watat, J. K., Olaleye, S. A., & Ukpabi, D. (2021). Recruit, retain and report: UK universities' strategic communication with stakeholders on Twitter. In *Strategic corporate communication in the digital age*. Emerald Publishing Limited.

Webb, R. M., Lubinski, D., & Benbow, C. P. (2007). Spatial ability: A neglected dimension in talent searches for intellectually precocious youth. *Journal of Educational Psychology, 99*(2), 397.

Whisenhunt, B. L., Cathey, C., Visio, M. E., Hudson, D. L., Shoptaugh, C. F., & Rost, A. D. (2019). Strategies to address challenges with large classes: Can we exceed student expectations for large class experiences? *Scholarship of Teaching and Learning in Psychology, 5*(2), 121.

World Bank. (2021). *World Bank country and lending groups*. [Online]. Retrieved May 5, 2021, from https://datahelpdesk.worldbank.org/knowledgebase/articles/906519

Yelkpieri, D., & Esia-Donkoh Kweku, W. (2011). Patronage of Educational Broadcasts and its Effects on Academic Growth of Students of Winneba and Apam Senior High Schools in the Central Region of Ghana. *Academic Leadership: The Online Journal, 9*(1), 40–54.

Zhou, M., & Li, Z. (2019). Blended mobile learning in theatre arts classrooms in higher education. *Innovations in Education and Teaching International, 56*(3), 307–317.

[illegible]

Index[1]

[1] Note: Page numbers followed by 'n' refer to notes.

E. Mogaji et al. (eds.), *Re-imagining Educational Futures in Developing Countries*,
https://doi.org/10.1007/978-3-030-88234-1

The manufacturer's authorised representative in the EU is Springer Nature Customer Service Centre GmbH, Europaplatz 3, 69115 Heidelberg, Germany. If you have any concerns regarding our products, please contact ProductSafety@springernature.com

Printed and bound by CPI Group (UK) Ltd, Croydon, CR0 4YY

30/09/2026

02225499-0020